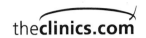

SURGICAL CLINICS
OF NORTH AMERICA

Benign Pancreatic Disorders

GUEST EDITOR
Stephen W. Behrman, MD

CONSULTING EDITOR
Ronald F. Martin, MD

December 2007 • Volume 87 • Number 6

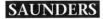

An Imprint of Elsevier, Inc.
PHILADELPHIA   LONDON   TORONTO   MONTREAL   SYDNEY   TOKYO

W.B. SAUNDERS COMPANY
A Division of Elsevier Inc.

1600 John F. Kennedy Blvd., Suite 1800, Philadelphia, PA 19103-2899

http://www.theclinics.com

SURGICAL CLINICS OF NORTH AMERICA
December 2007
Editor: Catherine Bewick

Volume 87, Number 6
ISSN 0039–6109
ISBN-10: 1-4160-5127-9
ISBN-13: 978-1-4160-5127-5

The ideas and opinions expressed in *The Surgical Clinics of North America* do not necessarily reflect those of the Publisher. The Publisher does not assume any responsibility for any injury and/or damage to persons or property arising out of or related to any use of the material contained in this periodical. The reader is advised to check the appropriate medical literature and the product information currently provided by the manufacturer of each drug to be administered to verify the dosage, the method and duration of administration, or contraindications. It is the responsibility of the treating physician or other health care professional, relying on independent experience and knowledge of the patient, to determine drug dosages and the best treatment for the patient. Mention of any product in this issue should not be construed as endorsement by the contributors, editors, or the Publisher of the product or manufacturers' claims.

Surgical Clinics of North America (ISSN 0039–6109) is published bimonthly by Elsevier Inc., 360 Park Avenue South, New York, NY 10010-1710. Months of publication are February, April, June, August, October, and December. Business and Editorial Offices: 1600 John F. Kennedy Blvd., Suite 1800, Philadelphia, PA 19103-2899. Customer Service Office: 6277 Sea Harbor Drive, Orlando, FL 32887-4800. Periodicals postage paid at New York, NY and additional mailing offices. Subscription prices are $238.00 per year for US individuals, $382.00 per year for US institutions, $119.00 per year for US students and residents, $292.00 per year for Canadian individuals, $466.00 per year for Canadian institutions, $309.00 for international individuals, $466.00 per year for international institutions and $154.00 per year for Canadian and foreign students/residents. To receive student/resident rate, orders must be accompanied by name of affiliated institution, date of term, and the *signature* of program/residency coordinator on institution letterhead. Orders will be billed at individual rate until proof of status is received. Foreign air speed delivery is included in all *Clinics* subscription prices. All prices are subject to change without notice. POSTMASTER: Send address changes to *Surgical Clinics*, Elsevier Periodicals Customer Service, 6277 Sea Harbor Drive, Orlando, FL 32887-4800. **Customer Service: 1-800-654-2452 (US). From outside of the US, call 1-407-345-1000.**

The Surgical Clinics of North America is also published in Spanish by McGraw-Hill Interamericana Editores S.A., P.O. Box 5-237 06500 Mexico D.F. Mexico; and in Portuguese by Interlivros Edicoes Ltda., Rua Comandante Coelho 1085, CEP 21250, Rio de Janeiro, Brazil; and in Greek by Paschalidis Medical Publications, Athens Greece.

The Surgical Clinics of North America is covered in *Index Medicus, EMBASE/Excerpta Medica, Current Contents/Clinical Medicine, Current Contents/Life Sciences, Science Citation Index*, and *ISI/BIOMED*.

Printed in the United States of America.

CONSULTING EDITOR

RONALD F. MARTIN, MD, Staff Surgeon, Marshfield Clinic, Marshfield; and Clinical Associate Professor, University of Wisconsin School of Medicine and Public Health, Madison, Wisconsin; Lieutenant Colonel, Medical Corps, United States Army Reserve

GUEST EDITOR

STEPHEN W. BEHRMAN, MD, Associate Professor of Surgery, University of Tennessee, Memphis, Memphis, Tennessee

CONTRIBUTORS

AYMAN M. ABDEL AZIZ, MD, FERCP, Fellow, Division of Gastroenterology/ Hepatology, Department of Medicine, Indiana University Medical Center, Indianapolis, Indiana

DAVID B. ADAMS, MD, Professor and Head, Section of Gastrointestinal and Laparoscopic Surgery, Medical University of South Carolina, Charleston, South Carolina

SIRIBOON ATTASARANYA, MD, FERCP, Fellow, Division of Gastroenterology/ Hepatology, Department of Medicine, Indiana University Medical Center, Indianapolis, Indiana

STEPHEN W. BEHRMAN, MD, Associate Professor of Surgery, University of Tennessee Memphis, Memphis, Tennessee

GREG J. BEILMAN, MD, Director, Surgical Critical Care Fellowship Program; and Professor and Chief, Division of Surgical Critical Care/Trauma, Department of Surgery, University of Minnesota, Minneapolis, Minnesota

MELENA BELLIN, MD, Fellow, Division of Pediatric Endocrinology, Department of Pediatrics, University of Minnesota, Minneapolis, Minnesota

SIMON BERGMAN, MD, Clinical Assistant Professor, Department of Surgery, Center for Minimally Invasive Surgery, The Ohio State University, Columbus, Ohio

JUAN J. BLONDET, MD, Postdoctoral Associate, Division of Surgical Critical Care/ Trauma, Department of Surgery, University of Minnesota, Minneapolis, Minnesota

ANNELISA M. CARLSON, MD, Surgery Resident, Department of Surgery, University of Minnesota, Minneapolis, Minnesota

CAITLIN S. CURTIS, PharmD, Clinical Pharmacist, Department of Pharmacy, University of Wisconsin-Madison Hospital and Clinics, Madison, Wisconsin

CHRISTOPHER J. DENTE, MD, FACS, Assistant Professor of Surgery, Emory University School of Medicine, Department of Surgery, Grady Memorial Hospital, Atlanta, Georgia

MOHAMMED ELFAR, MD, The Methodist Hospital, Houston, Texas

DAVID V. FELICIANO, MD, FACS, Professor of Surgery and Chief of Surgery, Grady Memorial Hospital, Emory University School of Medicine, Atlanta, Georgia

CRAIG P. FISCHER, MD, MPH, The Methodist Hospital, Houston, Texas

ERIC S. FOWLER, MS, CGC, Clinical Director of Genetics, Baptist Centers for Cancer Care, Baptist Memorial Hospital-Memphis, Memphis, Tennessee

MARTIN L. FREEMAN, MD, Professor of Medicine; Director, Pancreaticobiliary Endoscopy Fellowship; and Co-Director, Minnesota Pancreas and Liver Center, Department of Medicine, University of Minnesota, Minneapolis, Minnesota

A. OSAMA GABER, MD, The Methodist Hospital, Houston, Texas

LILLIAN W. GABER, MD, Houston, Texas

JOHN C. HANEY, MD, MPH, Resident, Program of General Surgery, Duke University Medical Center, Duke University School of Medicine, Durham, North Carolina

BERNHARD J. HERING, MD, Scientific Director, Diabetes Institute for Immunology and Transplantation; Director, Islet Transplant Program; and Professor, Division of Transplantation, Department of Surgery, University of Minnesota, Minneapolis, Minnesota

TUN JIE, MD, Fellow, Division of Transplantation, Department of Surgery, University of Minnesota, Minneapolis, Minnesota

DAVID H. KIM, MD, Assistant Professor, Department of Radiology, University of Wisconsin Medical School, Madison, Wisconsin

TAKASHI KOBAYASHI, MD, Postdoctoral Associate, Division of Transplantation, Department of Surgery, University of Minnesota, Minneapolis, Minnesota

KENNETH A. KUDSK, MD, Professor of Surgery, Department of Surgery, Veterans Administration Surgical Services, William S. Middleton Memorial Veterans Hospital; and Department of Surgery, University of Wisconsin-Madison Hospital and Clinics, Madison, Wisconsin

GLEN A. LEHMAN, MD, Professor of Medicine, Division of Gastroenterology/Hepatology, Department of Medicine, Indiana University Medical Center, Indianapolis, Indiana

JAMES A. MADURA, MD, J. Stanley Battersby Professor of Surgery, Emeritus, Indiana University School of Medicine, Indianapolis, Indiana

JAMES A. MADURA II, MD, Associate Professor of Surgery and Attending General Surgeon, Department of General Surgery, Rush University Medical Center; and Attending Surgeon, John Stroger Hospital of Cook County, Chicago, Illinois

MICHAEL D. MARION, MD, Resident in General Surgery, Department of Surgery, Marshfield Clinic and Saint Joseph's Hospital, Marshfield, Wisconsin

RONALD F. MARTIN, MD, Staff Surgeon, Marshfield Clinic, Marshfield; and Clinical Associate Professor, University of Wisconsin School of Medicine and Public Health, Madison, Wisconsin; Lieutenant Colonel, Medical Corps, United States Army Reserve

W. SCOTT MELVIN, MD, Professor of Surgery; and Director, Center for Minimally Invasive Surgery, Division of General Surgery, The Ohio State University, Columbus, Ohio

KATHERINE A. MORGAN, MD, Assistant Professor, Section of Gastrointestinal and Laparoscopic Surgery, Medical University of South Carolina, Charleston, South Carolina

THEODORE N. PAPPAS, MD, Professor of Surgery, Duke University Medical Center, Duke University School of Medicine, Durham, North Carolina

PERRY J. PICKHARDT, MD, Associate Professor, Department of Radiology, University of Wisconsin Medical School, Madison, Wisconsin

SUSHANTH REDDY, MD, Surgical Resident, Department of Surgery, University of Kentucky, Lexington, Kentucky; Postdoctoral Research Fellow, John L. Cameron Division of Surgical Oncology, Department of Surgery, The Johns Hopkins Medical Institutions, The Johns Hopkins Hospital, Baltimore, Maryland

OMAIMA SABEK, PhD, The Methodist Hospital, Houston, Texas

ANURADHA SUBRAMANIAN, MD, Assistant Professor of Surgery, Baylor College of Medicine, Department of Surgery, Michael E. DeBakey Veterans Affairs Medical Center, Houston, Texas

DAVID E.R. SUTHERLAND, MD, PhD, Director, Diabetes Institute for Immunology and Transplantation; Golf Classic "fore" Diabetes Research Chair; and Professor and Head, Division of Transplantation, Department of Surgery, University of Minnesota, Minneapolis, Minnesota

CHRISTOPHER L. WOLFGANG, MD, PhD, Assistant Professor, John L. Cameron Division of Surgical Oncology, Department of Surgery, The Johns Hopkins Medical Institutions, The Johns Hopkins Hospital, Baltimore, Maryland

CONTENTS

Although the most common causes of chronic pancreatitis have not changed, it has become clear that a host of modifying biochemical, inflammatory, neural, and genetic deviations allows the disease to progress. Alterations in biochemical composition allow calcific stone formation, whereas various toxins, cytokines, and neuro-peptides contribute to the progression of fibrosis and pain production. The basic cellular structure contributing to fibrosis of the pancreas has been elucidated and factors responsible for its activation delineated. Of most importance is the recent recognition of a set of genetic mutations that results in several aberrations of normal pancreatic physiology, which, in conjunction with other inciting insults or by themselves, allow the disease to begin and progress.

Acute pancreatitis is an inflammatory condition that is initiated by the intra pancreatic activation of proteases. Pancreatic enzyme activation triggers a local and systemic inflammatory response that is associated with recruitment of inflammatory cells into the pancreas and a widespread up-regulation of inflammatory markers in distant tissues.

FORTHCOMING ISSUES

RECENT ISSUES

SURGICAL
CLINICS OF
NORTH AMERICA

Surg Clin N Am 87 (2007) xiii–xv

Foreword

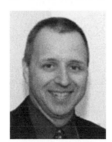

Ronald F. Martin, MD
Consulting Editor

Pancreatic surgery, and to some degree the surgeons who specialize in pancreatic surgery, has had an almost mythical—if not mystical—quality imbued to it. The oft quoted warnings about staying away from the pancreas and the general jitters that some people get when confronted with these problems have served to reinforce the idea that there is something fundamentally different about the pancreas. I cannot say that I have witnessed any concerted effort to dispel such notions, and I may have seen a few people try very hard to reinforce the idea. And in some ways that may have been a good thing.

Our understanding of how the pancreas works, how it fails to function properly, who is at greater risk for developing pancreatic disorders, and who is best capable of treating people who have pancreatic diseases continues to unfold at a refreshingly rapid pace. In this issue, an excellent series of reviews are provided that should well acquaint the reader with what we currently believe to be true regarding benign disorders of the pancreas. For those of you who like to hear the other shoe drop, we expect to include in a future issue a similarly comprehensive review of what we know about malignant disorders of the pancreas.

Over the past twenty years or so, there have been tremendous advances in our capacity to diagnose and treat patients who have pancreatic disorders. Along with this increase in knowledge, there has been a concerted effort to "centralize," (for lack of a better word) by some and to limit the care of these patients to certain locations. The motivations of those who have supported this effort, in my opinion, have been to maximize benefit to the

doi:10.1016/j.suc.2007.10.002   *surgical.theclinics.com*

individual patient and to the collective group of patients at large. Yet, there are some who could look upon this "centralization" as a "restraint of trade" issue. And since the practice of medicine and delivery of health care are still private industries, legislative fiat is limited in how much it can do to enforce such matters.

The evolution of thinking on who should deliver complex and unusual services for patients who have pancreatic diseases has moved along in parallel track to the development of our improved understanding. For a period of time it was suggested that institutional volume was the sole determinant of who could best provide care. Subsequently, it would appear that individual volume (of surgeons, at least) is probably a better predictor, though we don't really know what the actual volume of patients should be.

It never made sense to me that a surgeon who has a high volume pancreatic experience in one facility would become less capable if he or she moved to another facility. Nor did it make sense that if a hospital had a high overall volume of a given procedure that a "low volume" surgeon would derive "institutional benefit" for performing procedures infrequently unless the operative part of the patient's care was not really that important. It would therefore stand to reason that there are probably some features of surgeons that are important (something I think most people who perform these procedures often would agree with), and there are some institutional features that are important, as they may influence not only the care of the patient in "non-operative" situations but may also impact the ability of the surgeon to develop a high volume practice.

The traditional concept of the general surgeon has been one of an "incharge", individually responsible physician. We construct our training that way. The American Board of Surgery still instructs those of us who give the certifying exams to tell the candidates that "their consultants are all unavailable." But the more realistic viewpoint is that we are all parts of a system in which overall system performance is becoming, if not already, more important that individual performance. Surely, the weak link in the chain theory holds true in such cases, but one link does not make much of chain—strong link or otherwise. We as surgeons are most likely at a point where, if we want better operative outcomes for either individual patients or for collective groups of patients, we shall need to expend as much energy trying to improve the system lines that we work in as much as improve our own skill sets.

Pancreatic surgery lends itself well to these challenges. The discipline relies heavily on diagnostic imaging, endoscopic evaluation and treatment, metabolic and physiologic support, behavioral counseling, operative expertise (not just from the surgeon but from the entire operative team), anesthetic care, and, in some cases, perioperative critical care. Many of these associated disciplines have their own volume-to-expertise ratios that have to be considered as well. All of these disciplines are associated with fixed basal costs to maintain appropriate staffing and equipment capitalization to offer competitive quality services. The availability of adequate patient volume and revenue generation to sustain a full-time supra-critical mass of all the key clinical elements in a service-line model for the care of patients who have pancreatic diseases is probably the major determinant of where pancreatic surgery could be practiced. Maintaining adequate resources to achieve outcomes that are competitive with the "best practices" that are available at a finically acceptable burden will probably be the major barrier for most institutions to clear in order to participate in this type of care.

Individual focus and study as well as concentrating the challenging problems in the hands of fewer people who are willing to fully commit to their best solution for the patient has carried us a long way. As much as some of us might like to think that the discipline of pancreatic surgery is best characterized as "one riot, one ranger" (the motto of the Texas Rangers,) the reality is that we need to be a part—an important part, no doubt, but a part of a larger team if we expect to be competitive with the best performing groups.

The issue that Dr. Behrman has assembled should well familiarize the reader with the current state of understanding of benign pancreatic disorders. I am personally grateful to him for assuming the duties of editing this issue, as he did it on short notice as a favor. I would also like to acknowledge his other contributions to our country through his service in the United States Navy while activated as a reservist during the initial phases of this current military conflict. His efforts as well as those of his colleagues have helped countless suffering persons during tragic times.

Ronald F. Martin, MD
Department of Surgery
Marshfield Clinic
1000 North Oak Avenue
Marshfield, WI 54449, USA

E-mail address: martin.ronald@marshfieldclinic.org

SURGICAL
CLINICS OF
NORTH AMERICA

Surg Clin N Am 87 (2007) xvii–xviii

Preface

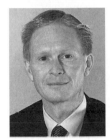

Stephen W. Behrman, MD
Guest Editor

The past decade has been noteworthy for incredible advances in the pathophysiology, diagnosis, and management of benign pancreatic disorders. The inflammatory cascade and genetics (or both) are now known to be intimately involved in the ravages associated with acute and chronic pancreatitis, respectively. Modern radiologic and endoscopic techniques allow precise imaging and physiologic assessment of pathologic pancreatic diseases. Tremendous advances in endoscopic and laparoscopic management of pancreatic disorders have simplified and hastened resolution and recovery of many benign conditions. Modern management of traumatic pancreatic injury has allowed improved diagnostic and therapeutic acumen in the operating room, which has translated to a decreased morbidity and mortality associated with this devastating injury. The role of islet cell transplantation to alleviate the complication of diabetes suffered by many patients who have benign pancreatic disorders has broadened, and progress in this field has been nothing less than spectacular. Finally, advances in the surgical management of benign pancreatic diseases have resulted in decreased procedure and pathologic-related complications and death.

To my knowledge, this is the first issue of the *Surgical Clinics of North America* devoted exclusively to benign pancreatic conditions—and rightly so. I can think of few areas in surgery where our decision-making and management have changed so rapidly in so short a period of time, and I offer a few examples. As Dr. David Sutherland pointed out to me when I asked him to contribute to this issue, the first islet cell transplant was reported in the *Surgical Clinics* in 1978. In 2007, this technique has reached the point

0039-6109/07/$ - see front matter © 2007 Elsevier Inc. All rights reserved.
doi:10.1016/j.suc.2007.10.001

where total pancreatectomy with auto islet cell transplantation can now safely be recommended to many with chronic pancreatitis as their *first* procedure. Necrotizing pancreatitis was almost a lethal event when I was in training, but refinements in diagnosis and operative management now mean that most will survive. Total parenteral nutrition previously utilized to "rest" the pancreas now largely plays a bridesmaid's role to enteral nutrition with its superior immune competence properties. In the past, Sphincter of Oddi dysfunction and pancreas divisum were diagnoses shrouded in mystery, but now both have defined diagnostic and therapeutic principles upon which to expect a satisfactory outcome. Modern nomenclature, diagnosis, and management of cystic neoplasms of the pancreas now allow superior nonoperative and operative outcomes.

I would like to sincerely thank all the contributors for their time and commitment to this endeavor. I value each as a surgical colleague, an expert in their respective field, and, after working with all, a friend. Their work and devotion on behalf of this issue I will not forget. I would like to specifically thank Ms. Catherine Bewick at Elsevier publications for her patience and expertise in helping this novice editor put this issue of the *Surgical Clinics of North America* together.

Finally, I was fortunate to be asked to take on the role of guest editor for this issue of the *Surgical Clinics of North America* by your regular consulting editor, Ronald F. Martin, MD. Ron has a wealth of experience in management of pancreatic diseases and truly should have edited this issue himself, except for the fact he was serving his *second* tour of duty in Iraq as an army reservist surgeon since the 2003 invasion. As a former military officer myself, I have a deep appreciation for this sacrifice and I know I speak on behalf of all the authors of this issue and the entire surgical community in thanking Ron for his commitment to our men and women in uniform and to our country.

Enjoy and savor this reading. It is my sincere hope that a future issue of the *Surgical Clinics of North America* on this very topic renders this issue a footnote to future advances.

Stephen W. Behrman, MD
University of Tennessee, Memphis
910 Madison Avenue
2nd Floor, Room 208
Memphis, TN 38163, USA

E-mail address: sbehrman@utmem.edu

SURGICAL
CLINICS OF
NORTH AMERICA

Surg Clin N Am 87 (2007) 1309–1324

Pathophysiology of Chronic Pancreatitis

Stephen W. Behrman, MD[a],*,
Eric S. Fowler, MS, CGC[b]

[a]Department of Surgery, University of Tennessee, Memphis, 910 Madison Avenue,
2nd Floor, Room 208, Memphis, TN 38163, USA
[b]Baptist Centers for Cancer Care, Baptist Memorial Hospital-Memphis,
55 Humphreys Center, Dr. Suite 301, Memphis, TN 38120, USA

Chronic pancreatitis (CP) is defined as the permanent destruction of the gland on a histologic level and a failure of the organ on a physiologic level. Inflammation and fibrosis of the pancreas eventually lead to destruction of acinar cells and the islets of Langerhans. Clinically, this process is associated with chronic abdominal pain in most patients, weight loss, steatorrhea, and diabetes. Economically, CP inflicts considerable damage in terms of lost wages, innumerable hospital visits, excessive medication (narcotic) usage, and the need for operative and nonoperative intervention. The diagnosis carries with it a higher risk for early mortality and an increased risk for the development of pancreatic carcinoma. In the Western world, the cause of the disease remains primarily one of self-indulgence with alcohol, although CP only affects a minority (approximately 10%) of individuals using alcohol in excess. To attribute the cause and progression of CP to any one given mechanism would be oversimplification. It has become increasingly recognized that although the inciting event of CP may be consistent, the pathophysiology of the disease is multifactorial and likely includes environmental, nutritional, chemical, and genetic abnormalities. For example, a genetic predisposition to the disease has become a not uncommonly recognized phenomenon and may partly explain why the minority of individuals abusing alcohol develop CP. This article reviews new concepts in the pathogenesis of CP.

Incidence and natural history

Defining the exact incidence of CP is difficult because autopsy findings of fibrosis may be seen as part of the aging process and there is poor

---

* Corresponding author.
E-mail address: sbehrman@utmem.edu (S.W. Behrman).

doi:10.1016/j.suc.2007.09.001 *surgical.theclinics.com*

correlation between histologic findings and either the symptoms of CP or evidence of organ dysfunction. The underlying cause of the disease varies, although most often alcohol is thought to represent the inciting event. Finally, definitions and diagnostic criteria used to define CP are variable. With these limitations in mind, CP is demonstrated in approximately 0.05% to 5% of autopsies, which most likely represents an overestimate [1]. The prevalence of the disease has been reported as high as approximately 1 per 830 in the orient and India, where tropical pancreatitis (TP) is common, to 27.4 per 100,000 in Scandinavia, where CP most commonly results from alcohol consumption [2,3].

Genetic abnormalities associated with CP include mutations of the cystic fibrosis transmembrane conductance regulator (CFTR), the Kazal type 1 serine protease inhibitor (SPINK1), and the protease serine 1 (PRSS1) genes. The incidence of one or more of these mutations in individuals who have CP varies from 0 to 100% depending on the cause of CP, as is discussed later in this article [4].

The natural history of CP is characterized by progressive pain and loss of glandular function. Pain, initially intermittent, becomes constant. Most often, exocrine and endocrine function is gradually lost, with endocrine dysfunction lagging behind that of the exocrine pancreas [5,6]. Evidence suggests that a progressive loss of pancreatic function with or without an increase in glandular calcification may lead to an alleviation of pain (pancreatic "burnout") [5,7]. In the study by Ammann and colleagues [5], 145 patients with alcoholic relapsing calcific pancreatitis were followed for a mean of 10.4 years. In this group, 85% of patients had lasting pain relief within a median time of 4.5 years. A gradual increase of pancreatic calcification and progressive pancreatic dysfunction was observed with increasing duration of disease. The observation of predictable nonoperative pain resolution given a certain disease duration remains controversial, and this conservative approach to the disease has not been universally followed [8]. Results in surgical series suggest that pancreatic ductal decompression not only relieves pain in most patients but also delays exocrine and endocrine dysfunction [9,10]. The impact of continued alcohol use on the progression of CP is also contentious. Some studies suggest that abstinence may decrease the severity and frequency of pain and reduce the progressive loss of pancreatic function [11,12]. In contrast, other studies have found that cessation from alcohol does not alter the course of the disease or that CP remains stable despite continued use [13].

The mortality rate associated with CP may approach 50% within 20 years of diagnosis, especially in persons whose disease is caused by alcohol abuse [5,6,11]. In this population, most deaths are caused by complications related to tobacco abuse, liver dysfunction, infection, and malnutrition. Approximately 20% of deaths are related to complications arising from CP itself, however. CP is a known risk factor for the development of pancreatic carcinoma. Approximately 3% to 4% of individuals who have CP develop carcinoma, a rate that is substantially higher than the general population [5,14]. The cumulative lifetime risk of pancreatic cancer in persons with hereditary pancreatitis (HP) approaches 40%. It is crucial to consider and diagnose this genetic disorder because earlier and more aggressive pancreatic resection might be considered (see later discussion) [15,16].

Chronic pancreatitis: defining normal function

A discussion of the pathophysiology of CP involves the interplay of several key components. A brief discussion of normal physiology is critical to understanding the aberrations that occur in this disease [17]. Pancreatic acinar cells are responsible for the production, storage, and release of digestive enzymes. Autodigestion in the normal pancreas is prevented by several mechanisms. Enzymes are synthesized as inactive precursors and segregated into membrane-bound organelles. Intracellular antiproteases prevent premature activation of these zymogens. The PRSS1 gene is important in maintaining the stability of pancreatic zymogens in their inactive form. PRSS1 gene mutations allow activation of trypsinogen to trypsin, which allows conversion of all proteolytic proenzymes to their active counterparts. The SPINK1 gene is responsible for maintaining the integrity of the serine protease inhibitor that binds with intrapancreatic trypsin, which maintains trypsin homeostasis within the acinar cell. Mutations of this gene allow abnormally high concentrations of trypsin to activate other proenzymes.

The duct cells are responsible for the volume and bicarbonate concentration in pancreatic juice, which are important in maintaining trypsin in its inactive state. A diminution of either or both increases the risk for protein precipitation, which can lead to obstruction, potential calcification, ductal hypertension, and trypsin activation. Low bicarbonate secretion leads to a compensatory increase in secretin release and an increased demand in the face of a relative obstruction that likely contributes to the pain of CP. In the pancreas, CFTR regulates ductal bicarbonate secretion and volume, because water flows passively in response to bicarbonate concentration because of an osmotic gradient. Mutations of this gene reduce bicarbonate secretion and allow these pathologic conditions to exist.

Pancreatic stellate cells (PSCs) are morphologically similar to hepatic stellate cells [18]. Both types are the principal cells responsible for fibrosis within their respective organs and are the predominant source of collagen. PSCs regulate the synthesis and degradation of the extracellular matrix proteins that comprise fibrous tissue and are usually quiescent. Activated PSCs have been demonstrated in tissue from persons who have alcoholic pancreatitis. Stellate cells are activated by acetaldehyde, the metabolite of ethanol (PSCs have alcohol dehydrogenase activity), and plasma lipopolysaccharides (increased in individuals with heavy ethanol use). Cytokines released during pancreatitis (eg, tumor necrosis factor-α, interleukins [IL]-1 and -6) have been demonstrated to activate PSCs in vitro. PSCs can synthesize cytokines that can perpetuate cell activation, extracellular matrix production, and fibrosis, even after the initial insult has subsided. Pain sensation in the pancreas is mediated by visceral afferent sympathetic fibers with transmission to the celiac plexus and splanchnic nerves. Any compromise to the pancreatic nervous system by inflammation or fibrosis may allow abnormal interaction with various pain-mediated neuropeptides and cytokines.

Histopathology of chronic pancreatitis

Although the causes of CP may differ, the histologic features of the disease are similar [19,20]. In sequential fashion, variable interlobular, lobular, and ductal fibrosis may be seen throughout the gland in the early stages of CP and become more diffuse as the disease progresses. As acinar cells within the lobules are destroyed by fibrosis, exocrine dysfunction ensues. The islets of Langerhans are generally preserved until CP is advanced, and endocrine dysfunction generally lags behind that of the exocrine pancreas. In advanced stages, subintimal fibrosis of blood vessels can be demonstrated and nerve fibers are drawn into the fibrotic process. Infiltrating into these areas of fibrosis are lymphocytes, plasma cells, and macrophages. The PSC has been demonstrated in vitro and in vivo to be primarily involved with collagen deposition and eventual fibrosis [18]. PSCs are activated by cytokines released during pancreatitis and the direct, toxic effects of alcohol. Chronic alcohol use is associated with pancreatic juice that is rich in protein from acinar cell secretion but low in volume and bicarbonate from the duct cell [21]. This favors the formation of eosinophilic protein plugs noted on microscopic examination. These plugs can calcify and obstruct both side branches and the main duct of Wirsung, which contributes to the pain associated with CP.

Pathophysiology of pain

Stone formation

Pancreatic duct stones found in alcoholic, hereditary, and TP are rich in calcium carbonate and glycoprotein-2 (GP-2). GP-2 is released from the apical surface of the acinar cell and is a protein analog of uromodulin, which contributes to nephrolithiasis [22]. Evidence suggests that a chemical imbalance contributes to calcific stone formation and ductal obstruction, which may help explain, in part, why CP affects only a minority of individuals who abuse alcohol. Pancreatic juice contains high concentrations of calcium and bicarbonate. Lithostathine, a glycoprotein secreted into pancreatic juice from the acinar cell, is an inhibitor of calcium carbonate precipitation [23]. The concentration of lithostathine in pancreatic juice is diminished in persons with calcific pancreatitis [24]. Although most patients with pancreatic calcifications may have pain presumably on the basis of ductal obstruction, this is by no means universal because other patients are completely asymptomatic, even with major ductal dilation.

Pancreatic hypertension

With or without major ductal obstruction by calcifications, increased intrapancreatic pressure, or "pancreatic hypertension," has been demonstrated in nearly every surgical patient who has CP [25,26]. Pancreaticoenterostomy and pancreatic resection are associated with an immediate reduction in pancreatic pressure, and the degree of pain relief typically correlates with the drop in pressure. Experimental animal models suggest that the pain associated with increased ductal pressure is on the basis of tissue ischemia [27]. Increased pressure in the pancreas is associated with a reduction in interstitial pH, tissue oxygen tension, and pancreatic blood flow. Cellular necrosis may ensue. Secretory stimulation of the pancreas in animals with CP paradoxically exacerbates the decrease in pancreatic blood flow contrary to what is observed in the normal pancreas. Alcohol, a known stimulant of pancreatic secretion, is associated with these abnormal physiologic changes [28]. Physiologic and histologic changes associated with pancreatic hypertension are thought to account for the "necrosis to fibrosis" theory of CP. Pancreatic hypertension and tissue ischemia are reversed in animal models by pancreaticojejunostomy [29]. This improved physiologic state with ductal decompression might explain the preservation of exocrine and endocrine function and the alleviation of pain noted in clinical studies [9,10].

Neural pathology

Changes in the neural innervation of the pancreas may explain potential contributions to pain encountered by persons who have CP. The pancreas receives nerve fibers from the sympathetic division of the autonomic nervous system via the splanchnic nerves and parasympathetic fibers from the vagus nerves. The nerves typically follow blood vessels and pancreatic ducts to reach the pancreatic acini. The splanchnic nerves also contain visceral afferent (pain) fibers. The splanchnic nervous system (greater, lesser, and least) is composed of preganglionic efferent fibers from the fifth through the eleventh thoracic segments. These nerves pierce the diaphragm to enter the celiac plexus and ganglion. Pain sensation is transmitted by visceral afferent sympathetic fibers within the pancreas to the celiac plexus and the splanchnic nerves and then moves on to the thoracic spinal cord. No clear evidence supports a vagal contribution to pancreatic pain.

Histologic changes to nerve sheaths within the pancreas in persons who have CP were reported by Bockman and colleagues [30]. Pancreatic tissue from 18 patients having duodenum-preserving resection of the pancreatic head for CP were analyzed and compared with 10 controls. In persons who had CP, the mean diameter of nerves was greater, although the mean area served per nerve was less because of parenchymal atrophy and fibrosis. There was no evidence of constriction of nerves by the fibrotic process. The integrity of the perineural sheath was altered by edema, however, which suggested that the normal microenvironment of the nerve may be compromised and allow substances to interact with nerves that would otherwise be excluded, including local neuropeptides. By immunostain technique, the pain neurotransmitters substance P and calcitonin gene-related peptide have been shown to be present in greater concentration in tissue from persons who have CP, which suggests an up-regulation of these neuropeptides [31]. The combination of a compromised perineurium with an up-regulation of pain-inducing neurotransmitters may represent not only an important pathway of pain production in CP but also a potential approach toward targeted therapy in pain reduction. Cytokines also may play a role in neural pain production. Substance P directly stimulates the release of (IL-8, a proinflammatory hyperalgesia mediator, from macrophages [32]. IL-8 stimulates postganglionic sympathetic neurons and is present in increased quantities in tissue recovered from individuals who have CP. IL-8 mRNA expression correlates with the inflammatory score associated with CP. These neuronal changes may help explain why splanchnicectomy for CP (and pancreatic carcinoma), by interrupting the sympathetic pathway, is associated with pain relief [33,34]. In all surgical series to date, however, pain relief after splanchnicectomy is neither universal nor reliably longstanding in all patients, which suggests that other factors contribute to the discomfort of CP.

Although the pathologic findings in CP are consistent, it is unlikely that the pain associated with this disease can be explained on the basis of one model alone. Not every patient with pancreatic calcifications or ductal obstruction has pain. Decompressive or resectional surgical procedures are not always associated with long-term pain relief. The interplay of physiologic, neural, anatomic, and chemical factors impacts on the dysfunction and pain involved in persons who have CP. Treatment of patients should be rendered only after thorough scrutiny of the pathways to pain production. Because of the multifactorial production of pain, a multimodality approach to pain resolution may be necessary.

The genetics of chronic pancreatitis

Historical perspective

In the early 1950s, Comfort and associates [35] described HP as a highly penetrant, autosomal dominant condition. It was not until the mid-1990s that several groups established linkage between chromosome 7q35 and the HP phenotype. A specific alteration in the cationic trypsinogen gene, PRSS1, was found to segregate with the disease in multiple HP kindreds [36]. In 1998, two separate reports found an increased incidence of CFTR gene mutations in patients who had idiopathic CP [37,38]. More recently,

Witt and colleagues [39] reported that mutations in the SPINK1 gene were associated with CP. The discovery of transheterozygotes—individuals with mutations in multiple genes—and the resultant additive or synergistic effect on disease underscores the complex nature of genotype and phenotype expression in CP.

Gene mutations associated with chronic pancreatitis

The complexities of the genetic factors that predispose to, modify, and impact upon CP are slowly being unraveled (Table 1). Molecular and clinical studies are beginning to delineate our understanding of the interrelationship between genetic and environmental influences on the development and progression of CP. The importance of interactions between genotype and environment is emphasized by variations in the penetrance and disease severity even among family members with the same mutation. Mutations that result in loss of protein function rather than diminished activity have been demonstrated to have a major impact even in the heterozygous state [40]. Environmental factors, such as smoking and alcohol consumption, may act to decrease the threshold for the development of CP or exacerbate disease progression. The current knowledge and understanding of the genetic components of CP are reviewed.

PRSS1

Digestive enzymes in the pancreas are stored in their inactive forms in pancreatic zymogen granules. Under most circumstances, enzyme activation is controlled, which prevents autodigestion of the pancreas [41]. PRSS1 is one of three genes that produce functional trypsinogen and specifically results in the production of cationic trypsinogen [17]. Certain mutations in the PRSS1 gene, most notably R122H and N29I, are frequently observed in patients who have HP and are thought to result in gain of function resulting in the intrapancreatic activation of trypsinogen to trypsin [41–43]. The R122H mutation blocks autolysis of trypsin and results in continuous

Table 1
Cause of chronic pancreatitis and recognized associated genetic mutations

Cause	Genetic mutation (may have 1 or more)
Alcoholic	SPINK 1
	CFTR
Tropical	SPINK1
Hereditary	PRSS1
	SPINK1
	CFTR
Idiopathic	SPINK1
	CFTR

trypsin activity. The N29I mutation may change the structure of trypsin and result in decreased binding to SPINK1 and lead to its increased stability and autoactivation [41]. By increasing transcription and gene dosage effects with the duplication of large segments of DNA, additional, less common PRSS1 mutations may lead to pancreatitis by the activation of other pancreatic enzymes [41,44–46].

PRSS1 mutations are inherited in an autosomal dominant manner, with 50% of the offspring of carriers inheriting the mutation. The onset of symptoms is early, with median age of onset being 13 years. More than 50% of families who have HP have PRSS1 mutations, and 70% to 80% of patients with the R122H and N29I mutations develop pancreatitis [47]. The explanation for incomplete penetrance is unclear, but it is hypothesized that modifier genes (protective and disease associated) and environmental factors impact phenotype [17].

SPINK1

The SPINK1 protein protects the pancreas from autodigestion by the inhibition of approximately 20% of trypsin activity. The pathologic effect of SPINK1 mutations remains controversial, with some hypotheses predicting a causal effect in pancreatitis and others proposing a modifier role in the development of disease [42]. Two recurrent mutations, N34S and 194+2T > C, have been observed in patients who develop CP. There is debate over whether the N34S mutation is pathogenic, and suspicion exists that a closely linked intronic sequence variant may be the deleterious mutation (may have 1 or more) [17,39]. The N34S mutation may lower the threshold for disease by interacting with other genes and environmental factors [41]. The 194+2TA > C mutation affects mRNA splicing, which leads to skipping of exon 3 and a truncated SPINK1 protein that results in a loss of function [48]. Research suggests that patients heterozygous for SPINK1 mutations are less likely to have CP than their homozygous counterparts, although this finding has not been duplicated in every study [38,41]. Disease penetrance may depend on the functional impact of the mutation, with severe mutations having a causal effect in a single dose and milder mutations having phenotypic impact when on both alleles or with the interaction of other loci [17,39].

Data gathered from multiple institutions in Europe and the United States have shown an association between SPINK1 mutations and CP. The N34S mutation is detected in the heterozygous and homozygous state in 12.6% and 3.6% of patients with CP, respectively. This rate compares with a 1.9% incidence in a control population [17]. The N34S mutation also has been implicated as a major risk factor in the development of tropical calcific pancreatitis and as a more minor susceptibility allele in cases of alcoholic and idiopathic CP [40,42]. Age of onset and likelihood of pancreatitis associated with SPINK1 mutations vary, although affected children and adolescents are widely reported in the literature [40].

Cystic fibrosis transmembrane conductance regulator

The CFTR gene produces a chloride channel protein essential in fluid, chloride, and bicarbonate secretion in the respiratory and digestive tracts. CF is an autosomal recessive condition that results from the inheritance of two pathogenic CFTR mutations, which contributes to respiratory dysfunction and pancreatic insufficiency. Only a minority of patients who have CF develop pancreatitis [17]. Abnormal CFTR channel proteins inadequately flush the digestive enzymes from the pancreatic duct and limit bicarbonate secretion, which helps maintain trypsin in its inactive form [49].

Approximately 25% to 30% of patients who have CP are single and compound CFTR heterozygotes with mutations detected at six times the expected rate of the normal population [50,51]. Compound heterozygotes, in whom one mutation is milder, may present with pancreatitis but not demonstrate the more severe manifestations of CF [52]. As in the case of SPINK1, CFTR mutations may act as disease modifiers and lower the threshold for the development of pancreatitis.

Genetic counseling and patient identification

Genetic counseling for HP is a multistep process that involves patient identification, pedigree analysis, pretest education and counseling, the provision of informed consent, the selection of genetic tests, the disclosure of results, and posttest counseling and follow-up. Genetic counselors, gastroenterologists, endocrinologists, surgeons, and oncologists are part of the multidisciplinary team that works with patients who have HP.

In 2001, during the Third International Symposium on Inherited Diseases of the Pancreas, a consensus conference was held to address genetic testing in HP. The result was the following criteria for genetic testing [53]:

- Recurrent (two or more separate, documented episodes with hyperamylasemia) attacks of acute pancreatitis for which there is no other explanation (eg, anatomic anomalies, ampullary or main pancreatic strictures, trauma, viral infection, gallstones, alcohol, drugs, hyperlipidemia)
- Unexplained (idiopathic) CP, particularly onset younger than age 25
- A family history of pancreatitis in a first-degree (parent, sibling, child) or second-degree (aunt, uncle, grandparent) relative
- Looser criteria in two close relatives with recurrent episodes of acute pancreatitis or CP
- An unexplained episode of documented pancreatitis occurring in a child that requires hospitalization and in cases in which there is significant concern that HP should be excluded

These guidelines were applicable only to genetic testing for mutations in the PRSS1 gene. In our practice, these parameters are also used in conjunction with genetic testing for SPINK1 and CFTR mutations.

A three-generation pedigree is an essential part of the initial information-gathering process, including information about the familial incidence of pancreatitis, abdominal pain, diabetes, and pancreatic cancer. The information provided in pretest genetic counseling should include a review of general genetics principles, the link between genetics and disease, a summary of the genes being evaluated, the possibility of informative and indeterminate results, and the implications of and management issues arising from the discovery of a mutation. Other issues to be addressed are the psychological ramifications of the test results, potential changes in family dynamics, and the current knowledge of the risks (albeit low and hypothetical) of genetic discrimination.

The selection of a laboratory for genetic testing should be based on test methodology, quality measures, cost, which genes are evaluated, and turn-around time. Determine the method of results disclosure with patients—whether in person or by more indirect means—before the testing is initiated. Posttest genetic counseling includes interpreting the meaning of the genetic test results in accessible terms, reviewing strategies for sharing results with family members, discussing medical management recommendations, and, if a mutation is detected, identifying other family members who would benefit from genetic testing.

Common causes of chronic pancreatitis

Defining its relationship to pathophysiology

Alcohol

By far, the most common cause of CP is alcohol consumption, which accounts for 70% to 90% of all cases in Western countries. Typically, the onset of CP correlates with the duration and amount of ethanol intake; however, the disease can occur even with relatively little consumption but almost never occurs in persons who consume alcohol for less than 5 years [54]. This factor, combined with the fact that few individuals who use alcohol in heavy amounts develop CP, suggests that other mediators are involved in the evolution of CP. Smoking and a diet high in fat and proteins in combination with alcohol abuse may allow the development of CP, with the latter being associated with more rapid development of pancreatic calcifications [54,55]. With respect to smoking, animal studies suggest that tobacco is a risk factor for the development of CP independent of alcohol [56]. Human studies that examined the development of CP in persons with idiopathic CP (in whom alcohol use was felt to be "minimal" and have little impact on disease initiation and progression) have confirmed these findings and suggested that disease onset and endocrine insufficiency may be hastened in individuals who abuse alcohol and tobacco [57,58]. Clearly, smoking imparts a synergistic effect to alcohol alone in the development of CP.

Perhaps the most intriguing cofactor responsible for the development of CP in persons who abuse alcohol involves genetic abnormalities. CFTR and SPINK1 gene mutations have been associated with alcohol-induced CP, and researchers have estimated that alcohol triples the risk of CP in carriers of these mutations [59]. CFTR mutations have been reported in approximately 8.5% of patients who have alcohol-induced CP [36]. In a similar population, two separate centers found a SPINK1 mutation in approximately 6% [60,61]. It seems plausible that future discovery of other mutations within these genes might significantly increase the number of patients susceptible to CP in this population.

Nearly all patients who have alcohol-induced CP develop calcification of the gland with resultant obstruction of the minor and major ducts. Pancreatic hypertension with subsequent ischemia-related phenomena follows and is associated with exocrine and endocrine dysfunction, changes that can be reversed by ductal decompression [9,10]. Inefficient secretion of digestive enzymes may allow activation of intrapancreatic trypsin and result in local tissue injury. By failing to maintain normal trypsin binding, inactivation, and release, SPINK1 and CFTR mutations exacerbate this local environment. Obstruction also causes a diminution in bicarbonate and enzyme release from the pancreatic duct and increased protein secretion from the acinar cell, which results in a concomitant exaggerated release of cholecystokinin and secretin and further increases pancreatic secretion in the face of a relative obstruction. A vicious cycle ensues that results in pancreatic tissue injury, PSC activation, and fibrosis.

Finally, alcohol or one of its metabolites may have a direct harmful effect on ductal acinar cells [17]. In vitro studies have demonstrated that the pancreas metabolizes ethanol into acetaldehyde and free fatty acid ethyl esters. Acetaldehyde has been demonstrated in animal models to cause direct morphologic damage to the pancreas and directly stimulates PSCs, which leads to gland fibrosis. Fatty acid ethyl esters have been demonstrated in a rat model to cause pancreatic edema, acinar vacuolization, and trypsinogen activation.

Tropical pancreatitis

TP is the most common form of CP in parts of India and the tropics, with a much higher prevalence than geographic areas in which alcohol predominates as the inciting event [62]. Its distribution is generally restricted to areas within 30 degrees of the equator. Most patients develop the disease before age 40, and almost universally the gland becomes diffusely calcified with dilation of the duct of Wirsung and associated gland atrophy. As such, pancreatic hypertension and ischemia-related phenomena undoubtedly exist. Clinically, these patients develop chronic abdominal pain and nutritional deficiencies. Diabetes develops not uncommonly before age 30.

The pathophysiology of this disease remains incomplete. Alcohol abuse, biliary disease, and metabolic disorders are not common in endemic areas.

Protein-calorie malnutrition is found not infrequently, but it is also found in other parts of the world where TP is not common, and the disease affects persons with higher income levels in whom malnutrition would not be prevalent. There has been an association with cassava (tapioca) intake, because the dietary intake of this food staple frequently—but not absolutely—correlates with the endemic distribution of TP [63]. Cassava is a source of cyanogenic glycosides, which have been associated with oxidative injury of the pancreas.

It has been previously recognized that TP frequently has a familial clustering [64]. Recent studies have demonstrated heterozygous and homozygous mutations of the SPINK1 gene in up to 47% of individuals who have TP [65,66]. In the study by Bhatia and colleagues [65], 29 (44%) of 69 unrelated Indian patients who have TP carried mutations of the SPINK1 gene. It may be that future genetic analysis will yield further mutations responsible for phenotypic expression of this disease.

Hereditary pancreatitis

In the broadest sense, HP in a patient may be defined as recurrent episodes of disease with an underlying germline mutation. The discovery of PRSS1, SPINK1, and CFTR mutations in patients with chronic disease and a negative family history has blurred the lines between the terms "hereditary" and "idiopathic" CP [17]. The strictest definition of HP was published in the EUROPAC study and included two first-degree relatives or three or more second-degree relatives in two or more generations with recurrent acute pancreatitis or CP for which there were no precipitating factors [43].

Patients who have HP typically present with a first episode of pancreatitis at an early age—frequently even before adolescence—that progresses to CP in early adulthood. Approximately 50% of individuals who have HP harbor a PRSS1 mutation, and patients with this disease may show defects in all three known genes. It is important to reiterate that any patient who has recurrent pancreatitis before age 25 without a discernible cause should be referred for genetic analysis to assess for HP. In our experience, although many of these patients may be amenable to surgical drainage procedures (pancreaticojejunostomy) or resection (pancreaticoduodenectomy or distal pancreatectomy), long-term results of these more common operations have not been satisfactory [16]. Although early pain relief may be anticipated, we have been impressed with a rapid progression of the disease and a high rate of recidivism. Our current approach is to recommend up-front total pancreatectomy. Scarring at the index procedure is significant, and reoperation for this disease has been particularly difficult. Pain relief after total pancreatectomy has been durable, and total pancreatectomy eliminates the concern in this population for the future development of pancreatic carcinoma. Ideally, identification of HP early in its course would allow these patients to be candidates for total pancreatectomy with auto islet cell transplantation before endocrine destruction ensues.

Idiopathic chronic pancreatitis

The cause of CP remains elusive in up to one third of patients with disease. These cases, grouped under the term idiopathic CP, have negative family histories and have been the focus of much research [42,52]. Smoking is likely a contributor to—and may be frankly responsible for—CP in this cohort [57]. Highly penetrant mutations in the PRSS1 gene are unlikely to be found in patients who have idiopathic CP. In contrast, germline mutations in the less penetrant SPINK1 and CFTR genes have been identified in patients who have idiopathic CP in multiple studies, with an incidence of SPINK1 mutations ranging from 6% to 40% of cases [47,61,67,68]. One recent study determined that 80% of patients who had idiopathic CP had mutations in either SPINK1 or CFTR or were transheterozygotes with mutations in both genes [52]. Like other forms of CP, this disease is associated with exocrine and endocrine dysfunction, although these physiologic derangements tend to progress slower than other more common forms of the disease, perhaps because of the lack of a contributing insult, such as alcohol. Approximately two thirds of these patients still ultimately require surgical intervention, however.

Summary

The cause of CP has not changed; however, our understanding of disease initiation and progression has expanded. Biochemical, environmental, physiologic, and neural abnormalities contribute to disease onset, progression, and pain. These disease modifiers help explain the susceptibility for the development of CP in only some individuals at risk. PSCs provide the matrix for gland fibrosis, and the pathogenesis for their activation has been ascertained. Without question, the most important contribution to our understanding of CP has been the elucidation of a series of genetic mutations that cause myriad physiologic derangements in normal pancreatic exocrine function. In some instances these mutations act as disease modifiers that amplify other inciting events, such as alcohol and smoking. These genetic abnormalities are also capable of causing CP independent of other risk factors, however. Future progress in this field likely will include further delineation of the cytokines involved with the disease, the neurotransmitters responsible for pain, factors involved with PSC stimulus and function, and identification of other genetic mutations that contribute to the development of CP.

References

[1] Olsen TS. The incidence and clinical relevance of chronic inflammation in the pancreas in autopsy material. Acto Pathol Microbiol Scand 1978;86(A):361–5.
[2] Copenhagen Pancreatitis Study: an interim report from a prospective multicentre. Scand J Gastroenterol 1981;16:305–12.

[3] Balaji LN, Tandon RK, Tandon BN, et al. Prevalence and clinical features of chronic pancreatitis in Southern India. Int J Pancreatol 1993;15:29–34.

[4] Rosendahl J, Bodeker H, Mossner J, et al. Hereditary chronic pancreatitis. Orphanet J Rare Dis 2007;2:1–10.

[5] Ammann RW, Akovbiantz A, Largiader F, et al. Course and outcome of chronic pancreatitis: longitudinal study of a mixed medical-surgical series of 245 patients. Gastroenterology 1984;86:820–8.

[6] Lankisch PG, Lohr-Happe A, Otto J, et al. Natural course in chronic pancreatitis: pain, exocrine and endocrine pancreatic insufficiency and prognosis of the disease. Digestion 1993;54:148–55.

[7] Kloppel G, Maillet B. The morphological basis for the evolution of acute pancreatitis into chronic pancreatitis. Virchows Arch A Pathol Anat Histopathol 1992;420:1–4.

[8] Warshaw AL. Pain in chronic pancreatitis: patients, patience, and the impatient surgeon. Gastroenterology 1984;86:987–9.

[9] Jalleh RP, Williamson RCN. Pancreatic exocrine and endocrine function after operations for chronic pancreatitis. Ann Surg 1992;216:656–62.

[10] Nealon WH, Thompson JC. Progressive loss of pancreatic function in chronic pancreatitis is delayed by main pancreatic duct decompression: a longitudinal prospective analysis of the modified puestow procedure. Ann Surg 1993;217:458–68.

[11] Hayakawa T, Kondo T, Shibata T, et al. Chronic alcoholism and evolution of pain and prognosis in chronic pancreatitis. Dig Dis Sci 1989;34:33–8.

[12] Ammann RW, Buehler H, Muench R, et al. Differences in the natural history of idiopathic (nonalcoholic) and alcoholic pancreatitis: a comparative long-term study of 287 patients. Pancreas 1987;2:368–77.

[13] Ammann RW, Muellhaupt B, Meyenberger C, et al. Alcoholic nonprogressive chronic pancreatitis: prospective long-term study of a large cohort with alcoholic acute pancreatitis (1976–1992). Pancreas 1994;9:365–73.

[14] Lowenfels AB, Maisonneuve P, Cavallini G, et al. Pancreatitis and the risk of pancreatic cancer. N Engl J Med 1993;328:1433–7.

[15] Lowenfuls AB, Maisonneuve P, DiMagno EP, et al. Hereditary pancreatitis and the risk of pancreatic cancer: international hereditary pancreatitis study group. J Natl Cancer Inst 1997;89:442–6.

[16] Behrman SW, Mulloy M. Total pancreatectomy for the treatment of chronic pancreatitis: indications, outcomes and recommendations. Am Surg 2006;72:297–302.

[17] Witt H, Apte MV, Keim V, et al. Chronic pancreatitis: challenges and advances in pathogenesis, genetics, diagnosis and therapy. Gastroenterology 2007;132:1557–73.

[18] Apte MV, Wilson JS. Stellate cell activation in alcoholic pancreatitis. Pancreas 2003;27: 316–20.

[19] Howard JM, Nedwich A. Correlation of the histologic observations and operative findings in patients with chronic pancreatitis. Surg Gynecol Obstet 1971;132:387–95.

[20] Kloppel G, Maillet B. Pathology of acute and chronic pancreatitis. Pancreas 1993;8:659–70.

[21] Sachel J, Sarles H. Modifications of pure human pancreatic juice induced by chronic alcohol consumption. Dig Dis Sci 1979;24:897–905.

[22] Freedman SD, Sakamoto D, Venu RP. GP2, the homologue to the renal cast protein uromodulin, is a major component of intraductal plugs in chronic pancreatitis. J Clin Invest 1993; 92:83–90.

[23] Bernard JP, Adrich Z, Montalto G, et al. Inhibition of nucleation and crystal growth of calcium carbonate by human lithostathine. Gastroenterology 1992;103:1277–84.

[24] Sarles H. Chronic pancreatitis and diabetes. Baillierres Clin Endocrinol Metab 1992;6: 745–75.

[25] Jalleh RP, Aslam M, Williamson RCN. Pancreatic tissue and ductal pressures in chronic pancreatitis. Br J Surg 1991;78:1235–7.

[26] Ebbehoj N, Borly L, Bulow J, et al. Evaluation of pancreatic tissue fluid pressure and pain in chronic pancreatitis. Scand J Gastroentereol 1990;25:462–6.

[27] Patal A, Toyama MT, Reber H, et al. Pancreatic interstitial pH in human and feline chronic pancreatitis. Gastroenterology 1995;109:1639–45.

[28] Toyama MT, Patal AG, Nguyen T, et al. Effect of ethanol on pancreatic interstitial pH and blood flow in cats with chronic pancreatitis. Ann Surg 1997;225:223–8.

[29] Patel AG, Reber PU, Toyama MT, et al. Effect of pancreaticojejunostomy on fibrosis, pancreatic blood flow and interstitial pH in chronic pancreatitis: a feline model. Ann Surg 1999; 230:672–9.

[30] Bockman DE, Buchler M, Malfertheiner P, et al. Analysis of nerves in chronic pancreatitis. Gastroenterology 1988;94:1459–69.

[31] Buchler M, Weihe E, Friess H, et al. Changes in peptidergic innervation in chronic pancreatitis. Pancreas 1992;7:183–92.

[32] DiSebastiano P, di Mola FF, DiFebbo C, et al. Expression of interleukin 8 (IL-8) and substance P in human chronic pancreatitis. Gut 2000;47:423–8.

[33] Mallet-Guy PA. Late and very late results of resections of the nervous system in the treatment of chronic relapsing pancreatitis. Am J Surg 1983;145:234–8.

[34] Buscher HC, Jansen JB, van Dongen R, et al. Long-term results of bilateral thoracoscopic splanchnicectomy in patients with chronic pancreatitis. Br J Surg 2002;89:158 62.

[35] Comfort MW, Steinberg AG. Pedigree of a family with hereditary chronic pancreatitis. Gastroenterology 1952,21.54–63.

[36] Whitcomb DC, Gorry MC, Preston RA, et al. Hereditary pancreatitis is caused by a mutation in the cationic trypsinogen gene. Nat Genet 1996;14:141–5.

[37] Cohn JA, Friedman KJ, Noone PG, et al. Relation between mutations of the cystic fibrosis gene and idiopathic pancreatitis. N Engl J Med 1998;339:653–8.

[38] Sharer N, Schwarz M, Malone G, et al. Mutations of the cystic fibrosis gene in patients with chronic pancreatitis. N Engl J Med 1998;339:645–52.

[39] Witt H, Luck W, Hennies HC, et al. Mutations in the gene encoding the serine protease inhibitor, Kazal type 1, are associated with chronic pancreatitis. Nat Genet 2000;25:213–6.

[40] Kiraly O, Boulling A, Witt H, et al. Signal peptide variants that impair secretion of pancreatic secretory trypsin inhibitor (SPINK1) cause autosomal dominant hereditary pancreatitis. Hum Mutat 2007;28(5):469–76.

[41] Hirota M, Ohmuraya M, Baba H. Genetic background of pancreatitis. Postgrad Med J 2006; 82(974):775–8.

[42] Chandak GR, Idris MM, Reddy DN, et al. Absence of PRSS1 mutations and association of SPINK1 trypsin inhibitor mutations in hereditary and non-hereditary chronic pancreatitis. Gut 2004;53(5):723–8.

[43] Howes N, Lerch MM, Greenhalf W, et al. European Registry of Hereditary Pancreatitis and Pancreatic Cancer (EUROPAC). Clinical and genetic characteristics of hereditary pancreatitis in Europe. Clin Gastroenterol Hepatol 2004;2:252–61.

[44] Teich N, Le Marechal C, Kukor Z, et al. Interaction between trypsinogen isoforms in genetically determined pancreatitis: mutation E79K in cationic trypsin (PRSS1) causes increased transactivation of anionic trypsinogen (PRSS2). Hum Mutat 2004;23:22–31.

[45] Nemoda Z, Sahin-Toth M. Chymotrypsin C (caldecrin) stimulates autoactivation of human cationic trypsinogen. J Biol Chem 2006;281:11879–86.

[46] Le Marechal C, Masson E, Chen JM, et al. Hereditary pancreatitis caused by triplication of the trypsinogen locus. Nat Genet 2006;38:1372–4.

[47] Witt H, Luck W, Becker M. A signal peptide cleavage site mutation in the cationic trypsinogen gene is strongly associated with chronic pancreatitis. Gastroenterology 1999;117:7–10.

[48] Kume K, Masamune A, Kikuta K, et al. [215G > A;IVS3 + 2T > C] mutation in the SPINK1 gene causes exon 3 skipping and loss of the trypsin binding site. Gut 2006;55:1214.

[49] Keiles S, Kammescheidt A. Identification of CFTR, PRSS1, and SPINK1 mutations in 381 patients with pancreatitis. Pancreas 2006;33(3):221–7.

[50] Audrezet MP, Chen JM, Le Marechal C, et al. Determination of the relative contribution of three genes—the cystic fibrosis transmembrane conductance regulator gene, the cationic

trypsinogen gene, and the pancreatic secretory trypsin inhibitor gene—to the etiology of idiopathic chronic pancreatitis. Eur J Hum Genet 2002;10:100–6.

[51] Noone PG, Zhou Z, Silverman LM, et al. Cystic fibrosis gene mutations and pancreatitis risk: relation to epithelial ion transport and trypsin inhibitor gene mutations. Gastroenterology 2001;121:1310–9.

[52] Tzetis M, Kaliakatsos M, Fotoulaki M, et al. Contribution of the CFTR gene, the pancreatic secretory trypsin inhibitor gene (SPINK1) and the cationic trypsinogen gene (PRSS1) to the etiology of recurrent pancreatitis. Clin Genet 2007;71:451–7.

[53] Ellis J, Lerch MM, Whitcomb DC, et al. Genetic testing for hereditary pancreatitis: guidelines for indications, counseling, content and privacy issues. Pancreatology 2001;1:405–15.

[54] Levy P, Mathurin P, Roqueplo A, et al. A multidimensional case-control study of dietary, alcohol, and tobacco habits in alcoholic men with chronic pancreatitis. Pancreas 1995;10:231–8.

[55] Cavallini G, Talamini G, Vaona B, et al. Effect of alcohol and smoking on pancreatic lithogenesis in the course of chronic pancreatitis. Pancreas 1994;9:42–6.

[56] Wittel UA, Pandey KK, Andrianifahanana M, et al. Chronic pancreatic inflammation induced by environmental tobacco smoke inhalation in rats. Am J Gastroenterol 2006;101:148–9.

[57] Maisonneuve P, Frulloni L, Mullhaupt B, et al. Impact of smoking on patients with idiopathic chronic pancreatitis. Pancreas 2006;33:163–8.

[58] Maisonneuve P, Lowenfels AB, Mullhaupt B, et al. Cigarette smoking accelerates progression of alcoholic chronic pancreatitis. Gut 2005;54:446–7.

[59] Whitcomb DC. Genetic predisposition to alcoholic chronic pancreatitis. Pancreas 2003;27:321–6.

[60] Threadgold J, Greenhalf W, Ellis I, et al. The N34S mutation of SPINK1 (PSTI) is associated with a familial pattern of idiopathic chronic pancreatitis but does not cause the disease. Gut 2002;50:675–81.

[61] Drenth JPH, te Morsche R, Jansen JBMJ. Mutations in serine protease inhibitor Kazal type 1 are strongly associated with chronic pancreatitis. Gut 2002;50:687–92.

[62] Mohan V, Pitchumoni CS, et al. Tropical calcific pancreatitis. In: Beger HG, Warshaw AL, Buchler MW, editors. The pancreas. Malden (MA): Blackwell Science; 1998. p. 688–97.

[63] McMillan DE, Geervarghese PJ. Dietary cyanide and tropical malnutrition diabetes. Diabetes Care 1979;2:202–8.

[64] Mohan V, Chari ST, Hitman GA, et al. Familial aggregation in tropical fibrocalculous pancreatic diabetes. Pancreas 1997;4:690–3.

[65] Bhatia E, Choudhuri G, Sikora SS, et al. Tropical Calcific Pancreatitis: strong association with SPINK1 trypsin inhibitor mutations. Gastroentereology 2002;123:1020–5.

[66] Chandek GR, Idris MM, Reddy DN, et al. Mutations in the pancreatic secretory trypsin inhibitor gene (PSTI/SPINK1) rather than the cationic trypsinogen gene (PRSS1) are significantly associated with tropical calcific pancreatitis. J Med Genet 2002;39:928–34.

[67] Chen JM, Mercier B, Audrezet MP, et al. Mutations of the pancreatic secretory inhibitor gene, alcohol use and chronic pancreatitis. JAMA 2001;285:2716–7.

[68] Pfutzer RH, Barmada MM, Brunskill APJ, et al. SPINK1/PST1 polymorphisms act as disease modifiers in familial and idiopathic chronic pancreatitis. Gastroenterology 2000;119:615–23.

SURGICAL
CLINICS OF
NORTH AMERICA

Surg Clin N Am 87 (2007) 1325–1340

The Inflammatory Cascade in Acute Pancreatitis: Relevance to Clinical Disease

Mohammed Elfar, MD[a], Lillian W. Gaber, MD[b],
Omaima Sabek, PhD[a], Craig P. Fischer, MD, MPH[a],
A. Osama Gaber, MD[a],*

[a]*Weill Cornell Medical College, Department of Surgery, The Methodist Hospital,
6550 Fannin Street, Suite SM1661A, Houston, TX 77030, USA*
[b]*Houston, TX, USA*

This article summarizes the current state of knowledge regarding the inflammatory cascade of acute pancreatitis (AP) and highlights the relevance of the laboratory findings to human disease onset, progression, and treatment.

AP is an inflammatory condition of the pancreas with variable incidence in different geographic regions of the world. Recent studies document a gradual rise in the incidence of acute pancreatitis and a stable case fatality rate [1–3]. AP is characterized clinically by the acute onset of abdominal pain and a rise in the activity of pancreatic enzymes in blood or urine. Most episodes of AP have a self-limiting course, but severe attacks can lead to shock, respiratory failure, and possibly death. Early mortality and most of the morbidities of the acute episode are caused by a systemic inflammatory response syndrome and to subsequent multiorgan failure. Later mortality is usually caused by sepsis and its consequences. The frequency of early death (first 2 weeks) varies between 5% and 50% of all deaths caused by AP [4,5].

Pathologically, AP usually presents with pancreatic swelling associated histologically with microscopic interlobular and intralobular edema, fat necrosis, particularly in the peripancreatic fat, and leukocyte infiltrates. The mostly neutrophilic infiltrate is found in the interstitial spaces and may extend to the pancreatic ducts and acini. In the more severe cases, confluent areas of necrosis are seen with macroscopic evidence of pancreatic necrosis and hemorrhage. In patients who have mild AP, the interstitial swelling of the gland

---

* Corresponding author.
E-mail address: aogaber@tmhs.org (A.O. Gaber).

recovers quickly, and the gland returns to histological normality. Endocrine function returns to normal soon after the acute phase, while exocrine function may take up to 1 year for full recovery [5,6]. In patients who have severe AP, the necrotizing inflammation may cause permanent exocrine and endocrine insufficiency in about one third to one half of patients [7].

Pancreatic physiology

The stimulus for pancreatic enzyme secretion is either vagal stimulation and/or the presence of fat and protein in the duodenum, which trigger the secretion of the duodenal hormone cholecystokinin, a powerful stimulant for enzyme secretion. The pancreas produces a viscous solution rich in hydrolytic enzymes that are used for breakdown of large food molecules and a watery solution rich in bicarbonate that neutralizes gastric acid in the duodenum. More than 98% of the pancreas is devoted to these exocrine functions. Some of the pancreatic enzymes, such as amylase, lipase, DNAase, and RNAase are secreted as active enzymes, but others, including most of the digestive enzymes (eg, trypsin, chymotrypsin, phospholipase, elastase, and carboxypeptidase) are synthesized as inactive proenzymes or zymogens. Both the proteases and lysosomal hydrolases are assembled on ribosomes attached to the rough endoplasmic reticulum [8]. Once secreted from the Golgi apparatus, proenzymes are packaged in secretory granules that transport the enzymes to the apex of the acinar cell facing the lumen of the pancreatic duct to prevent their premature activation inside the cell. Proteases then are excreted into the duct lumen by exocytosis of the zymogen granules and are activated only after they reach the gut lumen through the action of enteric enteropeptidases. Many of the lysosomal hydrolases also are synthesized as inactive proenzymes, but their activation is accomplished within the cell. To prevent intrapancreatic activation of digestive enzymes, the acinar cells segregate lysomal hydrolases such as cathepsin B in separate granules that are organized around the basolateral membrane.

In normal physiological situations, small amounts of trypsinogen may become activated spontaneously inside the pancreas into trypsin [8,9]. Should this happen, the pancreas has a set of intrinsic defense mechanisms to quickly counter and remove activated trypsin. These mechanisms include the secretion of the pancreatic secretory trypsin inhibitor (PSTI or SPINK1), which binds and inactivates about 20% of the trypsin activity [10]. Another defense mechanism involves autolysis of prematurely activated trypsin. Hereditary pancreatitis is thought to be caused by absence of this mechanism. Mesotrypsin and enzyme Y occur naturally in the pancreas and can lyse and inactivate trypsin inhibitors. To date, their role as protectors from pancreatitis is unclear [11]. The last mechanism for inactivation of prematurely or excessively secreted active trypsin is by means of the nonspecific antiproteases such as alpha-1-antitrypsin and alpha-2-macroglobulin, which are present in abundance in the pancreatic interstitium [12].

Evolution of acute pancreatitis and its systemic manifestations

AP results from autodigestion of the pancreas by its own proteases. Pancreatic hyperstimulation or injury causes intracellular activation of pancreatic enzymes by a process of colocalization of the lysosomal enzymes such as cathepsin B with the digestive zymogens including trypsinogen [13,14]. Alternatively, pancreatic injury may lead to altered secretion of activated proteases or their proenzymes through the basolateral membranes of the acinar cells followed by their leakage into the interstitium [15]. Enhanced pancreatic ductal permeability [16,17] allows activated enzymes to leak from the duct and initiate pancreatic autodigestion. In addition, oxygen radicals released secondary to pancreatic injury [18] cause inactivation of circulating protease inhibitors, thereby contributing to the accumulation of activated proteases in pancreatic tissue. As the stimulus persists, the normal defense mechanisms of the pancreas are overwhelmed by the released trypsin [10]. These changes can lead to an increase in the levels of intracellular calcium concentration, along with a decrease in the intracellular pH, both causing premature activation of trypsinogen by means of up-regulation of nuclear factor kβ [19]. Other pancreatic enzymes such as phospholipase, chymotrypsin, and elastase also are activated by trypsin. In addition, trypsin activates other cascades, including complement, kallikrein–kinin, coagulation, and fibrinolysis. The release of active pancreatic enzymes within the pancreatic tissue leads to pancreatic autodigestion and sets up a vicious cycle of active enzymes damaging cells, which then release more active enzymes. The destruction spreads along the gland and into the peripancreatic tissue [20,21]. Besides the activation of enzymatic cascade in animal models, trypsin also has demonstrated a documented role in stimulating cytokine production from resident intrapancreatic and circulating macrophages both in vivo and in vitro [22], and has been shown to induce cytokine production directly from acinar cells [23].

The role of activated proteases in the pathogenesis of AP is supported by the detection of activated trypsin and chymotrypsin in the pancreatic juice of patients with AP, and by their appearance in the ascites, urine, and serum of animals and people with AP [24,25]. Further, the pretreatment of rats with protease inhibitors ameliorates the progression of AP [26]. Trials employing protease inhibitors in AP, however, have failed to demonstrate reduction in systemic complications or improvement of overall patient survival [27], suggesting that proteases may be important in the early stages of the disease, while other mechanisms may mediate progression and systemic manifestations of AP.

Guise and colleagues [28] hypothesized 15 years ago that inflammatory cytokines are overproduced in AP and mediate the systemic manifestations and pathophysiological changes of the disease. Cytokines up-regulate adhesion molecules locally and in distant organs (eg, lung) and trigger a cascade of events that include leukocyte migration, PLA$_2$ production, activation of complement, degranulation of neutrophils, and production of nitric oxide and O_2 radicals. The authors' work since then has led to the demonstration of the central role of pancreatic autodigestion in stimulating an inflammatory cascade that results in dissemination of the systemic manifestations of AP. This work has been supported by other investigators [29–31] and is now the basis of current understanding of the disease progression.

Cause-specific mechanisms for acute pancreatitis

In Western countries, alcohol and gallstones account for more than 80% to 90% of cases. Other less common causes include: hyperlipidemia, hypercalcemia, trauma, medications, viral infections such as mumps, dysfunction of the sphincter of Oddi, congenital abnormalities of the pancreatic duct (pancreas divisum), and scorpion venom. A small percent of cases is ascribed to idiopathic or familial causes [12]. Despite the high association of AP with these etiologies, only 3% to 7% of patients who have gallstones [32], 10% of alcoholics, and a smaller percentage of patients who have hypercalcemia actually develop pancreatitis [33].

The exact mechanism of how alcohol induces pancreatic autodigestion is not elucidated fully. It is unclear, for example, why alcohol-induced pancreatitis occurs only after a prolonged period of alcohol abuse and not after a single binge [34]. It is postulated that a mixed ductular–acinar mechanism may be operative in alcoholic AP [35]. Alcohol ingestion causes an increase in intraductal pressure, duct permeability, and a direct toxic effect on the acinar cells that is mediated through acetaldehyde. Besides acute injury, acetaldehyde leads to activation of pancreatic stellate cells with subsequent increased production of collagen and other matrix proteins, an important step in promoting pancreatic fibrosis with alcohol intake [36]. CCK plays an important role in pathogenesis of alcohol-induced AP. Alcohol potentiates the effect of CCK on the activation of nuclear factor kappa-beta (NFKβ) of activating protein-1. Additionally, experimental data point to the fact that alcohol induces basolateral plasma membrane to become receptive to CCK-induced activation of aberrant exocytosis of zymogen granules into the interstitial spaces, leading to cytokine production and acute pancreatic inflammation [37,38].

In gallstone pancreatitis, the inciting event appears to be related to either reflux of bile into the pancreatic duct during the transient obstruction of the ampulla as a result of passage of gallstones, particularly smaller stones, or to increased pancreatic duct pressure secondary to obstruction of the ampulla by stone impaction and/or edema [39,40]. On the other hand, although the association between biliary sludge and AP has not been proven definitely [41], the results of uncontrolled studies suggest that biliary sludge can lead to pancreatitis [42]. In all cases, bile pancreatic duct obstruction leads to an increase in pancreatic ductal pressure and permeability with resultant premature enzyme activation [43] and cytokine production from acinar cells, probably by means of oxidant-activated signal transduction pathways [23]. This is followed by the up-regulation of adhesion molecules and recruitment of leukocytes into the pancreas [44], which then can be induced to produce more cytokines and initiate a cycle of further leukocyte recruitment and increased cytokine production.

Hypertriglyceridemia-induced AP occurs rarely when triglyceride levels are less than 20 mmol/L [45]. Mild-to-moderate elevations of triglycerides (2 to 10 mmol/L) are seen commonly in patients who have pancreatitis and at these levels are thought to be an epiphenomenon of AP rather than a causative agent [46]. True hypertriglyceridemia-induced AP usually is associated with appearance of chylomicrons in the blood stream. These lipid-rich particles may impair circulatory flow in the pancreatic capillary bed. The resultant ischemia of acinar cells may lead to cellular activation or disruption and may expose the chylomicrons to the pancreatic lipase. Pancreatic lipase releases free fatty acids from the triglycerides within pancreatic capillaries [47]. The release of free fatty acids further stimulates the ischemia-activated acinar cells to produce cytokines and to recruit inflammatory cells into the pancreas [48]. Hyperlipidemia may account for 1.3% to 3.8% of cases of AP [49].

Hypercalcemia can cause pancreatitis secondary to either the deposition of calcium in the pancreatic duct or to calcium-induced activation of trypsinogen within the pancreatic parenchyma [50,51]. In rat animal models, it was found that acute calcium infusions produced hyperamylasemia and dose-dependent morphological changes characteristic of AP [51]. The low incidence of pancreatitis in patients with chronic hypercalcemia, however, suggests the possible involvement of other factors. Similarly, the pathogenesis of drug-induced pancreatitis may be multifactorial. Pancreatitis is the result of an idiosyncratic response in some cases (eg, 6-mercaptopurine, aminosalicylates, and sulfonamides), or can be related to direct toxic effects of other drugs (eg, diuretics, sulfonamides) [12]. On the other hand, pancreatitis associated with angiotensin-converting enzyme inhibitors is thought to reflect angioedema of the gland. To determine a causal relationship between a particular drug and pancreatitis, pancreatitis should develop during treatment with the drug, in the absence of other likely causes of pancreatitis. Furthermore, pancreatitis should resolve upon discontinuing the drug and recur upon readministration of the drug [52].

Acute postsurgical pancreatitis represents one form of pancreatitis that is precipitated by microcirculatory disturbance of the pancreas. An impairment of pancreatic microcirculation appears to play a key role in the progression of edematous to necrotizing pancreatitis and is a component of all models of necrotizing pancreatitis. Causative factors include: poor blood fluidity by hemoconcentration and intravascular hypercoagulability; impairment of arteriolar inflow by vasospasms, endothelial injury, edema, and thrombosis; and direct toxic injury by activated enzymes, kinins, and other mediators [53].

Numerous genetic mutations causing premature activation of pancreatic zymogens within the pancreas also have been proposed as part of the pathogenetic mechanism for hereditary pancreatitis. Some genetic disorders are associated with a high penetrance such as mutations at codons 29 and 122 of the cationic trypsinogen gene. Other mutations have a low penetrance or are less frequent in the general population, such as mutations in codons 16, 22, and 23 of the cationic trypsinogen gene and mutations in serine protease inhibitor Kazal type 1 (SPINK1). In addition, certain mutations in cystic fibrosis genes have been associated with pancreatitis [54].

Pancreatitis that presents as acute and eventually progresses to chronic form may be inherited as autosomal dominant, autosomal recessive, or be a multigenetic disorder as a result of mutations in these genes or yet unidentified ones. Autosomal dominant forms of hereditary pancreatitis are thought to be caused by mutations in exon 2 (N29I) and exon 3 (R122H) of the cationic trypsinogen gene [55–58].

Other additional mutations such as: A16V, D22 G, and K23R also have been described in the cationic trypsinogen gene. These mutations, however, do not result in the autosomal dominant high-penetrance pancreatitis seen with the R122H and N29I mutations [12].

Mutations in the cystic fibrosis transmembrane conductance regulator (CFTR) and PSTI or SPINK1 have been identified in some patients with and without a family history of pancreatitis. Approximately 2% of the general population carries SPINK1 mutations. These mutations may act as disease modifiers [59].

Approximately 2% to 37% of patients who have chronic idiopathic and acute recurrent pancreatitis have demonstrated mutations in at least one allele of CFTR [54,60]. The prevalence of CFTR mutations in gallstone pancreatitis and alcohol-induced chronic pancreatitis (approximately 0% to 5%) is no greater than that seen in the general population [61].

It is unclear how CFTR mutations might produce AP. A possible explanation is that these mutations cause the production of a more concentrated, viscid, and acidic pancreatic secretion leading to ductal obstruction. Altered acinar cell functions caused by decreased intracellular pH or abnormal intracellular membrane transport also have been hypothesized.

Patients who have unexplained etiology for pancreatitis should undergo sequencing of the CFTR gene, as this may reveal additional mutations.

Animal models in the study of the pancreatic inflammatory cascade

Animal models of AP have been used widely to study onset, pathogenesis, progression, and consequences of AP [62,63]. It is important to note that despite the richness of the experimental literature on pancreatitis, none of the animal models are comparable or equivalent to the human condition. Gallstones and alcohol abuse, for example, are responsible for most cases of AP in people, but neither disease has been reproduced in the animal models. Despite these limitations, several models have been used to study AP, with quite a few models particularly well characterized. In models of diet- induced pancreatitis, mice are fed a choline-deficient diet supplemented by ethionine. In other models, intravenous infusion of supramaximal doses of the CCK agonist cerulein is used to overstimulate the pancreas and induce pancreatic inflammation. These two models generally are used to study nonsurgical AP. Other models of retrograde bile infusion and bile duct obstruction are used to mimic gallstone-induced pancreatitis.

Experimental models suggest that most pancreatitis-inducing stimuli prevent the extrusion of the zymogen granules from the apical part of acinar cells. This situation leads to fusion of the zymogen granules with intracellular lysosomes, activation of zymogen proenzyme trypsinogen, and generation of active intracellular trypsin, which is capable of cellular autodigestion [8].

Although this mechanism is not applicable to all models of pancreatitis, similarities in the structural and pathophysiological changes seen in early AP have been demonstrated between animal models and people. These early changes are fairly constant regardless of the offending agent, suggesting a common pathway from the injury to the disease.

Animal studies demonstrate that unless therapy is initiated within a few hours of the inciting event, the cascade of events leading to AP cannot be offset [64]. It is not clear, however, why some individuals experience only a mild form of the disease with interstitial or edematous pancreatitis, while others proceed to develop necrotizing inflammation. In animal models, the severity of pancreatitis can be titrated by adjusting the magnitude of the stimulus, as well as by increasing the concentration of the ethionine in the diet, or increasing the pressure of the bile duct injection. Whether human disease severity is related to the severity of the inciting event or to a predisposition to violent cytokine responses is not known [65]. Evidence is accumulating in various inflammatory diseases for a role for cytokine gene polymorphisms or other genetic mechanisms in determining the disease severity and outcome. Genetic polymorphisms have been associated with increased morbidities in dialysis [66,67], trauma [62], and renal transplant patients [67].

In animal models, trypsinogen activation within the pancreas can occur within 10 minutes of infusing rats with a supramaximally stimulating dose of the cholecystokinin analog cerulein [68]. The activation of trypsinogen occurs before any evidence of either biochemical or morphological injury to acinar cells. In humans, studies have shown that pancreatic enzyme secretion is reduced during AP, with the greatest reductions being observed in patients who have necrotizing disease. Despite the low rates of luminal secretion, trypsin continued to be synthesized in patients with AP without a change in the time of appearance of newly synthesized trypsin. In fact, in patients who had necrotizing pancreatitis, newly synthesized enzyme appeared more rapidly [69]. In an in vitro model, it was found that complete inhibition of cathepsin B activity with E-64 d (a specific and irreversible cathepsin B inhibitor) prevented trypsinogen activation by cerulein [70]. These results support the importance of cathepsin B in the activation of trypsinogen and the significance of colocalization of pancreatic digestive enzymes and lysosomal hydrolases. Furthermore, they also point out to the fact that inhibition of cathepsin B may be of potential utility for preventing or treating AP [21].

Progression of acute pancreatitis

At the tissue level, the biochemical changes resulting from premature digestive enzyme activation damage the acinar cells, pancreatic interstitium, and vascular endothelium [71,72]. In experimental models of acute pancreatitis, microcirculatory changes following acute pancreatic injury include vasoconstriction, capillary stasis, decreased oxygen saturation, and progressive ischemia. These microcirculatory changes lead to increased vascular permeability and edema of the gland (interstitial pancreatitis). Vascular injury could lead to amplification of the pancreatic injury by means of local microcirculatory failure, and through selective pancreatic ischemia [73], or ischemia–reperfusion injury.

Marked glandular invasion by macrophages and polymorphonuclear leukocytes in the early stages of animal and human pancreatitis has been shown in microscopic and radionuclide studies using Indium-111 tagged leukocytes [74,75]. Activation of complement and the subsequent release of C5a have a significant role in the recruitment of these inflammatory cells. There is, however, also some contradicting evidence that C5a has some anti-inflammatory effect in acute pancreatitis; thus, its net effect remains unclear [76].

The activation of granulocyte and macrophage leads to the release of proteolytic and lipolytic enzymes, reactive oxygen metabolites, proinflammatory cytokines as interleukins (IL) 1, 6, and 8, tumor necrosis factor (TNF), and arachidonic acid metabolites as prostaglandins, platelet-activating factor, and leukotrienes. Interestingly, cytokine activation is not limited to the intra- or peri-pancreatic tissue, but can be systemic in nature, as evidenced by the detection of significant up-regulation of TNF-α mRNA in splenic mononuclear cells in rat models following the induction of acute pancreatitis [77–79]. These local and systemic inflammatory substances overwhelm the scavenging capacity of endogenous antioxidant systems. They also damage the pancreatic microcirculation, leading to an increase in vascular permeability, thrombosis, hemorrhage, and eventually pancreatic necrosis.

The triad of activated pancreatic enzymes, microcirculatory impairment, and release of inflammatory mediators in its severe form can lead to a systemic insult and is associated with the development of systemic inflammatory response syndrome (SIRS). As a result, some patients develop systemic complications, including: acute respiratory distress syndrome (ARDS), pleural effusions, renal failure, shock, and myocardial depression [80,81]. In addition to this triad, ARDS also may be induced by the release of active phospholipase A (lecithinase), which digests lecithin, a major component of surfactant.

Lung injury in severe pancreatitis also can be mediated by the up-regulation of adhesion molecules. The authors' laboratory demonstrated that the production of inflammatory cytokines precedes up-regulation of P- and E-selectin, whose expression coincided with the increased infiltration of CD18-positive cells and neutrophil sequestration in lung tissue. Temporally, these events correlated with evidence of histologic pulmonary injury and the increased myeloperoxidase activity in the lung. Lung injury also has been associated with overexpression of VCAM 1 [56,57] and the increased expression of P-selectin triggered by a mechanism dependent on free radicals generated by xanthine oxidase released by the damaged pancreas [82]. In addition, trypsin-generated complement activation was shown to participate in the up-regulation of Mac-1 and shedding of L-selectin on neutrophils in AP [83].

Myocardial depression and shock are the result of decreased vascular tone from flow maldistribution in the peripheral microcirculation, which limits tissue oxygenation in the face of increased metabolic requirements of the hypercatabolic state [84]. Acute renal failure has been attributed to hypovolemia and hypotension. Metabolic complications such as diabetic ketoacidosis, hyperglycemia, hypoglycemia, hyperlipidemia, and hypocalcemia have been described. The pathogenesis of hypocalcemia is multifactorial and includes calcium soap formation, binding of calcium by free fatty acid–albumin complexes, hormonal imbalances (eg, parathormone, calcitonin, glucagon), and intracellular translocation of calcium.

During the course of AP, the gut barrier is compromised, leading to translocation of bacteria, which can result in local and systemic infection [85]. The breach in the gut barrier is thought to be secondary to pancreatitis-induced gut arteriovenous shunting and a consequence of ischemia caused by the hypovolemia [86]. Isolation of common enteric organisms from pancreatic infection supports the notion that these organisms have translocated from the gastrointestinal tract. In an animal model of AP, plasmid-labeled *Escherichia coli* colonizing the gut were isolated from the mesenteric lymph nodes and at distant sites [87]. Local bacterial infection of pancreatic and peripancreatic tissues occurs in approximately 30% of patients who have severe AP. Infection carries the potential of multiorgan failure and its consequences, which could be fatal.

Bacterial translocation and endotoxemia were proposed as mechanisms for the violent cytokine response observed in AP. In a mouse model of AP induced by choline-deficient ethionine-supplemented diet, however, the authors were able to demonstrate that the progression of AP into its fulminant form, the propagated cytokine response, and the resultant early deaths are independent of endotoxemia [88].

Treatment perspectives

Treatment of human AP has several goals. First, one must identify and correct predisposing factors, by performing endoscopic retrograde cholangiopancreatography in patients who have gallstone pancreatitis, by control of hypertriglyceridemia and hypercalcemia, and by withholding possible causative drugs. The second goal is to avoid further stimulation of the inflamed gland by adopting measures such as restricting food intake, bowel rest, and administration of Octreotide. The third goal is to compensate for the fluid deficit during the acute phase and support the patient through the hyperdynamic state. Adequate symptomatic treatment of pain, nausea, and emesis is also a priority. The next goal of clinical management is to prevent bacterial translocation and superimposed infection of the pancreatic debris by encouraging early enteral nutrition and careful use of antibiotics. The last part of the treatment regimens, which is still experimental, is the use of potential disease modifiers. AP is a medical disease; supportive medical therapy is the key. The surgical role is confined to management of surgically correctable etiologies and of the treatment of complications by performing pancreatic necrosectomy, and abscess drainage.

One of the most important intervention strategies involves the use of antiproteases in both animal and human disease. Protease inhibitors such as aprotinin, gabexate mesilate, nafamostat mesilate, and ulinastatin have been shown to inhibit the various enzymes and the inflammatory response in experimental and clinical studies. Thus, protease inhibitors have been considered as a potential treatment to inhibit the pancreatic inflammation in AP. In animal models, antiprotease treatment has been successful in ameliorating AP and decreasing the mortality of severe disease. The beneficial effects of antiproteases on experimental severe AP may be, in part, because of the modulation of inflammatory cytokine responses. The use of protease inhibitors in human AP has not been shown to be of value. Similarly the platelet activating factor antagonist, lexipafant, and somatostatin has been shown not to offer a survival benefit in AP [89,90]. There has been some evidence, however, from published meta-analyses of clinical trials, that gabexate mesilate and octreotide may reduce the incidence of complications in human disease [91,92].

The number of agents used in experimental animals to modify, ameliorate, or abort AP is too large to enumerate. The authors' laboratory embarked on a series of experiments to modify the disease using TNF α blockers [79,93–95]. These observations were reproduced by others [64,96], although TNF was not found routinely in plasma samples of patients who had AP [97]. TNF α is cleared from the bloodstream rapidly, and sensitivity and overall accuracy of its measurement seem to be time-dependent. Once released, TNF α stimulates a cascade of inflammatory responses that are less dependent on its persistence. This may explain why promising results seen in the laboratory, where anti-TNF therapy can be timed accurately in relationship to disease onset were not translated into clinical practice, where disease presentation and diagnosis may occur past the peak of TNF production and after other mediators have been activated. A similar pattern of success in treatment of animal disease has been reported with IL-1 [29,30,98–101].

Faced by these data, the authors' laboratory and others focused on attempting disease modification using therapies directed against later mediators of the inflammatory response. For example, the authors reported that blocking VCAM-1 on pulmonary vascular endothelium decreases leukocyte recruitment and adherence into lung, hence, reducing lung injury in severe AP. Clinically VCAM-1 antagonism may be an important adjunct to evolving therapy for distant organ injury in severe AP [102,103]. The adhesion molecules may offer a novel therapeutic option to ameliorate the systemic manifestations of AP [104]. Calcium channel blockade was associated with a significant reduction in serum TNF α levels and amelioration of pancreatitis by biochemical and pathological criteria. In one animal study, overall survival from bile-induced pancreatitis was improved dramatically in rats pretreated with diltiazem (80%) compared with untreated animals (40%) [105]. Recently, there have been reports of targeting the adhesion molecule junctional adhesion molecule C (JAM-C), which is involved in leukocyte transendothelial migration [106]. Also recently, several other interventions, including molecular targeting and ischemic preconditioning, have been reported [107–109].

AP is an inflammatory disease with a rising incidence in the last decade. Despite decades of experimental research, the clinical treatment of the disease remains unchanged. On the other hand, understanding of the etiology and pathogenesis of the disease have improved significantly, to where clinical breakthroughs may be imminent and certainly are needed. The next era hopefully will use the understanding of the pathophysiology of the disease to evolve therapeutic molecules that will change the natural history of AP.

References

[1] Yadav D, Lowenfels AB. Trends in the epidemiology of the first attack of acute pancreatitis: a systematic review. Pancreas 2006;33(4):323–30.
[2] Frey CF, Zhou H, Harvey DJ, et al. The incidence and case–fatality rates of acute biliary, alcoholic, and idiopathic pancreatitis in California, 1994–2001. Pancreas 2006;33(4): 336–44.
[3] Lindkvist B, Appelros S, Manjer J, et al. Trends in incidence of acute pancreatitis in a Swedish population: is there really an increase? Clin Gastroenterol Hepatol 2004;2(9):831–7.
[4] Gloor B, Muller CA, Worni M, et al. Late mortality in patients with severe acute pancreatitis. Br J Surg 2001;88(7):975–9.
[5] Mutinga M, Rosenbluth A, Tenner SM, et al. Does mortality occur early or late in acute pancreatitis? Int J Pancreatol 2000;28(2):91–5.
[6] Buechler MH, Hauke A, Malfertheiner P. Follow-up after acute pancreatitis–morphology and function. In: Beger H, Buechler M, editors. Acute pancreatitis—research and clinical management. Berlin: Springer-Verlag; 1987. p. 367.
[7] Scuro A, Angelini G, Cavallini G. Late outcome of acute pancreatitis. In: Gyr K, Singer MV, Sarles H, editors. Pancreatitis: concepts and classifications. Proceedings of the Second International Symposium on Classification of Pancreatitis in Marseille, France, March 28–30. Excerpta Medica; 1984. p. 403.
[8] Sherwood MW, Prior IA, Voronina SG, et al. Activation of trypsinogen in large endocytic vacuoles of pancreatic acinar cells. Proc Natl Acad Sci U S A 2007;104(13):5674–9.

[9] Lerch MM, Gorelick FS. Early trypsinogen activation in acute pancreatitis. Med Clin North Am 2000;84(3):549–63, viii.

[10] Hirota M, Ohmuraya M, Baba H. The role of trypsin, trypsin inhibitor, and trypsin receptor in the onset and aggravation of pancreatitis. J Gastroenterol 2006;41(9):832–6.

[11] Szmola R, Kukor Z, Sahin-Toth M. Human mesotrypsin is a unique digestive protease specialized for the degradation of trypsin inhibitors. J Biol Chem 2003;278(49):48580–9.

[12] Vege S, Chari ST. Pathogenesis of acute pancreatitis. Uptodate Online; (2007). Available at: http://www.utdol.com/utd/content/topic.do?topicKey=pancdis/4682&selectedTitle= 5~114&source=search_result.

[13] Bialek R, Willemer S, Arnold R, et al. Evidence of intracellular activation of serine proteases in acute cerulein-induced pancreatitis in rats. Scand J Gastroenterol 1991;26(2):190–6.

[14] Rinderknecht H. Activation of pancreatic zymogens. Normal activation, premature intrapancreatic activation, protective mechanisms against inappropriate activation. Dig Dis Sci 1986;31(3):314–21.

[15] Scheele G, Adler G, Kern H. Exocytosis occurs at the lateral plasma membrane of the pancreatic acinar cell during supramaximal secretagogue stimulation. Gastroenterology 1987; 92(2):345–53.

[16] Wedgwood KR, Adler G, Kern H, et al. Effects of oral agents on pancreatic duct permeability. A model of acute alcoholic pancreatitis. Dig Dis Sci 1986;31(10):1081–8.

[17] Harvey MH, Wedgwood KR, Austin JA, et al. Pancreatic duct pressure, duct permeability, and acute pancreatitis. Br J Surg 1989;76(8):859–62.

[18] Sanfey H, Bulkley GB, Cameron JL. The pathogenesis of acute pancreatitis. The source and role of oxygen-derived free radicals in three different experimental models. Ann Surg 1985; 201(5):633–9.

[19] Raraty MG, Murphy JA, McLoughlin E, et al. Mechanisms of acinar cell injury in acute pancreatitis. Scand J Surg 2005;94(2):89–96.

[20] Steer ML. Pathogenesis of acute pancreatitis. Digestion 1997;58(Suppl 1):46–9.

[21] Halangk W, Lerch MM, Brandt-Nedelev B, et al. Role of cathepsin B in intracellular trypsinogen activation and the onset of acute pancreatitis. J Clin Invest 2000;106(6): 773–81.

[22] Lundberg AH, Eubanks JW 3rd, Henry J, et al. Trypsin stimulates production of cytokines from peritoneal macrophages in vitro and in vivo. Pancreas 2000;21(1):41–51.

[23] Ramudo L, Manso MA, Sevillano S, et al. Kinetic study of TNF-alpha production and its regulatory mechanisms in acinar cells during acute pancreatitis induced by bile–pancreatic duct obstruction. J Pathol 2005;206(1):9–16.

[24] Sugimoto Y, Hayakawa T, Kondo T, et al. Peritoneal absorption of pancreatic enzymes in bile-induced acute pancreatitis in dogs. J Gastroenterol Hepatol 1990;5(5):493–8.

[25] Lankisch PG, Buschmann-Kaspari H, Otto J, et al. Correlation of pancreatic enzyme levels with the patient's recovery from acute edematous pancreatitis. Klin Wochenschr 1990; 68(11):565–9.

[26] Wilson C, Imrie CW. Effective intraperitoneal antiprotease therapy for taurocholate-induced pancreatitis in rats. Br J Surg 1990;77(11):1252–5.

[27] Leese T, Holliday M, Watkins M, et al. A multicentre controlled clinical trial of high-volume fresh- frozen plasma therapy in prognostically severe acute pancreatitis. Ann R Coll Surg Engl 1991;73(4):207–14.

[28] Guice KS, Oldham KT, Remick DG, et al. Anti-tumor necrosis factor antibody augments edema formation in caerulein-induced actue pancreatitis. J Surg Res 1991;51(6):495–9.

[29] Norman JG, Franz MG, Fink GS, et al. Decreased mortality of severe acute pancreatitis after proximal cytokine blockade. Ann Surg 1995;221(6):625–31 [discussion: 631–4].

[30] Norman J, Franz M, Messina J, et al. Interleukin-1 receptor antagonist decreases severity of experimental acute pancreatitis. Surgery 1995;117(6):648–55.

[31] Norman J. The role of cytokines in the pathogenesis of acute pancreatitis. Am J Surg 1998; 175(1):76–83.

[32] Moreau JA, Zinsmeister AR, Melton LJ 3rd, et al. Gallstone pancreatitis and the effect of cholecystectomy: a population-based cohort study. Mayo Clin Proc 1988;63(5):466–73.

[33] Bess MA, Edis AJ, van Heerden JA. Hyperparathyroidism and pancreatitis. Chance or a causal association? JAMA 1980;243(3):246–7.

[34] Purohit V, Russo D, Salin M, et al. Mechanisms of alcoholic pancreatitis: introduction and summary of a symposium. Pancreas 2003;27(4):281–355.

[35] Schmidt J, Klar E. [Etiology and pathophysiology of acute pancreatitis]. Ther Umsch 1996; 53(5):322–32 [in German].

[36] Bachem MG, Zhou Z, Zhou S, et al. Role of stellate cells in pancreatic fibrogenesis associated with acute and chronic pancreatitis. J Gastroenterol Hepatol 2006;21(Suppl 3):S92–6.

[37] Cosen-Binker LI, Gaisano HY. Recent insights into the cellular mechanisms of acute pancreatitis. Can J Gastroenterol 2007;21(1):19–24.

[38] Lam PP, Cosen Binker LI, Lugea A, et al. Alcohol redirects CCK-mediated apical exocytosis to the acinar basolateral membrane in alcoholic pancreatitis. Traffic 2007;8(5):605–17.

[39] Lerch MM, Saluja AK, Runzi M, et al. Pancreatic duct obstruction triggers acute necrotizing pancreatitis in the opossum. Gastroenterology 1993;104(3):853–61.

[40] Diehl AK, Holleman DR Jr, Chapman JB, et al. Gallstone size and risk of pancreatitis. Arch Intern Med 1997;157(15):1674–8.

[41] Garg PK, Tandon RK, Madan K. Is biliary microlithiasis a significant cause of idiopathic recurrent acute pancreatitis? A long-term follow-up study. Clin Gastroenterol Hepatol 2007;5(1):75–9.

[42] Ros E, Navarro S, Bru C, et al. Occult microlithiasis in idiopathic acute pancreatitis: prevention of relapses by cholecystectomy or ursodeoxycholic acid therapy. Gastroenterology 1991;101(6):1701–9.

[43] Lightner AM, Kirkwood KS. Pathophysiology of gallstone pancreatitis. Front Biosci 2001; 6:E66–76.

[44] Ramudo L, De Dios I, Yubero S, et al. ICAM-1 and CD11b/CD18 expression during acute pancreatitis induced by bile pancreatic duct obstruction: effect of N-acetylcysteine. Exp Biol Med (Maywood) 2007;232(6):737–43.

[45] Toskes PP. Hyperlipidemic pancreatitis. Gastroenterol Clin North Am 1990;19(4):783–91.

[46] Dominguez-Munoz JE, Juncmann F, Malfertheiner P. Hyperlipidemia in acute pancreatitis. Cause or epiphenomenon? Int J Pancreatol 1995;18(2):101–6.

[47] Dominguez-Munoz JE, Malfertheiner P, Ditschuneit HH, et al. Hyperlipidemia in acute pancreatitis. Relationship with etiology, onset, and severity of the disease. Int J Pancreatol 1991;10(3-4):261–7.

[48] Gan SI, Edwards AL, Symonds CJ, et al. Hypertriglyceridemia-induced pancreatitis: a case-based review. World J Gastroenterol 2006;12(44):7197–202.

[49] Fortson MR, Freedman SN, Webster PD 3rd. Clinical assessment of hyperlipidemic pancreatitis. Am J Gastroenterol 1995;90(12):2134–9.

[50] Mithofer K, Fernandez-del Castillo C, Frick TW, et al. Acute hypercalcemia causes acute pancreatitis and ectopic trypsinogen activation in the rat. Gastroenterology 1995;109(1): 239–46.

[51] Ward JB, Petersen OH, Jenkins SA, et al. Is an elevated concentration of acinar cytosolic free ionised calcium the trigger for acute pancreatitis? Lancet 1995;346(8981): 1016–9.

[52] Mallory A, Kern F Jr. Drug-induced pancreatitis: a critical review. Gastroenterology 1980; 78(4):813–20.

[53] Cuthbertson CM, Christophi C. Disturbances of the microcirculation in acute pancreatitis. Br J Surg 2006;93(5):518–30.

[54] Cohn JA, Friedman KJ, Noone PG, et al. Relation between mutations of the cystic fibrosis gene and idiopathic pancreatitis. N Engl J Med 1998;339(10):653–8.

[55] Le Bodic L, Bignon JD, Raguenes O, et al. The hereditary pancreatitis gene maps to long arm of chromosome 7. Hum Mol Genet 1996;5(4):549 54.

[56] Gorry MC, Gabbaizedeh D, Furey W, et al. Mutations in the cationic trypsinogen gene are associated with recurrent acute and chronic pancreatitis. Gastroenterology 1997;113(4): 1063–8.

[57] Whitcomb DC, Gorry MC, Preston RA, et al. Hereditary pancreatitis is caused by a mutation in the cationic trypsinogen gene. Nat Genet 1996;14(2):141–5.

[58] Whitcomb DC, Preston RA, Aston CE, et al. A gene for hereditary pancreatitis maps to chromosome 7q35. Gastroenterology 1996;110(6):1975–80.

[59] Pfutzer RH, Barmada MM, Brunskill AP, et al. SPINK1/PSTI polymorphisms act as disease modifiers in familial and idiopathic chronic pancreatitis. Gastroenterology 2000; 119(3):615–23.

[60] Sharer N, Schwarz M, Malone G, et al. Mutations of the cystic fibrosis gene in patients with chronic pancreatitis. N Engl J Med 1998;339(10):645–52.

[61] Choudari CP, Yu AC, Imperiale TF, et al. Significance of heterozygous cystic fibrosis gene (cystic fibrosis transmembrane conductance regulator mutations) in idiopathic pancreatitis. Gastroenterology 1998;114(10):A447.

[62] Rattner DW. Experimental models of acute pancreatitis and their relevance to human disease. Scand J Gastroenterol Suppl 1996;219:6–9.

[63] Granger J, Remick D. Acute pancreatitis: models, markers, and mediators. Shock 2005; 24(Suppl 1):45–51.

[64] Norman JG, Fink GW, Messina J, et al. Timing of tumor necrosis factor antagonism is critical in determining outcome in murine lethal acute pancreatitis. Surgery 1996;120(3): 515–21.

[65] Rinderknecht H. Genetic determinants of mortality in acute necrotizing pancreatitis. Int J Pancreatol 1994;16(1):11–5.

[66] Balakrishnan VS, Guo D, Rao M, et al. Cytokine gene polymorphisms in hemodialysis patients: association with comorbidity, functionality, and serum albumin. Kidney Int 2004;65(4):1449–60.

[67] Jaber BL, Rao M, Guo D, et al. Cytokine gene promoter polymorphisms and mortality in acute renal failure. Cytokine 2004;25(5):212–9.

[68] Grady T, Saluja A, Kaiser A, et al. Edema and intrapancreatic trypsinogen activation precede glutathione depletion during caerulein pancreatitis. Am J Physiol 1996;271(1 Pt 1): G20–6.

[69] O'Keefe SJ, Lee RB, Li J, et al. Trypsin secretion and turnover in patients with acute pancreatitis. Am J Physiol Gastrointest Liver Physiol 2005;289(2):G181–7.

[70] Saluja AK, Donovan EA, Yamanaka K, et al. Cerulein-induced in vitro activation of trypsinogen in rat pancreatic acini is mediated by cathepsin B. Gastroenterology 1997;113(1): 304–10.

[71] Prinz RA. Mechanisms of acute pancreatitis. Vascular etiology. Int J Pancreatol 1991;9: 31–8.

[72] Klar E, Messmer K, Warshaw AL, et al. Pancreatic ischaemia in experimental acute pancreatitis: mechanism, significance, and therapy. Br J Surg 1990;77(11):1205–10.

[73] Reilly PM, Toung TJ, Miyachi M, et al. Hemodynamics of pancreatic ischemia in cardiogenic shock in pigs. Gastroenterology 1997;113(3):938–45.

[74] Rinderknecht H. Fatal pancreatitis, a consequence of excessive leukocyte stimulation? Int J Pancreatol 1988;3(2–3):105–12.

[75] Kingsnorth A. Role of cytokines and their inhibitors in acute pancreatitis. Gut 1997;40(1): 1–4.

[76] Bhatia M, Saluja AK, Singh VP, et al. Complement factor C5a exerts an anti-inflammatory effect in acute pancreatitis and associated lung injury. Am J Physiol Gastrointest Liver Physiol 2001;280(5):G974–8.

[77] Grewal HP, Kotb M, el Din AM, et al. Induction of tumor necrosis factor in severe acute pancreatitis and its subsequent reduction after hepatic passage. Surgery 1994;115(2): 213–21.

[78] Hughes CB, Gaber LW, Kotb M, et al. Induction of acute pancreatitis in germ-free rats: evidence of a primary role for tumor necrosis factor-alpha. Surgery 1995;117(2):201–5.

[79] Hughes CB, Henry J, Kotb M, et al. Up-regulation of TNF alpha mRNA in the rat spleen following induction of acute pancreatitis. J Surg Res 1995;59(6):687–93.

[80] Agarwal N, Pitchumoni CS. Acute pancreatitis: a multisystem disease. Gastroenterologist 1993;1(2):115–28.

[81] Tenner S, Fernandez-del Castillo C, Warshaw A, et al. Urinary trypsinogen activation peptide (TAP) predicts severity in patients with acute pancreatitis. Int J Pancreatol 1997;21(2): 105–10.

[82] Folch E, Salas A, Panes J, et al. Role of P-selectin and ICAM-1 in pancreatitis-induced lung inflammation in rats: significance of oxidative stress. Ann Surg 1999;230(6):792–8 [discussion: 798–9].

[83] Hartwig W, Jimenez RE, Fernandez-del Castillo C, et al. Expression of the adhesion molecules Mac-1 and L-selectin on neutrophils in acute pancreatitis is protease- and complement-dependent. Ann Surg 2001;233(3):371–8.

[84] Cobo JC, Abraham E, Bland RD, et al. Sequential hemodynamic and oxygen transport abnormalities in patients with acute pancreatitis. Surgery 1984;95(3):324–30.

[85] Schmid SW, Uhl W, Friess H, et al. The role of infection in acute pancreatitis. Gut 1999; 45(2):311–6.

[86] Andersson R, Wang XD. Gut barrier dysfunction in experimental acute pancreatitis. Ann Acad Med Singapore 1999;28(1):141–6.

[87] Kazantsev GB, Hecht DW, Rao R, et al. Plasmid labeling confirms bacterial translocation in pancreatitis. Am J Surg 1994;167(1):201–6 [discussion 206–7].

[88] Eubanks JW 3rd, Sabek O, Kotb M, et al. Acute pancreatitis induces cytokine production in endotoxin-resistant mice. Ann Surg 1998;227(6):904–11.

[89] Kingsnorth AN, Galloway SW, Formela LJ. Randomized, double-blind phase II trial of Lexipafant, a platelet-activating factor antagonist, in human acute pancreatitis. Br J Surg 1995;82(10):1414–20.

[90] Johnson CD, Kingsnorth AN, Imrie CW, et al. Double blind, randomised, placebo-controlled study of a platelet activating factor antagonist, lexipafant, in the treatment and prevention of organ failure in predicted severe acute pancreatitis. Gut 2001;48(1):62–9.

[91] Andriulli A, Leandro G, Clemente R, et al. Meta-analysis of somatostatin, octreotide and gabexate mesilate in the therapy of acute pancreatitis. Aliment Pharmacol Ther 1998;12(3): 237–45.

[92] Messori A, Rampazzo R, Scroccaro G, et al. Effectiveness of gabexate mesilate in acute pancreatitis. A meta-analysis. Dig Dis Sci 1995;40(4):734–8.

[93] Grewal HP, Mohey el Din A, Gaber L, et al. Amelioration of the physiologic and biochemical changes of acute pancreatitis using an anti-TNF α polyclonal antibody. Am J Surg 1994;167(1):214–8 [discussion: 218–9].

[94] Hughes CB, Gaber LW, Mohey el-Din AB, et al. Inhibition of TNF α improves survival in an experimental model of acute pancreatitis. Am Surg 1996;62(1):8–13.

[95] Hughes CB, Grewal HP, Gaber LW, et al. Anti-TNF α therapy improves survival and ameliorates the pathophysiologic sequelae in acute pancreatitis in the rat. Am J Surg 1996; 171(2):274–80.

[96] Malleo G, Mazzon E, Genovese T, et al. Effects of thalidomide in a mouse model of cerulein-induced acute pancreatitis. Shock 2007 [epub ahead of print].

[97] Brivet FG, Emilie D, Galanaud P. Pro- and anti-inflammatory cytokines during acute severe pancreatitis: an early and sustained response, although unpredictable of death. Parisian Study Group on Acute Pancreatitis. Crit Care Med 1999;27(4):749–55.

[98] Denham W, Denham D, Yang J, et al. Transient human gene therapy: a novel cytokine regulatory strategy for experimental pancreatitis. Ann Surg 1998;227(6):812–20.

[99] Norman J, Yang J, Fink G, et al. Severity and mortality of experimental pancreatitis are dependent on interleukin-1 converting enzyme (ICE). J Interferon Cytokine Res 1997;17(2):113–8.

[100] Paszkowski AS, Rau B, Mayer JM, et al. Therapeutic application of caspase 1/interleukin-1beta-converting enzyme inhibitor decreases the death rate in severe acute experimental pancreatitis. Ann Surg 2002;235(1):68–76.

[101] Jaworek J, Bonior J, Pierzchalski P, et al. Leptin protects the pancreas from damage induced by caerulein overstimulation by modulating cytokine production. Pancreatology 2002;2(2):89–99.

[102] Callicutt CS, Sabek O, Fukatsu K, et al. Diminished lung injury with vascular adhesion molecule-1 blockade in choline-deficient ethionine diet-induced pancreatitis. Surgery 2003;133(2):186–96.

[103] Lundberg AH, Fukatsu K, Gaber L, et al. Blocking pulmonary ICAM-1 expression ameliorates lung injury in established diet-induced pancreatitis. Ann Surg 2001;233(2): 213–20.

[104] Lundberg AH, Granger DN, Russell J, et al. Quantitative measurement of P- and E-selectin adhesion molecules in acute pancreatitis: correlation with distant organ injury. Ann Surg 2000;231(2):213–22.

[105] Hughes CB, el-Din AB, Kotb M, et al. Calcium channel blockade inhibits release of TNF α and improves survival in a rat model of acute pancreatitis. Pancreas 1996;13(1):22–8.

[106] Vonlaufen A, Aurrand-Lions M, Pastor CM, et al. The role of junctional adhesion molecule C (JAM-C) in acute pancreatitis. J Pathol 2006;209(4):540–8.

[107] Bhatia M, Sidhapuriwala JN, Sparatore A, et al. Treatment with H2s-releasing diclofenac protects mice against acute pancreatitis-associated lung injury. Shock 2007 [epub ahead of print].

[108] Gultekin FA, Kerem M, Tatlicioglu E, et al. Leptin treatment ameliorates acute lung injury in rats with cerulein-induced acute pancreatitis. World J Gastroenterol 2007;13(21):2932–8.

[109] Yasuda T, Takeyama Y, Ueda T, et al. Protective effect of caspase inhibitor on intestinal integrity in experimental severe acute pancreatitis. J Surg Res 2007;138(2):300–7.

ELSEVIER
SAUNDERS

Surg Clin N Am 87 (2007) 1341–1358

SURGICAL
CLINICS OF
NORTH AMERICA

Radiologic Assessment of Acute and Chronic Pancreatitis

David H. Kim, MD*, Perry J. Pickhardt, MD

Department of Radiology, University of Wisconsin Medical School, E3/311 Clinical Science Center, 600 Highland Avenue, Madison, WI 53792-3252, USA

Imaging modalities have undergone tremendous advancements in underlying technology over the past several years, translating into increased capabilities in the assessment of pathologic processes. CT has evolved from axial imaging, to single-slice helical scanning, to multislice imaging capable of scanning the entire abdomen in a few seconds. MRI has also improved, including sequences leading to high-contrast breath-held images and sequences that better depict fluid-containing structures, such as biliary and pancreatic ducts. Current ultrasound equipment now generates images of surprising clarity and detail. In the realm of pancreatic imaging, these advancements allow an improved assessment of this organ for the surgeon and treating physician. This article outlines the current capabilities and role of imaging in the evaluation of acute and chronic pancreatitis.

Acute pancreatitis

Acute pancreatitis is defined as acute inflammation of the pancreatic gland and surrounding tissues and is thought to result from premature activation of pancreatic digestive enzymes. It encompasses a wide spectrum in disease severity, ranging from mild inflammation related to the gland alone, resulting in little morbidity and mortality, to severe cases of extensive pancreatic necrosis and surrounding inflammation in which mortality rates can reach 20% to 30% or higher with the presence of multiorgan failure [1,2]. Overall mortality is approximately 5% [1]. Once the diagnosis is established, the keys in management are related to the ability to determine the prognosis and detect complications. CT often plays a central role from an imaging standpoint. CT is helpful for diagnosis in complex clinical

* Corresponding author.
E-mail address: dkim@uwhealth.org (D.H. Kim).

0039-6109/07/$ - see front matter © 2007 Elsevier Inc. All rights reserved.
doi:10.1016/j.suc.2007.08.005

surgical.theclinics.com

presentations and aids in disease severity assessment during the acute presentation. It is also useful in the evaluation of potential subsequent complications. Other modalities, such as ultrasound and MRI, can provide much of the same information in specific clinical circumstances and are helpful adjuncts in the evaluation for underlying causes.

Imaging for diagnosis

CT may confirm the suspected diagnosis of acute pancreatitis in confusing clinical presentations. Perhaps more importantly, however, CT is helpful in assessing for alternative causes for the patient's clinical presentation that can mimic pancreatitis, such as duodenal ulceration/perforation, ruptured aortic aneurysm, and mesenteric ischemia. In the face of a typical clinical presentation and laboratory studies, routine use of CT for confirmation is likely not needed [1]. However, CT imaging is useful for confusing initial presentations, for failure of clinical improvement, for assessment of disease severity, and for the evaluation of complications. The imaging appearance of pancreatitis at CT is variable depending on the severity of the inflammation. In mild pancreatitis, the gland may appear normal without gross abnormalities detected. As the intensity of the inflammatory process increases, the pancreas can become enlarged and demonstrate decreased enhancement secondary to increasing edema infiltrating the parenchyma. The typical textured appearance of the pancreas is lost. The borders of the gland may become indistinct, with hazy soft tissue stranding consistent with inflammation surrounding the pancreas (Fig. 1). With more severe cases, the inflammatory stranding and fluid may extend distant from the gland proper along retroperitoneal interfascial planes and dissect into the lesser sac and various mesenteries (including small bowel mesentery and transverse mesocolon) [3,4]. Necrosis can result in severe pancreatitis presenting as zones of low attenuation representing nonenhancing parenchyma or as fluid-filled areas replacing the expected position of pancreatic parenchyma, representing liquefied necrosis (Fig. 2).

Our increased understanding of the vascular perfusion of this gland as it relates to the administration of iodinated contrast and the underlying technologic advancements in CT have significantly improved characterization of these pathologic processes. Initially, concerns regarding contrast administration in pancreatitis were raised. It was postulated that intravenous contrast could worsen pancreatic necrosis, as documented in one animal model [5]. This has not been corroborated in other animal models nor been demonstrated clinically in people [6]. It is generally accepted that contrast administration is a safe endeavor that does not exacerbate pancreatic necrosis. The additional information afforded by contrast is invaluable over a noncontrast examination. Normally, the pancreas enhances maximally with intravenous contrast to approximately 120 Hounsfield units (HU) from its baseline attenuation of 40 to 50 HU. This typically occurs

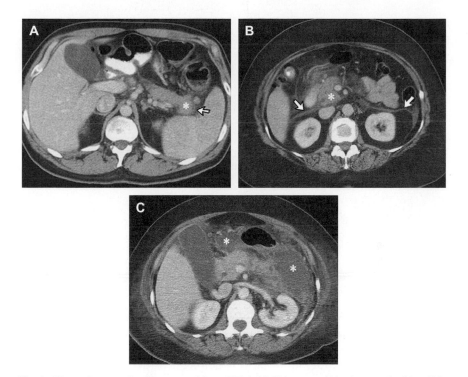

Fig. 1. Worsening severity of pancreatitis at CT. (*A*) Mild pancreatitis characterized by slight enlargement of the pancreatic body/tail (*asterisk*), with mild blurring of the border related to inflammation (*arrow*). (*B*) More severe pancreatitis in another patient who had inflammatory products and fluid around the pancreatic head (*asterisk*) tracking down retroperitoneal interfascial planes (*arrows*). (*C*) More extensive pancreatitis in a third patient with extrapancreatic fluid collections present (*asterisks*) and surrounding soft tissue inflammatory stranding.

40 to 45 seconds after contrast administration for persons with normal cardiac output [7–10]. Even at 70 seconds, when patients are typically scanned for routine CT (the optimal time for general assessment of the abdomen), there is good pancreatic enhancement (110 HU on average) [9]. In mild acute pancreatitis in which the parenchymal capillary network remains intact, there remains good uniform enhancement. With severe or necrotizing pancreatitis, areas of the pancreas can demonstrate decreased or no enhancement. The ability of increased contrast rate administration (typically 3–5 cc/s) versus previous rates (1–2 cc/s) and the ability to acquire images more quickly through the gland have translated to imaging of tighter contrast boluses and increased conspicuity between normal and abnormal enhancement. Consequently, subtle alterations related to edema or ischemia are depicted, whereas these changes were inapparent in the past. Fluid collections are now better defined from adjacent parenchyma, and the surrounding arterial and venous vasculature structures are better opacified. Sensitivity and characterization at CT have thus significantly improved.

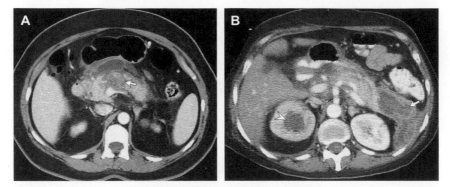

Fig. 2. Pancreatic necrosis. (*A*) Axial CT image demonstrates a zone of nonenhancement in the proximal pancreatic body (*arrow*). (*B*) CT in another patient demonstrates low attenuation in the pancreatic tail (*arrow*) consistent with extensive necrosis. Note the hydronephrosis of the right kidney (*arrowhead*) related to the retroperitoneal inflammation at a lower level (not shown). (*From* Lee AD, Pickhardt PJ. The pancreas. In: Pickhardt PJ, Arluk GM, editors. Atlas of gastrointestinal imaging: radiologic-endoscopic correlation. Philadelphia: WB Saunders; 2007. p. 405; with permission.)

Other imaging modalities play a lesser role for diagnosis establishment. Plain abdominal radiography may demonstrate suggestive findings, such as a localized ileus of the small bowel ("the sentinel loop") related to the pancreatic inflammation; however, it is neither sensitive nor specific. Ultrasound can certainly demonstrate an edematous swollen gland with reasonable sensitivity when the pancreas can be visualized, but the gland is often obscured by gas-filled bowel loops. In addition, evaluation of extrapancreatic extension of inflammatory stranding and fluid is limited for this modality, particularly when it is located in the transverse mesocolon [11]. MRI is extremely sensitive and can depict the findings as seen on CT. It also offers increased evaluation of the biliary system and gallbladder. MRI, however, is often difficult to perform in the acute setting related to the clinical status of the patient. Despite these limitations, ultrasound and MRI can be helpful in specific patients in establishing the diagnosis.

Imaging for severity assessment

After the diagnosis has been established, one of the most important contributions of imaging involves the evaluation for pancreatic necrosis. The early assessment of disease severity is a major determinant in predicting the future clinical course and directing potential treatment options. The most important identified factors include the presence of multiorgan failure and of pancreatic necrosis. In the absence of these factors, mortality is low, whereas it may increase to 35% to 50% with the presence of both [1]. It is important to note that pancreatic necrosis without associated organ failure has a low mortality rate unless complicated by infection. Again, CT with intravenous contrast has a primary role over other available imaging modalities for necrosis assessment. MRI could conceivably substitute for CT, but the lack of ready availability and difficulty of performance in agitated patients decrease its utility. In addition, for patients with depressed renal function, the use of gadolinium has recently been called into question because of the newly recognized link with nephrogenic systemic fibrosis (NSF) [12,13]. NSF is a progressive fibrosing cutaneous disorder with associated systemic manifestations. It is characterized by worsening fibrosis of the skin, leading to painful contractures and limited movement, and is often ultimately fatal. There is a postulated link to free gadolinium that has disassociated from its chelate in patients with poor renal function, resulting in heavy metal toxicity within the body.

The current classification scheme for acute pancreatitis (International Symposium on Acute Pancreatitis, Atlanta, GA, 1992) bases severity on organ failure through clinical and laboratory value assessment and on local complications (ie, pancreatic necrosis, abscess and pseudocyst formation) through imaging [14]. In addition, a Ranson score of 3 or greater and an Acute Physiology and Chronic Health Evaluation (APACHE) II score of 8 or greater are considered to demonstrate evidence of increased severity. Several definitions were standardized to allow valid comparisons between institutions. Mild acute pancreatitis is defined as pancreatitis that is associated with minimal or no organ dysfunction and leads to an uneventful recovery, whereas severe pancreatitis is defined as pancreatitis in association with organ failure or local complications. Interstitial pancreatitis is defined in terms of contrast-enhanced CT imaging as focal or diffuse enlargement of the pancreas with homogeneous enhancement of the parenchyma, whereas necrotizing pancreatitis is defined by imaging as the presence of nonenhanced parenchyma greater than 30% of the gland or greater than 3 cm in size. Interstitial pancreatitis is typically mild in severity, although a small percentage of cases may have a more severe course characterized by organ failure (typically transient) or by fluid collection/pseudocyst formation. Overall mortality in interstitial pancreatitis is low at 3% [1]. Necrotizing pancreatitis equates to severe pancreatitis (by definition), with an overall mortality of 17% [1]. In addition, the definitions for the terms *extrapancreatic fluid collection*, *pseudocyst*, *infected necrosis*, and *pancreatic abscess* were set (to be discussed in the following sections).

Pancreatic necrosis typically occurs within the first 24 to 48 hours of the disease course. The amount of pancreatic involvement is typically defined at this point without significant delayed extension. It presents at CT as zones of nonenhancing parenchyma and may evolve to fluid-filled spaces in the expected position of the pancreas ("organized necrosis"; see Fig. 2). Typically, the absolute HU measurements in areas of necrosis are 30 or less. Often, the diagnosis is made by a qualitative assessment in comparison to adjacent normal parenchyma and other organs, because the absolute Hounsfield measurements may be falsely decreased as a result of volume average artifact in a fatty gland. In addition, there is a normal variability of measurements between the head, body, and tail in some individuals related to the differing embryologic buds (ventral and dorsal anlage).

It is important to note that ischemia and necrosis may be difficult to detect within the first 12 hours and are much more evident on delayed imaging after the first 24 to 48 hours. Necrotizing pancreatitis accounts for approximately 15% of cases, with most remaining cases representing interstitial pancreatitis [1]. Some institutions use the CT severity index developed by Balthazar and colleagues [15], which combines pancreatic necrosis and local complications of fluid collection for a predictive score. As expected, as the extent of necrosis increases and the number of collections increases, morbidity and mortality significantly increase. The presence of infected necrosis is a serious finding, which correlates with a negative outcome that raises mortality from 12% in sterile necrosis to 30% with infected necrosis [1]. Infection may be suggested at CT by the development of air bubbles with the necrotic parenchyma (Fig. 3). Treatment of choice is surgical debridement, because percutaneous drainage is typically ineffective unless the infected necrosis is completely liquefied (which is often not the case).

In cases in which intravenous contrast cannot be given because of such contraindications as depressed renal function or severe allergy, predictive information can still be gleaned from noncontrast CT. Earlier CT classification systems were based on noncontrast examinations. Obviously, the assessment for pancreatic necrosis cannot be made; however, evaluation of diffuse gland enlargement, surrounding inflammation, and the presence of adjacent fluid collections or retroperitoneal air could be undertaken to categorize acute pancreatitis with stepwise worsening CT grades from A to E. Patients who have one or more fluid collections or retroperitoneal air have more severe pancreatitis (CT grade D and E), with a mortality

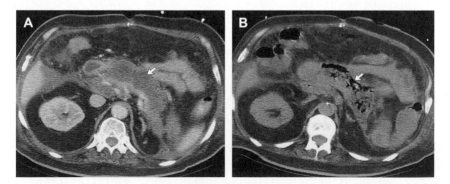

Fig. 3. Infected pancreatic necrosis. (*A*) Extensive area of nonenhancement throughout the pancreas consistent with necrosis (*arrow*). (*B*) Subsequent development of air (*arrow*) within the necrotic areas and clinical decline of the patient consistent with superinfection. (*From* Lee AD, Pickhardt PJ. The pancreas. In: Pickhardt PJ, Arluk GM, editors. Atlas of gastrointestinal imaging: radiologic-endoscopic correlation. Philadelphia: WB Saunders; 2007. p. 406; with permission.)

rate of 14% and morbidity rate of 54%, as compared with patients without these findings, with rates of 0% mortality and 4% morbidity [16].

Newer techniques currently under research include dynamic perfusion multidetector CT, in which perfusion color maps and curves of the pancreas are generated by measuring the change in attenuation with bolus injection of iodinated contrast over time. Parameters, such as perfusion (measured in mL/100 mL/min), peak enhancement intensity (in HU), time to peak (in seconds), and blood volume (in mL/100 mL), can be calculated. Potentially, information from such techniques may or may not prove useful in the future in the severity assessment of pancreatitis [17]. Such techniques currently are not ready for clinical use.

Imaging for etiology evaluation

Although not the typical choice for establishing diagnosis or disease severity assessment, other modalities (ie, ultrasound and MRI) are useful in the imaging evaluation of potential predisposing conditions for acute pancreatitis. The differential list for the underlying causes is extensive, including alcohol, gallstones, hypertriglyceridemia hypercalcemia, various drugs, infections, toxins, trauma, pregnancy, after endoscopic retrograde cholangiopancreatography (ERCP), and hereditary origins. From this list, ultrasound and MRI can detect potential structural causes. Biliary pancreatitis is a common cause of acute pancreatitis, accounting for approximately one third of cases [2]. Ultrasound has the advantage of being able to be undertaken in the acute setting and often is performed within the first 24 hours to assess for gallstones as a possible inciting agent (Fig. 4). It is highly sensitive for cholelithiasis and can be performed portably even in critically ill patients. It is postulated that small gallstones (<5 mm) are more likely causative than larger stones [18]. Although excellent for detection of calculi in the gallbladder, detection rates for choledocholithiasis are decreased typically because of an obscuring gas-filled bowel. For documented obstructing calculi, ERCP may then be helpful as a diagnostic and therapeutic option for a patient who has cholangitis or severe pancreatitis. However, it is not advocated for routine cases of suspected biliary pancreatitis [1].

In recent years, MRI has considerably advanced in underlying hardware and sequence development. Breath-held three-dimensional (3D) gradient echo images in multiple phases with dynamic gadolinium administration are a marked improvement over traditional T1-weighted spin echo sequences. Similar to CT, the dynamic instillation and improved contrast delivery and faster breath-held sequence acquisition allow for improved characterization of pancreatic enhancement. The development of specialized heavily T2-weighted sequences has allowed for improved depiction of the biliary ducts by using the fluid as an inherent contrast agent. These advancements have allowed magnetic resonance cholangiopancreatography (MRCP) to become a noninvasive diagnostic option to complement

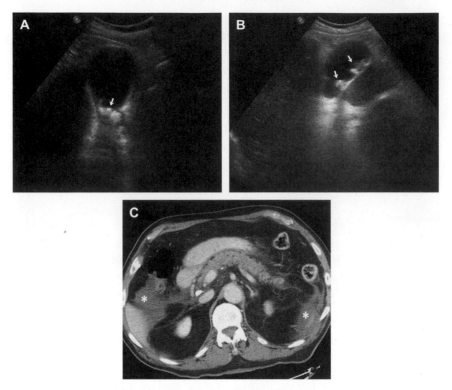

Fig. 4. Biliary pancreatitis. (*A*, *B*) Transverse and longitudinal ultrasound images demonstrate small shadowing gallstones (*arrows*) as the cause of this patient's pancreatitis. (*C*) Axial CT image in this patient demonstrates inflammatory stranding around the pancreas and fluid (*asterisks*) tracking down the right paracolic gutter and around the splenic tip.

ERCP for the evaluation of the biliary system. The sensitivity and specificity for MRCP have been shown to exceed 90% for choledocholithiasis [19]. The high negative predictive values are useful in the exclusion of calculi for suspected biliary pancreatitis [20]. In addition, MRCP is excellent at demonstrating other causes of biliary obstruction, given its ability to assess the extrabiliary surrounding structures. MRI is also able to depict pancreatic duct abnormalities, such as pancreatic divisum, which is a controversial predisposing cause for pancreatitis (Fig. 5). The specific technique of secretin injection with MRCP to improve pancreatic duct characterization is discussed in the section on chronic pancreatitis.

Imaging for complication assessment

A variety of complications can result from acute pancreatitis, including extrapancreatic fluid collections; pseudocyst development; infected pancreatic necrosis; pancreatic abscess formation; and vascular complications, such as splenic vein thrombosis and arterial pseudoaneurysm formation. Again,

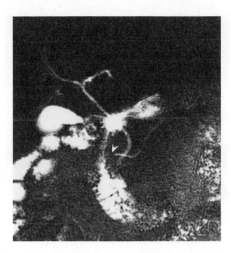

Fig. 5. Pancreatic divisum. Single-shot fast spin echo MRI scan depicts the pancreatic duct of the body and tail draining through the minor papilla (*arrowhead*). It is controversial as to whether this is a true cause of pancreatitis.

CT is a mainstay of evaluation because of its global assessment nature. MRI and ultrasound may also be useful depending on the specific clinical situation.

Extrapancreatic fluid collections occur early in the disease process, representing exudative collections of pancreatic fluid and enzymes. These collections may also contain fat necrosis, nonspecific inflammation, and hemorrhage. *Phlegmon* is an older discarded term included within extrapancreatic fluid collections as redefined by the international symposium [14]. Acute extrapancreatic fluid collections resolve spontaneously in approximately half of the cases [16], may become superinfected, or may progress into a pseudocyst. They initially present on CT as low-attenuation collections around the pancreas without a discrete border. They typically reside in the anterior pararenal space or lesser sac (Fig. 6). These fluid collections may dissect through various planes, including the gastrohepatic, gastrosplenic, and gastrocolic ligaments, and inferiorly along predetermined retroperitoneal fascial planes. They may also dissect into the root of the small bowel mesentery. Acute fluid collections and inflammation may cause significant mass effect, resulting in such sequelae as pain, biliary obstruction, or mechanical bowel obstruction. Suspicion of infection of extrapancreatic fluid collections may be confirmed by image-guided aspiration.

Superinfection of underlying pancreatic necrosis is a potential complication that may occur after several days and is a poor prognostic factor. It occurs in approximately one third of patients who have necrotizing pancreatitis [21]. As discussed previously, CT may demonstrate the presence of punctuate and coalescing foci of gas within the necrotic areas consistent with air, which is highly suggestive of superinfection in the appropriate clinical setting (see Fig. 3). Other nonspecific imaging signs that may point to

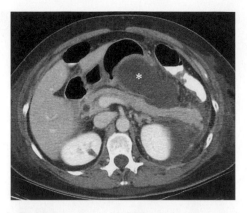

Fig. 6. Extrapancreatic fluid collections. Axial CT image in a patient who had ERCP-induced pancreatitis with acute fluid collections around the pancreas, including within the lesser sac (*asterisk*), with mass effect on the stomach. Note the lack of a defined wall as would be present in a pseudocyst. (*From* Lee AD, Pickhardt PJ. The pancreas. In: Pickhardt PJ, Arluk GM, editors. Atlas of gastrointestinal imaging: radiologic-endoscopic correlation. Philadelphia: WB Saunders; 2007. p. 405; with permission.)

infection, such as adjacent soft tissue stranding, overlap with the underlying inflammatory process seen with pancreatitis, and are therefore not particularly useful. It is important to note that imaging may be rather unremarkable despite the presence of significant infection that ultimately requires percutaneous sampling.

Pseudocysts represent extrapancreatic fluid collections that have developed surrounding a nonepithelialized capsule. This capsule forms as a result of the inflammatory process at its periphery and requires at least 4 weeks to develop. Thus, pseudocysts present at CT in the subacute time frame as low-attenuation fluid collections with a definable wall, typically rounded or oval in shape (Fig. 7). The wall can range from barely perceptible to a thick enhancing rind [7]. They are typically peripancreatic in nature and can dissect into the various extraperitoneal and mesenteric planes that acute fluid collections can inhabit. This terminology also includes intrapancreatic collections with a surrounding wall (typically, the result of varying amounts of liquefied pancreatic necrosis). In recent years, these collections have been recognized as distinct from peripancreatic pseudocysts, and the term *organized necrosis* has been applied, given their unique management difficulties [1,22]. Overall, approximately one half of all pseudocysts resolve spontaneously. Of the other half, most stabilize or remain asymptomatic. A few may progress with increasing pain, hemorrhage, infection, or gastrointestinal obstruction and may require intervention [23]. Bacteria can colonize pseudocysts with no clinical significance, but frank pus within the pseudocyst is compatible with a "pancreatic abscess." Percutaneous drainage with imaging guidance has become a viable treatment option in addition to surgical debridement and endoscopic drainage.

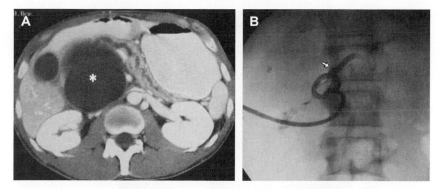

Fig. 7. Pancreatic pseudocyst. (*A*) Well-defined cystic structure (*asterisk*) consistent with a pseudocyst seen in a patient who had a known history of pancreatitis and now had worsening pain. (*B*) Percutaneous drainage of the pseudocyst with continued high output. Contrast injection demonstrates communication with the main pancreatic duct (*arrow*).

Image-guided percutaneous intervention is typically performed under CT, although in select cases, ultrasound guidance can be used. Simple collections can be drained with a smaller caliber pigtail catheter (8–10 French), whereas more complicated collections require larger bore catheters (12–14 French). Multiple catheter exchanges and additional catheters may be needed during the course of drainage. If output does not cease over a prolonged period, evaluation for connection to the pancreatic duct is indicated to exclude fistula formation driving the fluid output (see Fig. 7) [24].

Vascular sequelae are much less common but can result in significant morbidity and even mortality. The extravasated activated pancreatic enzymes can affect the adjacent vessels, leading to pseudoaneurysms of the splenic artery or branches of the pancreaticoduodenal arcade. If not treated, these may rupture, leading to significant intra-abdominal hemorrhage. A pseudoaneurysm can be easily detected with contrast-enhanced CT, presenting as a focal, rounded, enhancing collection in communication with the adjacent artery (Fig. 8). The presence of rupture is characterized by adjacent stranding and high-attenuation fluid, which can be diagnosed on noncontrast examinations if contrast cannot be given because of contraindications. The intense inflammatory process of acute pancreatitis may also result in splenic vein thrombosis. This can ultimately lead to collateral formation and gastric varices. In fact, the presence of isolated gastric varices (with the absence of esophageal varices) raises the high likelihood of splenic vein thrombosis.

MRI can be used to assess for these potential complications with equivalency to CT. MRI does not use ionizing radiation, which is advantageous, because many of these patients receive several scans related to this disease process over their lifetime. Disadvantages include difficulty in obtaining quality examinations in debilitated or agitated patients and the newly described risks for NSF for gadolinium contrast administration in patients

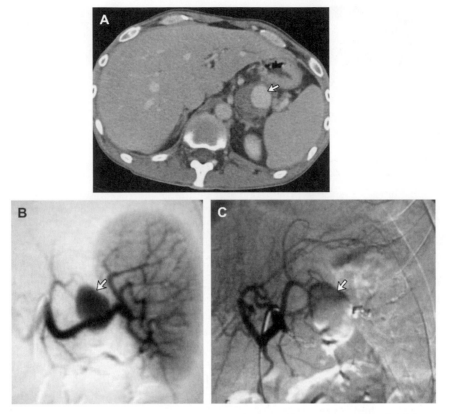

Fig. 8. Pseudoaneurysm of the splenic artery. (*A*) CT image demonstrates a large brightly enhancing splenic artery pseudoaneurysm with mural thrombus (*arrow*) from pancreatitis. (*B*, *C*)
Pseudoaneurysm (*arrow*) seen at contrast angiography with subsequent embolization. (*From*
Lee AD, Pickhardt PJ. The pancreas. In: Pickhardt PJ, Arluk GM, editors. Atlas of gastrointestinal imaging: radiologic-endoscopic correlation. Philadelphia: WB Saunders; 2007. p. 407;
with permission.)

with renal insufficiency. Ultrasound may be used in select situations; however, air-filled bowel may act as an acoustic block, precluding adequate evaluation. One instance in which ultrasound is useful is in the detection of
pseudoaneurysms of the splenic artery near the splenic hilum, wherein the
spleen itself can be used as an acoustic window to visualize this area
(Fig. 9). The application of Doppler techniques can then confirm the swirl-
ing blood within the pseudoaneurysm.

Chronic pancreatitis

Chronic pancreatitis is characterized by progressive fibrosis of the pancreas, resulting in exocrine and endocrine insufficiency. Previously, it was

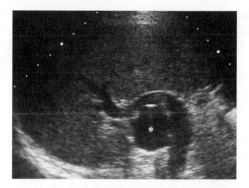

Fig. 9. Splenic artery pseudoaneurysm at ultrasound. Gray-scale ultrasound image demonstrates a rounded anechoic structure at the splenic hilum suspicious for a pseudoaneurysm (*asterisk*). Use of Doppler imaging may confirm active flow within the pseudoaneurysm.

thought to be a clinical entity distinct from acute pancreatitis, with few cases of acute pancreatitis progressing to chronic pancreatitis [25]. More recently, there is gaining consensus that chronic pancreatitis results from repeated episodes of acute necroinflammation causing damage and the resultant fibrosis [26]. After a variable subclinical phase, chronic pancreatitis may present with repeated bouts of abdominal pain and, ultimately, with exocrine and endocrine insufficiency. The most common cause of chronic pancreatitis is alcohol-related disease. Other cited causes include hereditary pancreatitis, tropical pancreatitis, autoimmune pancreatitis, and idiopathic pancreatitis. It is thought that many cases of idiopathic pancreatitis have genetic underpinnings and that this group is likely to decrease as the specific abnormalities are delineated. Aside from ERCP, MRI plays a more central role from an imaging standpoint over the other cross-sectional modalities, such as CT or ultrasound. Although not discussed in this article, it is important to realize that there are several functional studies in use to help in the diagnosis and severity assessment of chronic pancreatitis.

Imaging for diagnosis

There are some limitations to the use of imaging for chronic pancreatitis for diagnosis confirmation. Imaging relies on morphologic changes of the gland to confirm the diagnosis. Such changes are often evident in advanced disease, and the diagnosis is easily made in these cases. However, such changes do not typically appear in early disease, decreasing imaging sensitivity during the time when the clinical presentation may be equivocal or not suspected. Also, it is important to note that structural changes do not correlate well with level of gland functioning [27].

Central to chronic pancreatitis is the presence of parenchymal loss and replacement with fibrosis. Key histopathologic features include acinar atrophy, pancreatic fibrosis, distorted ducts with eosinophilic protein plugs, and calcium deposits. Consequently, in advanced cases, the gland may appear atrophic, with secondary changes to the ductal anatomy related to fibrosis. The fibrosis can create beading and ectasia of the side branches and, ultimately, enlargement of the main pancreatic duct. There can be secondary intraductal deposition of dystrophic calcification [28,29]. Potential early changes may range from normal imaging studies to a relatively normal-appearing nonatrophic gland with only minor T1-weighted signal changes at MRI and mild beading of a few pancreatic side branches. As the disease process progresses, the changes become more evident, characterized by an atrophic gland with deposition of calcifications in the ducts. The main pancreatic duct may dilate, with beaded side branches seen throughout the pancreas. Chronic pancreatitis is typically a diffuse process but occasionally manifests with a more focal appearance that can be difficult to distinguish from carcinoma.

Useful imaging modalities include ERCP, MRI, and CT. ERCP is useful in evaluating for the presence of ductal changes associated with chronic pancreatitis, whereas CT better depicts the parenchyma changes, including atrophy and the presence of calcifications. MRI has the advantage of evaluating the ductal anatomy and the parenchyma, and thus can allow a more global assessment. On MRI, the normal pancreas appears relatively bright in signal intensity on fat-suppressed T1-weighted noncontrast images. The loss of this normal bright signal may be seen with the presence of fibrosis and points to chronic pancreatitis [30]. Although calcifications are poorly seen at MRI, breath-held dynamic postcontrast fat-saturated T1-weighted sequences can clearly depict atrophy and duct dilation. In addition, the use of specialized heavily T2-weighted sequences in MRCP has improved the noninvasive evaluation of the pancreatic ducts, even more so with the administration of secretin.

MRCP with secretion injection is a relatively new technique that is useful in the evaluation of chronic pancreatitis. It involves the standard MRCP techniques of multiplanar heavily T2-weighted sequences, with the addition of intravenous secretin to promote distention of the pancreatic ducts. No intravenous gadolinium is required for the examination, wherein the T2 bright fluid within the pancreatic duct is used for intrinsic contrast. Secretin is a polypeptide hormone with numerous physiologic effects, including increasing the volume of bicarbonate-rich pancreatic secretions and increasing contraction of the sphincter of Oddi [31]. Consequently, these combined effects of secretin distend the pancreatic ducts and result in better visualization as compared with the standard MRCP examination without secretin [32,33]. The maximal effect occurs 5 to 10 minutes after administration. The main duct typically increases by at least 1 mm with secretin. There is little effect on the appearance of the biliary system with this agent [34].

ERCP has been considered the reference standard for pancreatic duct assessment. Standard MRCP typically has more difficulty in visualizing the small-caliber pancreatic ducts in the tail and side branches, leading to an increased false-negative rate [35]. The use of secretin with increased ductal distention is helpful in closing the gap between the diagnostic capabilities of MRCP and ERCP, although side branches may remain difficult to visualize at MRCP [33]. It is important to note that minor change within the side branches themselves is a difficult issue at ERCP, with fairly high intra- and inter observer variability and overlap in appearance in these branches with senescence [36]. Both modalities do well with advanced changes with dilation of the main duct and ectatic beading of multiple side branches (Fig. 10).

Other imaging modalities that may help with diagnosis confirmation include conventional radiography, which can depict diffuse pancreatic calcifications when extensive. Ultrasound and CT can be helpful in detecting gland atrophy, duct dilation, and more subtle calcification deposits, although, again, these stigmata of chronic pancreatitis are typically best identified in advanced cases (Fig. 11).

Imaging for severity assessment

Morphologic changes to the ductal anatomy and pancreatic gland are also used as a surrogate for the severity of chronic pancreatitis. It is important to note that structural changes may correlate poorly with clinical severity. The Cambridge classification can be used by ERCP and MRCP in grading chronic pancreatitis based on structural changes to the main pancreatic duct and side branches [37]. As the number of involved side branches increases and the main pancreatic duct is involved, the severity grade

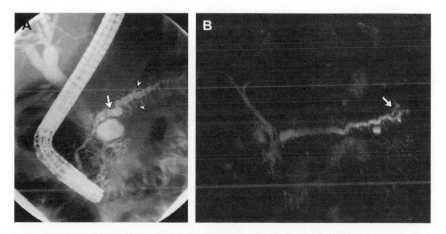

Fig. 10. Chronic pancreatitis. (*A*) Advanced structural changes seen at ERCP with massive main pancreatic duct (*arrow*) dilation, numerous dilated and beaded side branches (*arrowheads*), and pancreatic calcifications (difficult to separate from side branches because of contrast injection). (*From* Lee AD, Pickhardt PJ. The pancreas. In: Pickhardt PJ, Arluk GM, editors. Atlas of gastrointestinal imaging: radiologic-endoscopic correlation. Philadelphia: WB Saunders; 2007. p. 408; with permission.) (*B*) Heavily T2-weighted MRCP image depicting more mild changes with pancreatic duct prominence and a few beaded side branches (*arrow*) in the pancreatic tail.

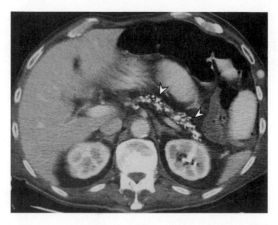

Fig. 11. Advanced chronic pancreatitis at CT. Axial postcontrast CT image demonstrates diffuse calcifications (*arrowheads*) stippling an atrophic gland.

increases. MRCP with secretin injection has also been shown to provide limited functional information. Gross qualitative assessment of exocrine function may potentially be made by the amount of induced pancreatic fluid detected in the duodenum. Reduced duodenal filling is noted in patients who have severe chronic pancreatitis [32].

Imaging for complication assessment

Complications seen in chronic pancreatitis mirror the sequelae that may occur in acute pancreatitis, including pseudocyst formation, pseudoaneurysms of the visceral arteries, and splenic vein thrombosis. When present, pseudocysts can be a source of pain, bleeding, and gastrointestinal or biliary obstruction. CT with intravenous contrast is perhaps the most useful imaging modality in evaluating for these potential complications because of its global assessment nature.

In addition to these complications, patients who have chronic pancreatitis are at higher risk for the development of ductal adenocarcinoma, with an overall lifetime risk of 4% [38]. Unfortunately, the imaging appearances of focal chronic pancreatitis and ductal adenocarcinoma demonstrate significant overlap, making diagnosis difficult. Both may present as focal masses with obstruction of the pancreatic or biliary ducts. If prior cross-sectional imaging studies are available, a significant change in the appearance of the pancreas would be highly concerning for interval development of carcinoma. Often, a biopsy is needed to make this diagnosis.

Summary

Imaging advances have considerably increased the noninvasive capability for the assessment of acute and chronic pancreatitis. In acute pancreatitis, the most important contributions from imaging (more so than the confirmation of diagnosis) involve assessment for pancreatic necrosis and for potential complications. CT with intravenous contrast plays a major role in this assessment. Other modalities, such as MRI and US, may help to evaluate for potential causes. In chronic pancreatitis, ERCP and MRCP play larger roles in diagnosis and severity assessment. Although morphologic changes are used for this evaluation, it is important to note that such changes may not be evident early in the disease course and may not correlate with disease severity clinically. CT remains a useful modality to assess for potential complications, including the development of adenocarcinoma.

References

[1] Banks PA, Freeman ML. Practice guidelines in acute pancreatitis. Am J Gastroenterol 2006; 101:2379 400.
[2] Pandol SJ, Saluja AK, Imrie CW, et al. Acute pancreatitis: bench to the bedside. Gastroenterology 2007;132:1127–51.
[3] Molmenti EP, Balfe DM, Kanterman RY, et al. Anatomy of the retroperitoneum: observations of the distribution of pathologic fluid collections. Radiology 1996;200:95 103.
[4] Meyers MA, Evans JA. Effects of pancreatitis on the small bowel and colon: spread along mesenteric planes. AJR Am J Roentgenol 1973;119:151–65.
[5] Foitzik T, Bassi DG, Schmidt J, et al. Intravenous contrast medium accentuates the severity of acute necrotizing pancreatitis in the rat. Gastroenterology 1994;106:207–14.
[6] Uhl W, Roggo A, Kirschstein T, et al. Influence of contrast-enhanced computed tomography on course and outcome in patients with acute pancreatitis. Pancreas 2002;24:191–7.
[7] Balthazar EJ, Freeny PC, vanSonnenberg E. Imaging and intervention in acute pancreatitis. Radiology 1994;193:297–306.
[8] Lu DS, Vedantham S, Krasny RM, et al. Two-phase helical CT for pancreatic tumors: pancreatic versus hepatic phase enhancement of tumor, pancreas, and vascular structures. Radiology 1996;199:697–701.
[9] McNulty NJ, Francis IR, Platt JF, et al. Multi-detector row helical CT of the pancreas: effect of contrast-enhanced multiphasic imaging on enhancement of the pancreas, peripancreatic vasculature, and pancreatic adenocarcinoma. Radiology 2001;220:97–102.
[10] Fletcher JG, Wiersema MJ, Fidler JL, et al. Pancreatic malignancy: value of arterial, pancreatic, and hepatic phase imaging with multi-detector row CT. Radiology 2003;229:81–90.
[11] Jeffrey RB, Laing FC, Wing VW. Extrapancreatic spread of acute pancreatitis: new observations with real-time US. Radiology 1986;159:707–11.
[12] Grobner T. Gadolinium: a specific trigger for the development of nephrogenic fibrosing dermopathy and nephrogenic systemic fibrosis? Nephrol Dial Transplant 2006;21:1104–8.
[13] Sadowski EA, Bennett LK, Chan MR, et al. Nephrogenic systemic fibrosis: risk factors and incidence estimation. Radiology 2007;243:148–57.
[14] Bradley EL. 3rd. A clinically based classification system for acute pancreatitis. Summary of the International Symposium on Acute Pancreatitis. Atlanta (GA); September 11–13, 1992. Arch Surg 1993;128:586–90.
[15] Balthazar EJ, Robinson DL, Megibow AJ, et al. Acute pancreatitis: value of CT in establishing prognosis. Radiology 1990;174:331–6.
[16] Balthazar EJ, Ranson JH, Naidich DP, et al. Acute pancreatitis: prognostic value of CT. Radiology 1985;156:127–32.
[17] Bize PE, Platon A, Becker CD, et al. Perfusion measurement in acute pancreatitis using dynamic perfusion MDCT. AJR Am J Roentgenol 2006;186:114–8.

[18] Diehl AK, Holleman DR Jr, Chapman JB, et al. Gallstone size and risk of pancreatitis. Arch Intern Med 1997;157:1674–8.

[19] Soto JA, Barish MA, Alvarez O, et al. Detection of choledocholithiasis with MR cholangiography: comparison of three-dimensional fast spin-echo and single- and multisection half-Fourier rapid acquisition with relaxation enhancement sequences. Radiology 2000; 215:737–45.

[20] Reinhold C, Taourel P, Bret PM, et al. Choledocholithiasis: evaluation of MR cholangiography for diagnosis. Radiology 1998;209:435–42.

[21] Perez A, Whang EE, Brooks DC, et al. Is severity of necrotizing pancreatitis increased in extended necrosis and infected necrosis? Pancreas 2002;25:229–33.

[22] Baron TH, Harewood GC, Morgan DE, et al. Outcome differences after endoscopic drainage of pancreatic necrosis, acute pancreatic pseudocysts, and chronic pancreatic pseudocysts. Gastrointest Endosc 2002;56:7–17.

[23] Yeo C, Bastidas J, Lynch-Nyhan A, et al. The natural history of pancreatic pseudocysts documented by computed tomography. Surg Gynecol Obstet 1990;170:411–7.

[24] vanSonnenberg E, Wittich G, Casola G, et al. Percutaneous drainage of infected and noninfected pancreatic pseudocysts: experience in 101 cases. Radiology 1989;170:757–61.

[25] Singer MV, Gyr K, Sarles H. Revised classification of pancreatitis. Report of the second International Symposium on the Classification of Pancreatitis in Marseille. France. March 28–30, 1984. Gastroenterology 1985;89:683–5.

[26] Witt H, Apte MV, Keim V, et al. Chronic pancreatitis: challenges and advances in pathogenesis, genetics, diagnosis, and therapy. Gastroenterology 2007;132:1557–73.

[27] Bozkurt T, Braun U, Leferink S, et al. Comparison of pancreatic morphology and exocrine functional impairment in patients with chronic pancreatitis. Gut 1994;35:1132–6.

[28] Luetmer PH, Stephens DH, Ward EM. Chronic pancreatitis: reassessment with current CT. Radiology 1989;171:353–7.

[29] Owens JL, Howard JM. Pancreatic calcification: a late sequel in the natural history of chronic alcoholism and alcoholic pancreatitis. Ann Surg 1958;147:326–38.

[30] Semelka RC, Shoenut JP, Kroeker MA, et al. Chronic pancreatitis: MR imaging features before and after administration of gadopentetate dimeglumine. J Magn Reson Imaging 1993;3: 79–82.

[31] Chey WY, Chang TM. Secretin, 100 years later. J Gastroenterol 2003;38:1025–35.

[32] Manfredi R, Costamagna G, Brizi MG, et al. Severe chronic pancreatitis versus suspected pancreatic disease: dynamic MR cholangiopancreatography after secretin stimulation. Radiology 2000;214:849–55.

[33] Hellerhoff KJ, Helmberger H, Rosch T, et al. Dynamic MR pancreatography after secretin administration: image quality and diagnostic accuracy. AJR Am J Roentgenol 2002;179: 121–9.

[34] Akisik MF, Sandrasegaran K, Aisen AA, et al. Dynamic secretin-enhanced MR cholangiopancreatography. Radiographics 2006;26:665–77.

[35] Takehara Y, Ichijo K, Touama N, et al. Breath-hold MR cholangiopancreatography with a long echo train fast spin-echo sequence and a surface coil in chronic pancreatitis. Radiology 1994;192:73–8.

[36] Forsmark CE, Toskes PP. What does an abnormal pancreatogram mean? Gastrointest Endosc Clin N Am 1995;5:105–23.

[37] Axon AT, Classen M, Cotton PB, et al. Pancreatography in chronic pancreatitis: international definitions. Gut 1984;25:1107–12.

[38] Lowenfels AB, Maisonneuve P, Cavallini G, et al. Pancreatitis and the risk of pancreatic cancer. N Engl J Med 1993;328:1433–7.

SURGICAL
CLINICS OF
NORTH AMERICA

ELSEVIER
SAUNDERS

Surg Clin N Am 87 (2007) 1359–1378

Benign Pancreatic Tumors

Sushanth Reddy, MD[a,b],
Christopher L. Wolfgang, MD, PhD[b,*]

[a]*Department of Surgery, University of Kentucky, 800 Rose Street,
MN-264, Lexington, KY 40536, USA*
[b]*John L. Cameron Division of Surgical Oncology, Department of Surgery,
The Johns Hopkins Medical Institutions, 600 North Wolfe Street, Blalock 604,
The Johns Hopkins Hospital, Baltimore, MD 21287, USA*

The management of a patient who has a tumor of the pancreas can be a challenging endeavor. Differentiating benign from malignant or premalignant tumors of the pancreas often poses a diagnostic challenge. Moreover, the stakes for making the correct determination are high. The resection of pancreatic lesions is associated with high morbidity and a slight risk for mortality. An unnecessary resection of a benign lesion places the patient at risk for lifelong morbidity that may significantly affect his or her quality of life. At the other extreme, pancreatic adenocarcinoma is a highly lethal disease with an incidence-to-death ratio approaching 1 [1]. The only chance for cure of patients diagnosed with pancreatic adenocarcinoma is through surgical resection of early-stage cancers. Pancreatic adenocarcinoma is associated with specific neoplastic lesions that are similar in radiographic appearance to some benign lesions. The correct differentiation of these malignant and premalignant lesions from their benign counterpart is paramount to their proper management.

The goal of this article is to describe the different types of benign pancreatic neoplasms, methods to distinguish between them, and treatment options. It should be noted that it is difficult to discuss benign neoplasms of the pancreas without discussing pancreatic malignancy, because many benign neoplasms are associated with malignancy. Therefore, although this review focuses on benign pancreatic tumors, they are discussed in the context of malignant disease.

---

* Corresponding author.
E-mail address: cwolfga2@jhmi.edu (C.L. Wolfgang).

Classification scheme for benign pancreatic tumors

Classification of benign pancreatic tumors is helpful because it serves to dictate their subsequent management. Box 1 demonstrates a paradigm for the classification of pancreatic tumors based on cause. These lesions can generally be divided into inflammatory and neoplastic tumors. Inflammatory tumors have no malignant potential, whereas neoplastic tumors have varying degrees of propensity to become malignant. It is often difficult to differentiate among the various types of these tumors. Therefore, because benign lesions account for less than 10% of all pancreatic masses [2], all pancreatic tumors should be considered malignant until proved otherwise. The following section describes the benign tumors listed in Box 1. The relative incidences of these tumors are shown in Table 1.

Inflammatory pancreatic tumors

Pseudocysts

Pseudocysts make up approximately 75% of all pancreatic masses and have no malignant potential. They are discussed briefly in this article because they must be considered in the evaluation of cystic pancreatic tumors but are discussed in detail elsewhere [3,4]. As their name implies, they are false cysts because they have a nonepithelial granulation tissue lining. They most often form after acute pancreatitis, which causes disruption of the parenchyma and ductal system, resulting in the release of digestive enzymes. These pancreatic hydrolases are thought to digest nearby tissue. A fluid collection forms in the lesser sac as a product of the process. Routine CT scanning has shown peripancreatic fluid collections in 30% to 50% of all

---

Box 1. Classification scheme for benign pancreatic tumors

Benign tumors
    Inflammatory
        Pseudocyst
        Lymphoplasmacytic sclerosing pancreatitis (LPSP)
    Neoplastic
        Solid (benign)
            Pancreatic neuroendocrine tumor (PNET)
            Solid pseudopapillary tumor (SPT)
    Cystic
        Serous cystadenoma
        Mucinous cystic neoplasm (MCN)
        Intraductal papillary mucinous neoplasm (IPMN)
    Microscopic
        Pancreatic intraepithelial neoplasm (PanIN)

Table 1
Incidence of pancreatic neoplasms

Name	Incidence
Pseudocysts	1:20,000
Endocrine tumors	1:100,000
Solid pseudopapillary tumors	1:3,200,000
Lymphoplasmacytic sclerosing pancreatitis	1:1,600,000
Serous cystadenomas	1:3,500,000
Mucinous cystic neoplasms	1:50,000
Intraductal papillary mucinous neoplasms	1:150,000
Pancreatic intraepithelial neoplasms	1:5
Pancreatic adenocarcinoma	1:700

patients who have acute pancreatitis. Most of these resolve; however, some persist and develop a wall of granulation tissue. If present for more than 4 weeks, these collections are considered pseudocysts [5]. In addition to acute pancreatitis, trauma that disrupts the pancreatic parenchyma and ductal anatomy can produce pseudocysts.

Cystic neoplasms often have radiographic characteristics similar to pseudocysts. The clinician should be aware of a patient's history leading to the presumed pseudocyst. The likelihood of malignancy increases in patients who do not have a history of pancreatitis or pancreatic trauma.

Lymphoplasmacytic sclerosing pancreatitis

LPSP is a newly recognized disease. It is thought to be an autoimmune disorder resulting in the formation of a pancreatic mass seen on routine imaging (Fig. 1). This variant of chronic pancreatitis occurs in the absence of gallstones, alcohol use, or other common causes of pancreatitis. It is characterized by a dense lymphoplasmacytic infiltrate that surrounds the main pancreatic duct and interlobular branches of the pancreatic duct with venulitis and is associated with an elevated serum IgG4 level [6]. The clinical presentation of obstructive jaundice and enlargement or a mass of the head of the pancreas is similar to that of pancreatic head adenocarcinoma. As such, many of these patients are approached as though they have pancreatic cancer. In contrast to pancreatic adenocarcinoma, CT in LPSP often shows sausage-like diffuse enlargement without a discrete mass [7]. Patients who have LPSP have a similar age of presentation as patients who have pancreatic cancer but are more likely to be male (2:1 ratio). Patients who have LPSP also have a greater likelihood of having a prior atopic or autoimmune disease. The diagnosis of LPSP is often made pathologically after resection for a presumed cancer. Indeed, the finding of LPSP in pancreatic specimens resected for all indications ranges from 5% to 23% [6].

Surgical resection of LPSP is associated with a 46% overall complication rate [8]. Many different investigators have described effective steroid therapy for LPSP obviating the need for surgical resection. Successful steroid

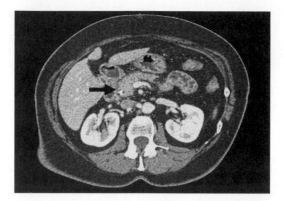

Fig. 1. LPSP. This CT scan shows diffuse enlargement of the pancreas without an associated mass. The head of the pancreas is shown by the arrow.

treatment requires 6 to 8 weeks of therapy [9]. This approach, of course, requires accurate diagnosis before any surgical intervention.

LPSP has been characterized primarily in the Japanese literature. The Japanese Pancreas Society created diagnostic criteria in 2002 that were modified in 2006. First, imaging studies should demonstrate narrowing of the main pancreatic duct with enlargement of the pancreas. Unlike a stricture, the pancreatic duct is diffusely narrowed with one third or more of the duct involved and proximal dilatation. The second criterion is the presence of autoantibodies or elevated serum gamma globulin, IgG, or IgG4. None of these findings are specific for LPSP but do implicate the autoimmune nature of this disease. Finally, histology reveals fibrosis with plasma cell and lymphocyte infiltration. Diagnosis requires the first criterion with the second or third and exclusion of malignancy. It is estimated that 10% to 20% of patients who have LPSP still undergo surgical resection after applying these criteria [7].

Solid neoplastic pancreatic tumors

Endocrine tumors

PNETs are rare neoplasms that arise from the endocrine portion of the pancreas. The overall incidence is roughly 1 in every 100,000 people [10]. Pancreatic neuroendocrine cells are members of amine precursor uptake decarboxylase (APUD) cells [11]. Endocrine tumors are categorized by the cell type from which they originate and their functional status. They include insulinomas, gastrinomas, vasoactive intestinal peptide-omas (VIPomas), glucagonomas, somatostatinomas, and nonfunctioning endocrine tumors. Although classically associated with multiple endocrine neoplasia (MEN) syndromes, von Hippel-Lindau disease, or von Recklinghausen's disease, most of these tumors are sporadic rather than familial [10]. Tables 2 and 3

Table 2
Incidence of endocrine tumors

Name	Incidence
Insulinomas	1:1,000,000
Gastrinomas	1:2,000,000
VIPomas	1:10,000,000
Glucagonomas	1:20,000,000
Somatostatinomas	1:40,000,000
Nonfunctioning	1:500,000

demonstrate the incidences and presentations of functional PNET, respectively. Malignancy is not determined by histopathologic examination but by the presence of metastasis. Between 60% and 80% of these tumors are metastatic at the time of presentation [11,13]. Most patients survive beyond 5 years with aggressive surgical therapy, however [10].

Preoperative imaging should precede any intervention. Investigators previously advocated somatostatin receptor scintigraphy, commonly known as the octreotide scan. Octreotide scans make use of the molecular properties of these tumors. Many endocrine lesions have a high density of somatostatin

Table 3
Symptoms and familial syndromes associated with pancreatic neuroendocrine tumors

Type of tumor	Clinical findings		Associated familial disorder
Insulinoma	Whipple's triad	• Symptoms of hypoglycemia • Serum glucose < 50 mg/dL • Relief of symptoms with glucose administration	MEN I (10%)
Gastrinoma	Zollinger-Ellison syndrome	• Peptic ulcer disease • Multiple ulcers • Ulcers that do not respond to medical treatment • Ulcers in unusual locations • Watery diarrhea	MEN I (25%)
VIPoma	WDHA syndrome	• Watery diarrhea • Hypokalemia • Achlorhydria	
Somatostatinoma	Cholelithiasis, diabetes mellitus type 2, steatorrhea		Neurofibromatosis type I (von Recklinghausen disease)
Glucagonoma	Diabetes, migratory necrolytic erythema		

Abbreviation: WHDA, watery diarrhea, hypokalemia, and achlorhydria.

receptors. These receptors are found on gastrinomas and, to some extent, on somatostatinomas, VIPomas, and glucagonomas. Only 17% to 50% of insulinomas carry this receptor, however, and the octreotide scan is of questionable utility in these patients [10,11].

Early reports showed that octreotide scans were superior to other imaging modalities for endocrine tumors. In a National Institutes of Health (NIH) prospective analysis of patients who had Zollinger-Ellison syndrome, octreotide scans had a higher sensitivity (70%) for localizing the primary tumor than CT (31%) or MRI (30%) ($P < .001$). Octreotide scans were also better at finding metastases, with a sensitivity of 92% compared with CT (42%) and MRI (71%) ($P = .004$) [12]. An NIH follow-up prospective study showed the superiority of octreotide scans in locating smaller tumors (<2 cm) and those in the duodenum [13]. Technologic advances during the past decade are changing these initial findings. A recent prospective study from France found that MRI was superior to CT ($P = .02$) and octreotide scanning ($P < .0001$) at detecting liver metastasis. Additionally, CT was superior to octreotide scanning ($P < .0001$) [14]. A smaller retrospective series showed that multidetector CT was equivalent to octreotide scans for pancreatic and duodenal endocrine tumors [15]. Improved biologic imaging using a [68]gadolinium-octerotide–based positron emission tomography (PET) scan for PNET has shown impressive results (97% sensitivity, 92% specificity, and 96% accuracy) [16]. To date, there has not been an extensive cost analysis of these different modalities.

The authors therefore recommend a multidetector CT scan (without a routine octreotide scan) as an initial study. CT can give important information about the surrounding vasculature and other structures and about metastases. In the event that CT fails to locate a lesion, one should proceed to MRI or an octreotide scan. All these measures should be used before angiography. Selective angiography with portal venous sampling of hormone levels seldom identifies lesions not seen on CT or MRI [12] and subjects the patient to an invasive procedure requiring a skilled interventional radiologist.

For functional PNETs, surgical therapy in general is directed at improving the abnormal physiology from hormone secretion through removing any tumors and associated metastasis. Resection of all intra-abdominal lesions does improve survival of these patients [17]. The presence of bony metastasis or extra-abdominal lesions is a contraindication to resection, and these patients should be managed medically. Local resection with enucleation is favored for small tumors away from the pancreatic duct [11]. Diabetes is noted in nearly 10% of patients who undergo distal pancreatectomy for PNETs, underscoring the need to preserve the pancreatic parenchyma. For this reason, we do not favor blind resection without proper preoperative localization. There is a growing body of literature demonstrating success with laparoscopic local resection of these lesions. Laparoscopy does seem to have improved morbidity rates compared with open enucleation, with similar cure rates [18]. Lesions greater than 2 cm are generally associated with malignancy and should be formally resected.

Insulinomas are the most common PNET. Their incidence is approximately 1 in every 1 million people. Most series have shown a slight female predominance, and patients are usually in their 40s [17,19]. These lesions are found with equal proclivity throughout the pancreas [10]. Approximately 5% of patients have an associated MEN I syndrome. Insulinomas are clinically characterized by the Whipple's triad: hypoglycemia with fasting or exercise, plasma glucose of less than 50 mg/dL, and relief of symptoms after glucose supplementation. Symptoms of hypoglycemia are varied and can lead to coma and death. The literature is replete with case reports of patients who had insulinoma and were misdiagnosed with psychiatric conditions. Surreptitious hypoglycemia can mimic insulinoma but can be differentiated by the lack of serum C-peptide and proinsulin. Diagnosis of insulinomas may be achieved in two ways. One is a 72-hour monitored fast in which plasma glucose and insulin concentrations are measured periodically while fasting until symptoms of hypoglycemia occur. A diagnosis is established if the insulin concentration is greater than 5 mU/mL with a glucose level of less than 40 mg/dL. A faster and more sensitive test is to determine the insulin-to-glucose ratio. After an overnight fast, a ratio greater than 0.4 is conclusive of the diagnosis (values less than 0.3 are considered normal) [20]. Approximately 13% of insulinomas are malignant [21]. As with all PNETs, malignancy is defined by evidence of distant spread rather than histopathologic findings. A retrospective analysis found that 89% of insulinomas smaller than 2 cm were benign, whereas 71% of insulinomas larger than 2 cm were malignant ($P < .05$) [22]. The authors therefore recommend that tumors greater than 2 cm in size or in close proximity to the pancreatic duct undergo a formal curative resection (pancreaticoduodenectomy or distal pancreatectomy). Lesions less than 2 cm in size without proximity to the pancreatic duct should undergo pancreatic parenchymal preservation (enucleation). With resection, patients who have benign lesions have a 10-year survival rate of 98.4%. Even patients who have malignant insulinomas (those with intra-abdominal metastases) have favorable prognoses (10-year survival rate of 75.7%) [21].

Gastrinomas follow insulinomas as the second most common PNET. Their incidence is roughly 1 in every 2 million people. Approximately 25% of patients have an associated MEN I syndrome [10]. Gastrinomas are slightly more common in men. Approximately 60% are malignant at diagnosis [10]. The most common presentation is abdominal pain, usually attributable to associated peptic ulcer disease or gastroesophageal disease from acid hypersecretion (Zollinger-Ellison syndrome) [23]. Fasting serum gastrin levels greater than 1000 pg/mL are diagnostic of a gastrinoma. Diagnosis can also be made using a secretin stimulation test; after administration of intravenous secretin, an increase in serum gastrin levels more than 200 pg/mL is diagnostic of a gastrinoma. Ninety percent of gastrinomas are found in the gastrinoma triangle: the confluence of the cystic and common bile ducts, the junction of the neck and body of the pancreas, and the junction of the second and third portions of the duodenum. Lesions in the pancreas are almost exclusively found in the gland's head. In addition to peptic ulcer disease, diarrhea can be a symptom of gastrinomas. The acidic environment leads to inactivation of pancreatic enzymes and subsequent steatorrhea and malabsorption. Diarrhea is a presenting symptom in 20% of gastrinomas [23]. Patients who have pancreatic lesions fare worse than those who have duodenal lesions because these lesions are more likely to have liver metastases [24]. In patients undergoing complete resection without metastases the 5-year and 10-year survival rates are 98% and 96%, respectively. Patients who have liver metastases have 5- and 10-year survival rates of 56% and 31%, respectively, underscoring the slow indolent nature of this disease. Lesions that are greater than 1 to 2 cm in size have a greater risk for hepatic metastasis [10,24,25]. Because of the malignant nature of this disease, the authors recommend formal resection at the time of presentation of the primary lesion and any resectable metastases.

VIPomas are next most common PNET. Their incidence is approximately 1 in every 10 million people. VIPomas classically present with watery diarrhea, hypokalemia, and achlorhydria (WDHA syndrome). Patients may also present with flushing, weakness, lethargy, and nausea. Symptoms tend to be intermittent, with lengthy asymptomatic periods. A fasting serum VIP level greater than 200 pg/mL is diagnostic. Most VIPomas are located in the tail of the pancreas, although 10% of these patients also have an extrapancreatic lesion, usually in the retroperitoneum or chest. Thus, the authors recommend CT of the chest while working up VIPomas. Treatment should initially revolve around correcting any electrolyte and fluid disturbances before intervention. VIPomas are metastatic at presentation 60% to 80% of the time [26]. Resection (usually a distal pancreatectomy) with debulking has proved effective even with metastasis. The 4-year survival rate is nearly 75% for all VIPomas [27] after resection.

Glucagonomas present in 1 in 20 million people. They are typically characterized by necrolytic migratory erythema, anemia, and weight loss. The necrolytic migratory erythema (present in 75% of cases) usually starts in the groin and perineum and is later found on the extremities. The etiology of this rash is unknown. Glucagonomas are typically located in the tail of the pancreas. The 5-year survival rate after resection is 83% [28]. Unfortunately, most are metastatic at presentation [11]. Still, these patients have a 5-year survival rate of 50% without resection [28]. This is probably attributable to the slow progression of the disease [28]. These lesions are typically large at presentation [29]. Because of the overwhelming malignant nature of glucagonomas, the authors recommend formal pancreatic resection when disease is confined to the pancreas.

Somatostatinomas are rare tumors (1 in 40 million people). These lesions are frequently metastatic at presentation, large (5 cm), and located in the head of the pancreas [10]. Somatostatinomas can present with hyperglyce-mia, diarrhea, steatorrhea, hypochloridia, and cholelithiasis. More than 70% are metastatic at presentation, but aggressive resection remains the mainstay of therapy. The overall 5-year survival rate is 75%. Metastatic dis-ease is associated with a 5-year survival rate of 60%. Eighty-five percent of pancreatic lesions are larger than 2 cm [30]. Again, the malignant nature and favorable survival statistics of these lesions lead to a recommendation to re-sect all these tumors whenever possible.

Care for patients who have hepatic metastases remains controversial. House and colleagues [31] showed that patients who underwent complete re-section of hepatic metastases had a trend toward better survival than those who did not have tumors amenable to metastectomy ($P = .06$). This finding, however, could be attributable to tumor biology, because patients who had widespread hepatic metastases probably had more aggressive disease. Other options for treatment are hepatic artery embolization and medical therapy for palliation of functional symptoms. Chamberlain and colleagues [32] demonstrated that surgery and hepatic artery embolization were superior to medical therapy in prolonging survival ($P < .05$). This same study also noted improved palliation with the resection of a dominant liver metastasis recalcitrant to medical therapy [32]. Because many PNETs are malignant, medical therapy should be geared toward alleviating symptoms and elimi-nating the tumor. With the advent of proton pump inhibitors and somato-statin analogues, the most common cause of death is liver failure from tumor burden [10]

Approximately 20% to 50% of all PNETs are classified as nonfunction-ing tumors. This nomenclature is misleading, because most nonfunctioning PNETs secrete a hormone at a subclinical level. Diagnosis is made by immu-nohistochemistry. Presentation is typically associated with tumor size and location, such as abdominal pain, jaundice, or weight loss, although 16% are found incidentally [10]. Most are found in the head, neck, or uncinate process. It is important to distinguish these tumors from the more aggressive pancreatic adenocarcinomas. Almost all nonfunctional PNETs have ele-vated chromogranin A and enhance on the arterial phase of CT. Although 60% to 92% of nonfunctional PNETs are malignant lesions [33,34], their 5-year survival rate is substantially better than that of pancreatic adenocarci-noma (52%–65%) [35].

Solid pseudopapillary tumors

SPTs have many different names, including solid and papillary tumors, papillary cystic tumors, solid cystic tumors, Franz tumors, and Hamoudi tu-mors. Although classified as a solid tumor, larger SPTs have been known to develop cystic degeneration. These are rare pancreatic lesions (less than 1% of all pancreatic neoplasms). SPTs are far more common in women and tend to occur in younger patients in their middle 20s. These lesions most commonly present with pain (47%) or a palpable mass (35%) [36]. SPTs have been reported up to 30 cm in size, although the median size is 6 to 7 cm [36,37]. They are commonly located in the body and tail of the pancreas.

CT scans show SPTs as hypodense lesions with a fibrous wall sharply demarcating them from the surrounding normal pancreas (Fig. 2). Almost all the recommendations regarding SPTs are based on small retrospective single-institution series. These lesions have low malignant potential. Those that are malignant and even have metastases still have favorable outcomes [36]. There are case reports of favorable outcomes after metastectomy or debulking procedures. A single patient with peritoneal spread has remained disease-free 10 years after distal pancreatectomy [38]. Another patient is disease-free 10 years after hepatic metastectomy [39].

Given their unique appearance on CT, we recommend proceeding with surgery after imaging. A large number of these patients undergo endoscopic ultrasound with fine-needle aspiration before surgical evaluation, however. SPT has been diagnosed in 52 patients in a meta-analysis by needle aspiration cytology [36]. In the same report, however, cytopathologic findings could not be generalized. Larger tumors develop a fibrous pseudocapsule, allowing for simple excision, although one series did note increased pancreatic fistula formation with enucleation [40]. In their practice, the authors have found that large tumor size necessitates a formal pancreatic resection (distal pancreatectomy or pancreaticoduodenectomy).

Cystic neoplastic pancreatic tumors

Serous cystadenoma

Cystic neoplasms make up approximately 10% to 15% of all cystic pancreatic lesions [5]. Compared with pseudocysts, serous cystadenomas are true cysts with an epithelial wall. They were previously called microcystic

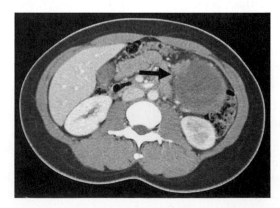

Fig. 2. SPT. Note the fibrous capsule demarcating the tumor from the remainder of the pancreatic tail (*arrow*).

adenomas or glycogen-rich cystadenomas. Serous cystadenomas are benign lesions. They usually present in older patients (seventh decade) with a 2:1 female-to-male ratio and are common in patients who have von Hippel-Lindau syndrome. Less than 15% cause biliary or pancreatic obstruction; therefore, serous cystadenomas can grow to large sizes [2]. The average size at presentation is 5 to 8 cm, and most are found incidentally [41,42]. When symptoms do occur, they tend to be nonspecific pain or nausea and vomiting from compression of surrounding structures [2].

Serous cystadenomas do not have a penchant for any particular anatomic location in the pancreas [42]. Imaging findings usually show a sharp demarcation from the remainder of the pancreas in contrast to MCNs. Serous cystadenomas do not communicate with the pancreatic duct. CT scanning shows a cluster of grapes or honeycomb pattern (many small cysts coalesced together) (Fig. 3). Additionally, a central calcified stellate scar is present one third of the time [41].

If an MCN or intraductal papillary neoplasm can be excluded, the authors recommend expectant management with serial CT scans for all patients without symptoms. Serous cystadenomas typically have low levels of carcinoembryonic acid (CEA) but can have variable levels of CA 19-9 [43]. If these lesions become symptomatic or enlarge by more than a centimeter in size over a 6-month period, the authors recommend an oncologic resection (eg, pancreaticoduodenectomy, distal pancreatectomy) rather than enucleation. Unless histopathologic findings are concerning for malignancy, no further radiographic follow-up is needed.

Mucinous cystic neoplasms

MCNs make up approximately 30% of all pancreatic cystic lesions. They are also frequently termed *mucinous cystadenomas*. They are noted for their thick wall lined with an ovarian-type stroma. MCNs have a 2-to-1 female

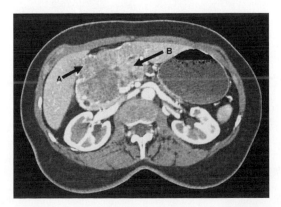

Fig. 3. Serous cystadenoma. Characteristic honeycomb pattern of these lesions from coalescing multiple smaller cysts (*arrow A*) and the stellate scar seen in one third of cases (*arrow B*).

preponderance in the fourth or fifth decade of life [2]. Like serous cystadenomas, MCNs usually present (most commonly) incidentally or with nonspecific pain related to their size and compression of adjacent structures. MCNs have a predilection for the body and tail of the pancreas [2]. MCNs usually appear on CT scans as unilocular cysts (Fig. 4). Similar to serous cystadenomas, they do not communicate with the pancreatic ductal system.

The differential diagnosis of MCNs includes pancreatic pseudocysts. If there is suspicion of malignancy, the authors recommend aspiration of the cystic structure. Endoscopic ultrasound (EUS) is the modality of choice for aspiration of these structures because of its safety and ability to obtain cyst fluid [43]. The presence of mucin in the aspirate indicates MCN, IPMN, or adenocarcinoma. Tumor markers in cystic fluid can also delineate these different cystic lesions. MCNs do have elevations in cyst CEA, whereas IPMNs have elevated cyst amylase [43]. Two recent series have shown the superiority of cyst mucin compared with other tumor markers [44,45]. MCNs are premalignant conditions. Their biology is similar to that of an adenomatous colon polyp with progression from atypia to mucinous cystadenocarcinoma. As such, all MCNs should be resected in an oncologic manner (usually a distal pancreatectomy). With a large portion of pancreatic pseudocysts being managed endoscopically, the authors stress the need for collection of cyst material for mucin staining. After resection in these patients who have benign MCNs, no further follow-up is necessary, because there is no risk for recurrence [46]. Patients who have malignant MCNs do have a risk for recurrence and should be followed with serial CT scans [47].

Intraductal papillary mucinous neoplasms

IPMNs are a relatively newly recognized disease entity. They were first classified by the World Health Organization in 1996. They have previously

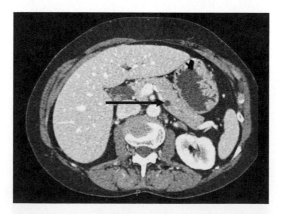

Fig. 4. MCN. This lesion, as indicated by the arrow, has a predilection for the pancreatic body and tail. Note that the MCN is unilocular and cannot be distinguished from a pancreatic pseudocyst from imaging alone.

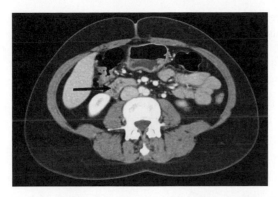

Fig. 5. Main duct IPMN. The arrow shows a cystic lesion in communication with the main pancreatic duct. This is pathognomonic of a main duct IPMN (in contrast to a branch duct IPMN, as seen in Fig. 7).

gone by several names, including intraductal papillary mucinous tumors, mucinous ductal ectasia, papillary hyperplasia, villous adenoma of the pancreas, intraductal carcinoma, and papillary mucinous tumor. Patients who have IPMNs tend to be in their 60s, and there is a slight male predominance [2]. A little more than half of patients present with abdominal pain [48]. Most IPMNs are located in the head of the pancreas [48]. IPMNs are considered to be a premalignant condition, with nearly one third of all resected specimens showing invasive cancer [48].

As their name implies, these are lesions of the pancreatic ductal system. There are two distinct forms: main duct IPMNs and branch duct IPMNs. The differences can often be appreciated on CT scans (Figs. 5 and 6). Dilation of the main pancreatic duct to more than 7 mm is a strong indicator of a main duct lesion. EUS and endoscopic retrograde cholangiopancreaticography (ERCP) can also be of assistance in differentiation of these two types

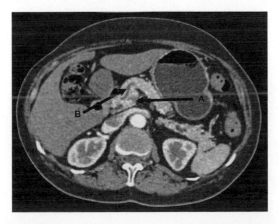

Fig. 6. Branch duct IPMN: lesion (A arrow) and main pancreatic duct (B arrow). The lesion is clearly separate from the main pancreatic duct, indicating a branch duct IPMN.

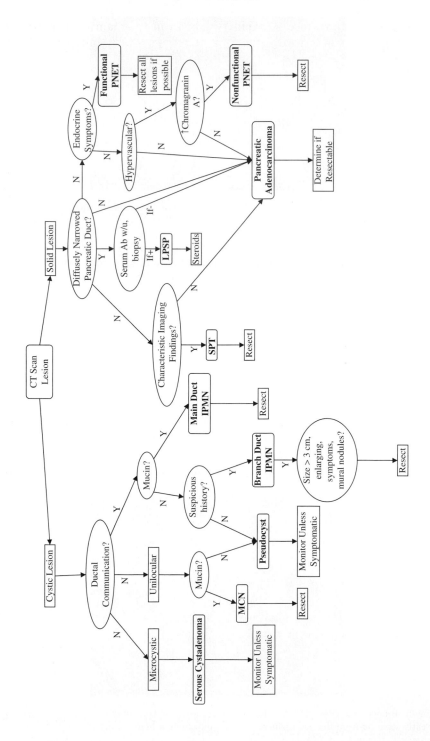

by detailing the presence of papillary growth in the main duct or branch pancreatic ducts [47]. Mucin found in secretions at the ampulla of Vater on ERCP is pathognomonic for IPMN. Disease associated with small branch ducts may not demonstrate this finding.

Carcinoma in situ or invasive disease is found in 60% to 92% of all main duct IPMNs. The prevalence of malignancy in branch duct IPMNs varies greatly from 0% to 41%. Multivariate analysis from a Japanese study shows that lesions sized greater than 3 cm and the presence of mural nodules were the greatest risk factors for malignancy in branch duct IPMNs [49]. Invasive carcinoma associated with IPMN has a significantly higher survival rate compared with pancreatic ductal adenocarcinoma (60% versus 15% at 5 years) [48]. Given these findings, the authors advocate the criteria developed by Tanaka and colleagues [47] for management of IPMNs. All main duct IPMNs should be resected when feasible. Branch duct IPMNs greater than 3 cm in size, associated with mural nodules, enlarging by more than 2 cm every 6 months, or causing symptoms should be resected as well. Any lesion with mucin-positive cytology should be considered malignant and resected [47]. Most (70%) resections are by means of pancreaticoduodenectomy, with 22% through total pancreatectomy and 8% by distal pancreatectomy [48].

There have been some reports of using intraoperative pancreatoscopy effectively in finding disease that ERCP and EUS could not identify. In one study, 10 of 24 patients were found to have disease not seen on conventional modalities, leading to extended resection for 3 patients [50]. The advent of high-resolution multidetector CT scanning has reduced the need for intraoperative pancreatoscopy, although it is still performed in some centers [51].

IPMNs are considered to be a field defect disease of the pancreas, and the entire pancreas is at risk for recurrence. Some practitioners therefore advocate total pancreatectomy [52–54]. Although total pancreatectomy may be performed safely, the long-term complication of brittle diabetes has led most surgeons to follow a more conservative approach to IPMNs (especially with elderly patients and patients with high operative risk). This includes close surveillance of the pancreatic remnant with high-resolution CT scans to look for changes in the size of the lesion, size of the main pancreatic duct, and presence of intramural nodules [47].

Fig. 7. Management flow diagram of a pancreatic cystic lesion found on a CT scan. In this decision algorithm, the ovals represent clinical questions to be addressed in each stage of management. After a pancreatic lesion is found on a CT scan, it may be classified as cystic or solid. CT findings should also delineate the relation between the lesion and the pancreatic ductal system. For example, a solid lesion with diffuse ductal involvement is suggestive of LPSP. If serum markers or the biopsy is nondiagnostic of LPSP, however, pancreatic adenocarcinoma is the likely diagnosis. Conversely, a solid lesion that does not involve the pancreatic duct, does not produce classic endocrine symptoms, is hypervascular, and is associated with elevated chromogranin A is suggestive of a nonfunctioning PNET.

Regardless of the initial management strategy, IPMNs warrant close long-term follow-up. Any remaining pancreatic duct remains at risk for new lesions, even if margins were negative after initial resection. Current adjuvant therapy for invasive cancer has offered marginal improvement in survival at best [55].

Neoplastic: microscopic

Pancreatic intraepithelial neoplasms

PanINs were first described by Hulst [56] in 1905. The authors have included a brief discussion of these lesions because they are benign neoplasms but are thought to be precursors to invasive ductal carcinoma. PanINs are thought to be relatively prevalent in the general population. Large autopsy series have demonstrated PanINs in 18% to 29% of noncancerous pancreata [57,58].

PanINs are a series of histologic changes from normal cuboidal to columnar epithelium. They are graded from PanIN-1A to PanIN-3. PanIN-1A is mucinous hypertrophy: flat columnar cells form with basally located nuclei and abundant cytoplasmic mucin located above the nuclei. PanIN-1B has similar intracellular changes as PanIN-1A but also demonstrates architectural changes to a papillary, micropapillary, or basally pseudostratified epithelium. PanIN-2 lesions are characterized by flat or papillary epithelia with associated mild to moderate nuclear atypia. PanIN-3 lesions have the aforementioned architectural changes with severe nuclear atypia. PanIN-3 lesions are thought to have the greatest risk for pancreatic adenocarcinoma [59–61].

There is a growing body of evidence suggesting that PanINs are precursor lesions to pancreatic adenocarcinomas. This includes case reports describing patients who had documented PanINs and went on to develop ductal adenocarcinoma [62]. In addition, PanINs are more common in adjacent pancreata of patients who have ductal adenocarcinoma than in normal pancreata resected for benign conditions [63]. Finally, and most convincingly, PanINs exhibit many of the molecular changes associated with ductal adenocarcinoma [60]. As a result of these observations, it has been proposed that PanINs are to pancreatic cancer what adenomatous polyps are to colon cancer.

The presence of PanINs themselves is not necessarily an indication for resection. The resection of PanIN lesions should be performed based on the context of the clinical situation. For example, at the time of pancreaticoduodenectomy, a PanIN-1 or PanIN-2 lesion at the neck margin in the face of a resected pancreatic adenocarcinoma does not necessarily warrant further resection. What to do with the finding of a PanIN-3 at the neck margin is less clear. Achieving a margin free of PanIN can be attempted but is not carried to the extent of performing a total pancreatectomy. Conversely, a high-grade PanIN at the neck margin during the resection of a low-grade tumor, such as a serous cystadenoma, is typically resected. This algorithm is

Table 4
Characteristic CT findings of benign pancreatic neoplasms

Name	CT characteristic
Pseudocyst	Unilocular with ductal connection
Solid pseudopapillary tumor	Hypodense lesion, demarcated by fibrous wall
Lymphoplasmacytic sclerosing pancreatitis	Pancreatic enlargement without definite mass, pancreatic ductal dilation
Serous cystadenoma	Microcystic clustering, stellate scar
Mucinous cystic neoplasm	Unilocular cyst without ductal communication in pancreatic tail
Intraductal papillary mucinous neoplasm	Unilocular cyst with ductal communication or pancreatic ductal dilation, with or without mural nodules
Pancreatic endocrine tumor	Distinct mass in pancreatic head, with or without metastatic lesions in liver

based on the premise that the most malignant lesion dictates the overall outcome of the patient.

Summary

An overall theme of the management of benign pancreatic neoplasms is their malignant potential. Most of the lesions described here require operative management. The authors have combined the diagnostic strategies presented here for each lesion to create a simplified decision flow diagram in Fig. 7. As one can see, the management of these lesions can still be quite complex. The characteristic CT findings are summarized in Table 4. It is paramount that the practitioner caring for the patients regards any pancreatic lesion with a high degree of suspicion. Similarly, surgeons treating these patients should understand the biologic properties of these tumors so that they know when to operate and what type of operation to perform.

References

[1] American Cancer Society. Cancer facts and figures 2007. Available at: http://www.cancer.org/downloads/STT/CAFF2007PWSecured.pdf. Accessed October 24, 2007.
[2] Nealon W. Unusual pancreatic tumors. In: Cameron JL, editor. Current surgical therapy. 8th edition. Philadelphia: Elsevier Mosby; 2004. p. 510–6.
[3] Baillie J. Pancreatic pseudocysts (part II). Gastrointest Endosc 2004;60:105–13.
[4] Baillie J. Pancreatic pseudocysts (part I). Gastrointest Endosc 2004;59:873–9.
[5] Shamamian P. Pancreatic pseudocysts. In: Cameron J, editor. Current surgical therapy. 8th edition. Philadelphia: Elsevier Mosby; 2004. p. 480–5.
[6] Abraham SC, Wilentz RE, Yeo CJ, et al. Pancreaticoduodenectomy (Whipple resections) in patients without malignancy: are they all 'chronic pancreatitis'? Am J Surg Pathol 2003;27:110–20.
[7] Okazaki K, Uchida K, Matsushita M, et al. How to diagnose autoimmune pancreatitis by the revised Japanese clinical criteria. J Gastroenterol 2007;42(Suppl 18):32–8.

[8] Hardacre JM, Iacobuzio-Donahue CA, Sohn TA, et al. Results of pancreaticoduodenectomy for lymphoplasmacytic sclerosing pancreatitis. Ann Surg 2003;237:853–8.

[9] Ito T, Nakano I, Koyanagi S, et al. Autoimmune pancreatitis as a new clinical entity. Three cases of autoimmune pancreatitis with effective steroid therapy. Dig Dis Sci 1997;42: 1458–68.

[10] Oberg K, Eriksson B. Endocrine tumours of the pancreas. Best Pract Res Clin Gastroenterol 2005;19:753–81.

[11] Muscarella P, Ellison EC. Pancreatic islet cell tumors excluding gastrinomas. In: Cameron JL, editor. Current surgical therapy. 8th edition. Philadelphia: Elsevier Mosby; 2004. p. 520–5.

[12] Gibril F, Reynolds JC, Doppman JL, et al. Somatostatin receptor scintigraphy: its sensitivity compared with that of other imaging methods in detecting primary and metastatic gastrinomas. A prospective study. Ann Intern Med 1996;125:26–34.

[13] Alexander HR, Fraker DL, Norton JA, et al. Prospective study of somatostatin receptor scintigraphy and its effect on operative outcome in patients with Zollinger-Ellison syndrome. Ann Surg 1998;228:228–38.

[14] Dromain C, de BT, Lumbroso J, et al. Detection of liver metastases from endocrine tumors: a prospective comparison of somatostatin receptor scintigraphy, computed tomography, and magnetic resonance imaging. J Clin Oncol 2005;23:70–8.

[15] Rappeport ED, Hansen CP, Kjaer A, et al. Multidetector computed tomography and neuroendocrine pancreaticoduodenal tumors. Acta Radiol 2006;47:248–56.

[16] Gabriel M, Decristoforo C, Kendler D, et al. 68Ga-DOTA-Tyr3-octreotide PET in neuroendocrine tumors: comparison with somatostatin receptor scintigraphy and CT. J Nucl Med 2007;48:508–18.

[17] Fendrich V, Langer P, Celik I, et al. An aggressive surgical approach leads to long-term survival in patients with pancreatic endocrine tumors. Ann Surg 2006;244:845–51.

[18] Sa CA, Beau C, Rault A, et al. Laparoscopic versus open approach for solitary insulinoma. Surg Endosc 2007;21:103–8.

[19] Tucker ON, Crotty PL, Conlon KC. The management of insulinoma. Br J Surg 2006;93: 264–75.

[20] Ritzel RA, Isermann B, Schilling T, et al. Diagnosis and localization of insulinoma after negative laparotomy by hyperinsulinemic, hypoglycemic clamp and intra-arterial calcium stimulation. Rev Diabet Stud 2004;1:42–6.

[21] Soga J, Yakuwa Y, Osaka M. Insulinoma/hypoglycemic syndrome: a statistical evaluation of 1085 reported cases of a Japanese series. J Exp Clin Cancer Res 1998;17:379–88.

[22] Schindl M, Kaczirek K, Kaserer K, et al. Is the new classification of neuroendocrine pancreatic tumors of clinical help? World J Surg 2000;24:1312–8.

[23] Fisher WE, Brunicardi FC. Zollinger-Ellison syndrome. In: Cameron JL, editor. Current surgical therapy. 8th edition. Philadelphia: Elsevier Mosby; 2004. p. 76–9.

[24] Yu F, Venzon DJ, Serrano J, et al. Prospective study of the clinical course, prognostic factors, causes of death, and survival in patients with long-standing Zollinger-Ellison syndrome. J Clin Oncol 1999;17:615–30.

[25] Weber HC, Venzon DJ, Lin JT, et al. Determinants of metastatic rate and survival in patients with Zollinger-Ellison syndrome: a prospective long-term study. Gastroenterology 1995;108: 1637–49.

[26] Perry RR, Vinik AI. Clinical review 72: diagnosis and management of functioning islet cell tumors. J Clin Endocrinol Metab 1995;80:2273–8.

[27] Soga J, Yakuwa Y. VIPoma/diarrheagenic syndrome: a statistical evaluation of 241 reported cases. J Exp Clin Cancer Res 1998;17:389–400.

[28] Chu Q, Al-Kasspooles M, Smith J, et al. Is glucagonoma of the pancreas a curable disease? Int J Gastrointest Cancer 2001;29:155–62.

[29] Doherty GM. Rare endocrine tumours of the GI tract. Best Pract Res Clin Gastroenterol 2005;19:807–17.

[30] Soga J, Yakuwa Y. Somatostatinoma/inhibitory syndrome: a statistical evaluation of 173 reported cases as compared to other pancreatic endocrinomas. J Exp Clin Cancer Res 1999;18:13–22.

[31] House MG, Cameron JL, Lillemoe KD, et al. Differences in survival for patients with resectable versus unresectable metastases from pancreatic islet cell cancer. J Gastrointest Surg 2006;10:138–45.

[32] Chamberlain RS, Canes D, Brown KT, et al. Hepatic neuroendocrine metastases: does intervention alter outcomes? J Am Coll Surg 2000;190:432–45.

[33] Vinik AI, Strodel WE, Eckhauser FE, et al. Somatostatinomas, PPomas, neurotensinomas. Semin Oncol 1987;14:263–81.

[34] Lo CY, van Heerden JA, Thompson GB, et al. Islet cell carcinoma of the pancreas. World J Surg 1996;20:878–83.

[35] Phan GQ, Yeo CJ, Hruban RH, et al. Surgical experience with pancreatic and peripancreatic neuroendocrine tumors: review of 125 patients. J Gastrointest Surg 1998;2:472–82.

[36] Papavramidis T, Papavramidis S. Solid pseudopapillary tumors of the pancreas: review of 718 patients reported in English literature. J Am Coll Surg 2005;200:965–72.

[37] de Castro SM, Singhal D, Aronson DC, et al. Management of solid-pseudopapillary neoplasms of the pancreas: a comparison with standard pancreatic neoplasms. World J Surg 2007;31:1130–5.

[38] Ng KH, Tan PH, Thng CH, et al. Solid pseudopapillary tumour of the pancreas. ANZ J Surg 2003;73:410–5.

[39] Hashimoto L, Walsh RM, Vogt D, et al. Presentation and management of cystic neoplasms of the pancreas. J Gastrointest Surg 1998;2:504–8.

[40] Sun CD, Lee WJ, Choi JS, et al. Solid-pseudopapillary tumours of the pancreas: 14 years experience. ANZ J Surg 2005;75:684–9.

[41] Galanis C, Zamani A, Cameron JL, et al. Resected serous cystic neoplasms of the pancreas: a review of 158 patients with recommendations for treatment. J Gastrointest Surg 2007;11:820–6.

[42] Compton CC. Serous cystic tumors of the pancreas. Semin Diagn Pathol 2000;17:43–55.

[43] Brugge WR, Lauwers GY, Sahani D, et al. Cystic neoplasms of the pancreas. N Engl J Med 2004;351:1218–26.

[44] Sedlack R, Affi A, Vazquez-Sequeiros E, et al. Utility of EUS in the evaluation of cystic pancreatic lesions. Gastrointest Endosc 2002;56:543–7.

[45] Walsh RM, Henderson JM, Vogt DP, et al. Prospective preoperative determination of mucinous pancreatic cystic neoplasms. Surgery 2002;132:628–33.

[46] Zamboni G, Scarpa A, Bogina G, et al. Mucinous cystic tumors of the pancreas: clinicopathological features, prognosis, and relationship to other mucinous cystic tumors. Am J Surg Pathol 1999;23:410–22.

[47] Tanaka M, Chari S, Adsay V, et al. International consensus guidelines for management of intraductal papillary mucinous neoplasms and mucinous cystic neoplasms of the pancreas. Pancreatology 2006;6:17–32.

[48] Sohn TA, Yeo CJ, Cameron JL, et al. Intraductal papillary mucinous neoplasms of the pancreas: an increasingly recognized clinicopathologic entity. Ann Surg 2001;234:313–21.

[49] Sugiyama M, Izumisato Y, Abe N, et al. Predictive factors for malignancy in intraductal papillary-mucinous tumours of the pancreas. Br J Surg 2003;90:1244–9.

[50] Kaneko T, Nakao A, Nomoto S, et al. Intraoperative pancreatoscopy with the ultrathin pancreatoscope for mucin-producing tumors of the pancreas 2. Arch Surg 1998;133:263–7.

[51] Fernandez-del CC. Surgical treatment of intraductal papillary mucinous neoplasms of the pancreas: the conservative approach 1. J Gastrointest Surg 2002;6:660–1.

[52] Tanaka M. Intraductal papillary mucinous neoplasm of the pancreas: diagnosis and treatment. Pancreas 2004;28:282–8.

[53] Inagaki M, Obara M, Kino S, et al. Pylorus-preserving total pancreatectomy for an intraductal papillary-mucinous neoplasm of the pancreas. J Hepatobiliary Pancreat Surg 2007;14:264–9.

[54] Yamaguchi K, Konomi H, Kobayashi K, et al. Total pancreatectomy for intraductal papil-lary-mucinous tumor of the pancreas: reappraisal of total pancreatectomy. Hepatogastroen-terology 2005;52:1585–90.

[55] Fernandez-del Castillo C. Intraductal papillary mucinous neoplasms. In: Cameron JL, editor. Current surgical therapy. 8th edition. Philadelphia: Elsevier Mosby; 2004. p. 517–9.

[56] Hulst SPL. Zur Kenntnis der Genese des Adenokarzinoms und Karzinoms des Pankreas. Virchows Arch 1905;180:288–316.

[57] Birnstingl M. A study of pancreatography. Br J Surg 1959;47:128–39.

[58] Kozuka S, Sassa R, Taki T, et al. Relation of pancreatic duct hyperplasia to carcinoma. Cancer 1979;43:1418–28.

[59] Sharif S, Plevy S, Finn OJ, et-al. Hereditary pancreatitis and its link to pancreatic cancer. In: Von Hoff DD, Evans DB, Hruban RH, editors. Pancreatic cancer. Studbury (MA): Jones and Bartlett; 2005. p. 119–32.

[60] Hruban RH, Wilentz RE, Kern SE. Genetic progression in the pancreatic ducts. Am J Pathol 2000;156:1821–5.

[61] Hruban RH, Adsay NV, bores-Saavedra J, et al. Pancreatic intraepithelial neoplasia: a new nomenclature and classification system for pancreatic duct lesions. Am J Surg Pathol 2001; 25:579–86.

[62] Wilentz RE, Geradts J, Maynard R, et al. Inactivation of the p16 (INK4A) tumor-suppres-sor gene in pancreatic duct lesions: loss of intranuclear expression. Cancer Res 1998;58: 4740–4.

[63] Cubilla AL, Fitzgerald PJ. Morphological lesions associated with human primary invasive nonendocrine pancreas cancer. Cancer Res 1976;36:2690–8.

ELSEVIER
SAUNDERS

SURGICAL
CLINICS OF
NORTH AMERICA

Surg Clin N Am 87 (2007) 1379–1402

Endoscopic Management of Acute and Chronic Pancreatitis

Siriboon Attasaranya, MD, FERCP,
Ayman M. Abdel Aziz, MD, FERCP,
Glen A. Lehman, MD*

*Division of Gastroenterology/Hepatology, Department of Medicine,
Indiana University Medical Center, 550 North University Boulevard,
UH 4100, Indianapolis, IN 46202, USA*

Patients who have acute pancreatitis or chronic pancreatitis (CP) may benefit from diagnostic and therapeutic endoscopic maneuvers. Certain etiologies of acute pancreatitis, such as biliary stones or microlithiasis, sphincter of Oddi dysfunction (SOD), pancreatic duct anomalies like pancreas divisum (PD), and ampullary tumors, can be definitively diagnosed by means of endoscopic retrograde cholangiopancreatography (ERCP) and sphincter manometry. Diagnosis of CP can be made and graded based on pancreatic ductal changes per the pancreatogram. Endoscopic approaches have been increasingly recognized as the effective therapy of certain etiologies, including biliary stones and SOD, and disease complications, such as pancreatic duct disruption, pseudocysts, pancreatic duct stones, and pancreatic duct stricture.

Endoscopic management related to the etiology of acute pancreatitis

Idiopathic acute/recurrent acute pancreatitis

Approximately 10% to 30% of patients who have acute/recurrent acute pancreatitis have an undefined etiology after a careful history, routine laboratory tests, and abdominal imaging studies (transabdominal ultrasound [US] and CT scan) [1]. Because a portion of patients who have acute (idiopathic) pancreatitis never experience the recurrent attack [2] and patients

---

S. Attasaranya and A.M. Abdel Aziz contributed equally to this work.
* Corresponding author.
E-mail address: glehman@iupui.edu (G.A. Lehman).

younger than 40 years of age rarely have a pancreatic tumor [3], those who present with a first episode of mild pancreatitis when they are younger than 40 years of age can therefore be managed expectantly. Further evaluation may be considered in patients who had multiple episodes, those who had a severe first attack, or those older than 40 years of age. Although less invasive imaging tests, such as magnetic resonance cholangiopancreatography (MRCP) and endoscopic ultrasound (EUS), may uncover the potential etiology, such as microlithiasis, common duct stones, PD, and annular pancreas, ERCP is still required, given its advantage of providing diagnostic and potential therapeutic value, as shown in Table 1. Further investigations with ERCP and sphincter manometry in patients who have idiopathic

Table 1
Summary of endoscopic management in patients who have acute or recurrent pancreatitis

Etiology	Role of endoscopic management	
	Diagnostic	Therapeutic
Biliary microlithiasis	Endoscopic ultrasound Aspirated bile for microcrystal analysis	Biliary sphincterotomy and stone removal
Sphincter of Oddi dysfunction	Sphincter of Oddi manometry	Endoscopic biliary or pancreatic sphincterotomy Prophylactic stent placement
Pancreas divisum	Endoscopic ultrasound	Minor papilla sphincterotomy
	Endoscopic retrograde pancreatography (ventral and dorsal ductogram)	Dorsal duct stenting
Anomalous pancreatobiliary junction	Endoscopic retrograde cholangiopancreatography	Major papilla sphincterotomy
Ampullary tumors	Endoscopic ultrasound	Ampullectomy
	Endoscopic retrograde cholangiopancreatography	Major papilla sphincterotomy Prophylactic pancreatic stent
Autoimmune pancreatitis	Endoscopic ultrasound with core biopsy or fine-needle aspiration	Stricture dilation and stenting
	Endoscopic retrograde cholangiopancreatography (suggestive)	Biliary or pancreatic sphincterotomy
Intraductal papillary mucinous tumor	Endoscopic ultrasound with fine-needle aspiration cytology and cyst fluid analysis	Pancreatic sphincterotomy facilitating mucus passage (if definitive surgery not being considered)
	Endoscopic retrograde pancreatography with juice cytology	
	Intraductal pancreatoscopy with or without biopsy	

acute/acute recurrent pancreatitis can discover the underlying causes in a significant portion of patients. One recent large series showed that SOD is the most common "hidden" etiology and accounts for 42% and 45% of patients presenting with acute and acute recurrent pancreatitis, respectively, whereas underlying CP was noted in 15% and 36% in these two groups, respectively (Table 2) [4].

Acute biliary pancreatitis

Gallstone disease is a common cause of acute pancreatitis (34%–54% of cases) in Western countries [5]. Clinically, biliary pancreatitis is generally suspected in the clinical setting of concurrent abnormal liver test results and the presence of gallbladder stones or bile duct dilation. One meta-analysis showed that elevated alanine aminotransferase (ALT) three times or greater the upper limit of normal measured within 1 to 2 days after onset of symptoms was the strongest predictor (with a positive predictive value of 95%) of biliary pancreatitis [6]. Given the significant risk of ERCP, its use is generally reserved for patients who likely require therapy based on suggestive/definite diagnosis of bile duct stones by other noninvasive tests, such as MRCP or EUS.

Table 2
Endoscopic retrograde cholangiopancreatography and manometric findings in 1343 patients who had idiopathic pancreatitis

	Preprocedure diagnosis					
	Acute pancreatitis		Acute recurrent pancreatitis		Chronic pancreatitis	
Endoscopic retrograde cholangiopancreatography/ sphincter manometry findings	N	% of 281 patients	N	% of 758 patients	N	% of 304 patients
Sphincter of Oddi dysfunction	117	41.6	343	45.2	76	26
Chronic pancreatitis	41	14.6	277	36.5	184	60.5
Pancreas divisum	38	13.5	155	20.4	43	14.1
Choledocholithiasis	35	12.4	18	2.4	8	2.7
Intraductal papillary mucinous tumor	6	2.1	44	5.8	5	1.6
Papilla of Vater adenoma/cancer	1	0.4	3	0.4	0	0
Anomalous pancreatobiliary junction	2	0.7	4	0.5	1	0.3
Cholelithiasis[a]	14	5	8	1.1	4	1.3
Periampullary diverticulum	21	7.5	52	6.9	9	3

[a] Without concurrent bile duct stones.

From Fischer M, Sipe BW, Sherman S, et al. ERCP/Manometry findings based upon preprocedure diagnosis: a sub-group analysis of 1,343 idiopathic pancreatitis patients. Gastrointest Endosc 2007;65(5):A242; with permission. Copyright © 2007, American Society for Gastrointestinal Endoscopy.

Most patients who have acute biliary pancreatitis (ABP) have self-limited mild to moderate disease, and the stone spontaneously passes into the duodenum in 70% of patients [7]. Routine preoperative ERCP is therefore not recommended. Because one third to two thirds of patients experience recurrent attacks as early as within 3 months unless gallstones are removed [8], it is currently recommended that cholecystectomy be performed during the same hospital stay (when pancreatitis subsides) if possible or shortly after discharge [9]. Patients with less evidence of persistent ductal stones (serum liver chemistries fully normalized) may directly proceed with laparoscopic cholecystectomy and an intraoperative cholangiogram. If any retained bile duct stones are documented, they can be addressed by laparoscopic bile duct exploration or during or after surgical ERCP depending on the local expertise.

Urgent endoscopic retrograde cholangiopancreatography in patients who have acute biliary pancreatitis

There are four initial randomized trials comparing urgent ERCP (within 72 hours after admission) with elective ERCP (Table 3) [10–13]. Biliary therapy was only performed if bile duct stones presented. The first two studies from the United Kingdom and Hong Kong demonstrated a significantly lower rate of complications in patients who had predicted severe pancreatitis and underwent early ERCP [10,11]. The third study, only presented in preliminary form to date, showed significant reduction of morbidity and mortality in patients who had predicted mild or severe ABP and underwent early ERCP [12]. The impressive treatment outcome seems to be attributable to the early intervention performed in this study. The fourth study from the Germany [13], conversely, showed a significantly higher rate of mortality and more severe complications, including respiratory failure, in patients undergoing early ERCP. This study has been criticized because of its higher rate of mortality in comparison to the prior three studies and an unclear association of early ERCP and respiratory distress. Expertise of the participant centers was also questioned, because 19 of 22 centers contributed less than an average of 2 patients per year to the trial [14]. A report on the fifth randomized control trial has been published recently [15]. A total of 103 patients who had ABP with persistent ampullary obstruction (defined by distal bile duct diameter larger than 8 mm with total bilirubin ≥ 1.2 mg/dL) were randomized, and patients who had cholangitis were excluded. This study, however, showed no significant benefit on disease severity, morbidity, and mortality in patients who underwent urgent ERCP. Two subsequent meta-analyses (at which time, the fifth study was still unreported) concluded that early endoscopic therapy significantly reduces morbidity (but not mortality) only in patients who have predicted severe ABP [16,17].

Cumulatively, in selected patients presenting with ABP, the earlier ERCP is performed, the better is the outcome that can be achieved. Currently, most experts agree that urgent ERCP (performed within 12–48 hours after

Table 3
Randomized trials of early endoscopic retrograde cholangiopancreatography in patients who had acute biliary pancreatitis

Studies	N	Timing of early ERCP	Bile duct stones found at the early ERCP	Complications (%)		Mortality (%)		Exclusion
				ERCP	Control	ERCP	Control	
Neoptolemos et al [10]	121	≤72 hours after admission	25% in mild cases 63% in severe cases	17[a]	34[a]	2	8	Other causes of pancreatitis
Fan et al [11]	195[b]	≤24 hours after admission	38%	18[a]	29[a]	5	9	Prior ABP, B-II surgery, ERCP pancreatitis
Nowak et al [12]	280	≤24 hours after admission	Not mentioned	17[a]	36[a]	2[a]	13[a]	75 patients with impacted stones at ampulla
Folsch et al [13]	238	≤72 hours after symptom onset	46%	46	51	11[a]	6[a]	Patients with bilirubin ≥5 mg/dL
Oria et al [15]	103	≤72 hours after admission	68% in mild cases 65% in severe cases	21	18	6[a]	2[a]	Patients with cholangitis

Abbreviation: B-II, Billroth-II gastrojejunostomy.
[a] Statistically significant difference.
[b] Included 127 patients who had biliary pancreatitis.

admission) should be performed in patients who have predicted severe ABP and in those who have concurrent cholangitis or suspected retained/impacted bile duct stones (Fig. 1). Clinically, several predicting factors of retained common duct stones during the episode of acute pancreatitis have been reported, including increasing bilirubin greater than 1.35 mg/dL on day 2 of hospitalization [7] and progressive increase in liver function test results and persistent dilation of the common duct [18].

Sphincter of Oddi dysfunction with acute/acute recurrent pancreatitis

SOD refers to benign abnormalities of the sphincter of Oddi (SO) and can result in outflow obstruction. The definitive diagnosis of SOD is made with sphincter of Oddi manometry (SOM); during this procedure, the basal sphincter pressure is determined. Abnormal SOM is defined by an elevated basal sphincter pressure greater than 40 mm Hg and has been variably observed in 15% to 72% of patients who have idiopathic pancreatitis [19]. It is important that pancreatic SOM be obtained in these patients, because the biliary SOM can be normal despite high pancreatic sphincter pressure [20].

Given its less invasiveness compared with surgery, endoscopic therapy is considered the preferable treatment option of sphincter therapy in patients who have SOD. At present, surgical approaches are generally reserved for patients with refractory stenotic papilla or when endoscopic therapy is technically infeasible (eg, in patients who have long limb roux-Y gastric bypass). In selected patients (who have abnormal pancreatic SOM) presenting with acute recurrent pancreatitis, pancreatic sphincterotomy seems to be more efficacious than biliary sphincterotomy alone [21]. Pancreatic sphincterotomy can be performed by using a "pull" sphinctetome or "needle-knife"

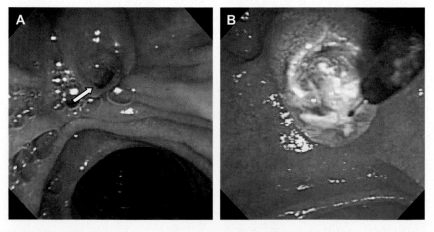

Fig. 1. (*A*) Impacted stone (*arrow*) at the ampulla. (*B*) Needle-knife sphincterotomy over the impacted stone.

papillotome. There are no available data to support whether one technique is more efficacious than the other. Overall, endoscopic pancreatic sphincterotomy provides clinical improvement in 70% of patients who have pancreatic SOD during mean follow-up periods ranging from 14 to 36 months [22]. This treatment outcome seems to be comparable with those of the surgical approach (open sphincteroplasty/pancreatic septoplasty), although a longer term of follow-up is lacking.

It is well known that post-ERCP pancreatitis rates in patients suspected of having SOD are relatively high and are reported at 10% to 30 % regardless of whether ERCP includes ductography alone, sphincter manometry, or therapy [23]. One meta-analysis showed that prophylactic (short-term) pancreatic stent placement significantly reduces the post-ERCP pancreatitis rate from 15.5 % to 5.8% in patients who have SOD and other high-risk patients, such as those who have difficult cannulation or precut papillotomy [24]. In patients who have suspected or documented SOD, it is currently agreed among most experts that prophylactic pancreatic stent placement is mandatory in these patients when performing diagnostic or therapeutic procedures.

Pancreas divisum

PD is the most common congenital anomaly of the pancreas, occurring in approximately 7% to 10% of the white population. PD occurs when ventral and dorsal pancreatic buds fail to join and communicate at the sixth or seventh week of gestation. Most patients who have PD are asymptomatic, and it has been estimated that less than 5% of patients who have PD ever become symptomatic [25]. In addition to the tiny minor papilla orifice that leads to inadequate drainage of pancreatic fluid during active secretion, other factors, such as genetic predisposition, may play a role in pathogenesis. Such patients may present with acute recurrent pancreatitis, CP, or chronic abdominal pain without pancreatitis.

The diagnosis of PD can be made by a helical CT scan, MRCP with/without secretin, and EUS. Secretin, with an enhancing effect on pancreatic secretion, leading to more accurate visualization of fluid-filled ducts, has been shown to increase the sensitivity of MRCP in detection of PD and "Santorinicele" [26,27], with a reported sensitivity rate of 73% [28]. Secretin-MRCP with quantification has been found to correlate with pancreatic exocrine function (eg, steatorrhea, fecal elastase) in one recent study [29]. The value of secretin-MRCP or secretin with any other imaging techniques to look for duct dilation to predict which patients who have PD may benefit from minor papilla therapy has not been well defined. The authors do not use this test clinically. ERCP, with an optimal pancreatogram, remains the most sensitive study to identify PD.

Generally, patients who have PD and a mild episode of acute pancreatitis can be managed expectantly. Those with a dilated dorsal duct per CT scan or MRI/MRCP and those with more frequent or severe episodes warrant further evaluation of the dorsal pancreas with potential minor sphincter therapy, however.

Endoscopic minor papilla therapy

Patients who have PD and present with acute/acute recurrent pancreatitis generally have a normal dorsal ductogram. Decompression of excessive intraductal pressure of the dorsal duct is the primary goal for therapy in patients who have PD. Endoscopic decompression may be achieved by balloon dilation, dorsal duct stenting, and minor papilla sphincterotomy. Use of minor papilla orifice balloon dilation has not been adequately evaluated to recommend its use. Long-term dorsal duct stenting has been shown to provide a favorable outcome, particularly in a subgroup of patients who presented with recurrent acute pancreatitis [30,31]. This (even a short-term trial of stenting), however, should be discouraged in patients with a normal dorsal duct because of the concerns of irreversible stent-induced pancreatic ductal and parenchymal changes, which are documented to occur as early as early as 2 months within placement of a 5-French stent in the normal canine pancreas [32]. The authors have observed such changes in patients as early as 2 weeks after placement.

Endoscopic minor papilla sphincterotomy is considered the procedure of choice for minor papilla therapy in symptomatic PD with a normal dorsal duct. Previous studies reported a favorable response (fewer attacks of pancreatitis and hospitalizations) in 76% to 94% of patients who have PD with recurrent acute pancreatitis after minor papilla sphincterotomy during medium-term follow-up (mean of 22–44 months) [32]. The benefit seems to be less obvious in patients who have CP and chronic pain alone.

Minor papilla sphincterotomy (papillotomy) can be performed by needle-knife sphincterotomy or standard pull-type sphincterotomy. Prior retrospective studies reported no difference in treatment outcomes between the two techniques [33,34]. The choice of techniques largely depends on the individual endoscopist's preference and the patient's anatomy. Because of the relative small size of minor papilla and the less obvious limits of the duodenal wall, the incision is typically made approximately 4 to 6 mm in length.

The post-ERCP pancreatitis rate seems to be similar to that of major papilla sphincterotomy and can be minimized by prophylactic pancreatic stent placement [24]. In the long term, restenosis of minor papilla has been estimated at 10% to 20% [32]. High-grade strictures of the terminal dorsal duct extending beyond the duodenal wall, which may require surgical correction, can be found in 2% to 3% of patients.

Anomalous pancreatobiliary duct junction

This entity is defined by a junction of the common bile duct and main pancreatic duct (MPD) joining outside the duodenal wall to form a common channel of greater than 15 mm in length. Anomalous pancreatobiliary duct junction (APBDJ) is a rare entity, with a reported incidence of 0.25% in the American population undergoing ERCP in a large referral center [35] and 1.5% to 3.2% in the Asian population [8]. Endoscopic sphincterotomy in patients who have APBDJ showed a decreased frequency of pancreatitis or pain in a previous reported series [35].

Choledochocele

Patients who have choledochoceles can present with acute pancreatitis or abdominal pain. Surgical resection is generally recommended for most patients who have choledochal cysts. In patients who have type III choledochoceles, in which a cystic dilation of the intraduodenal segment of the common duct occurs, biliary sphincterotomy has been recognized as the treatment of choice, providing a satisfactory long-term outcome [36]. The risk for subsequent cancer in patients who underwent endoscopic therapy seems to be low and does not warrant long-term surveillance.

Ampullary tumors

Patients who have major (or minor) papillary tumors can be diagnosed and treated with ERCP (Fig. 2). EUS to determine the tumor's depth and tumor invasion may be considered in selected patients. Typically, a small (<3 cm) tumor without ductal invasion is considered a good candidate for endoscopic resection. Patients who have larger or cancerous lesions and are at high risk for surgery may also be considered for endoscopic therapy, however. Snare ampullectomy with biliary or pancreatic sphincterotomy provides complete removal in 80% to 90% of cases if there is absence of intraductal invasion [37]. Procedure-related pancreatitis was reported to be as high as 20% to 33% [37,38], however, and has been shown to be reduced by prophylactic pancreatic stent placement (see Fig. 2) [38]. Endoscopic surveillance is mandatory to ensure complete tumor removal and to detect recurrence.

Endoscopic management of complications attributable to acute pancreatitis

Management of the complications of pancreatitis is complex and best accomplished with a multidisciplinary approach with expertise in all pancreatic specialties. Endoscopic therapy for a pancreatic pseudocyst (PP) and pancreatic disruption/fistula has been well recognized, whereas its role in other conditions, such as pancreatic necrosis and abscess, is less well established and it has only been performed in selected patients.

Pancreatic pseudocyst

Acute fluid collections are commonly found in patients who have acute pancreatitis, and most cases spontaneously resolve, although up to 15%

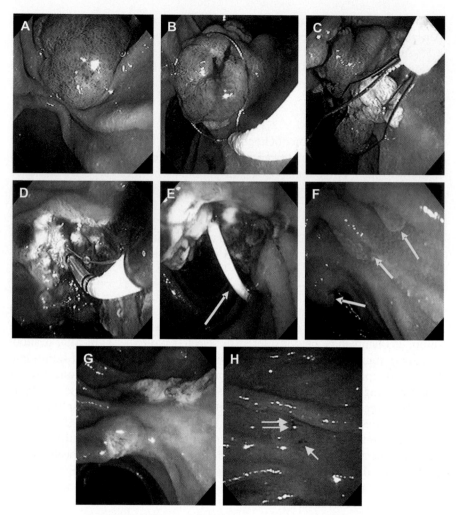

Fig. 2. (*A*) Ampullary adenoma. (*B*) Piecemeal snare resection. (*C*) Specimen retrieval using basket. (*D*) Biliary sphincterotomy. (*E*) Postpancreaticobiliary sphincterotomy with prophylactic pancreatic stenting (*arrow*). (*F*) Four months later showing scattered residual small adenoma (*arrows*). (*G*) Residual lesions were cauterized. (*H*) No adenoma was found at the 1-year follow-up. Patent pancreatic (*one arrow*) and biliary (*two arrows*) sphincterotomy orifices are noted.

develop into acute pseudocysts [9]. Specific interventions are considered only in symptomatic patients. The choice of therapy (surgical, radiographic, or endoscopic approach) is based on multiple factors, such as cyst size/location, pancreatic ductal anatomy, and local expertise. It is important to note that differentiating a pseudocyst from liquefied pancreatic necrosis is crucial, because more solid components are likely to require a more aggressive approach. MRI or EUS (rather than CT) is the preferable technique to serve this purpose. The authors generally wait 2 to 3 weeks to allow pancreatitis to diminish and the pseudocyst capsule to begin to mature. Further details of endoscopic therapy are noted in the section in this article on chronic pseudocysts.

Pancreatic duct disruption

Approximately one third of patients who have pancreatic necrosis have pancreatic duct disruption [18]. The clinical presentation includes a pancreatic fluid collection/pseudocyst, pancreatic ascites, pleural effusion, or a pancreaticocutaneous fistula. Definite diagnosis can be established by endoscopic retrograde pancreatography (ERP). Endoscopic therapy is discussed further in the section in this article on CP.

Pancreatic necrosis/abscess

Pancreatic necrosis defined as a diffuse or localized area of nonviable pancreatic parenchyma [39] and can be found approximately 20% of patients who have acute pancreatitis. Two to 3 weeks after acute necrosis, when the inflammatory process is becoming partially liquefied, a fibrotic capsule begins to surround the necrotic area and is called organized pancreatic necrosis (OPN). A pancreatic abscess is defined by a circumscribed collection of purulent material that contains bacteria in proximity to the pancreas, with little or no pancreatic necrosis [39]. This may be caused by superimposed infection in the necrotic pancreatic parenchyma or pseudocysts.

Generally, sterile necrosis requires no specific interventions. In patients who have intractable symptoms or infected necrosis (proved by CT-guided needle aspiration for Gram's stain and culture), however, surgical debridement is generally required and considered as the standard therapy. Nonsurgical therapy (radiographic or endoscopic approach) may be considered in selected patients who have documented OPN or abscess.

Endoscopic therapy for OPN and abscesses has been reported in a few series [40–46]. Most series recruited patients who had well-defined, organized, partially liquefied collections and those who were at high risk for surgery. To perform transmural drainage (without EUS guidance), extrinsic compression of the gastric/duodenal lumen with a close proximity (<1 cm) to the collection is required. Drainage is generally accomplished by transmural stenting and placement of a nasocystic catheter for aggressive irrigation. Transpapillary drainage was only performed in selected cases with pancreatic duct leak or obstruction. Resolution was achieved in 72% to 92% of patients. Complications, including infection and need for surgery, were as high as 37%, however, with a recurrent rate of 29% in one study [42]. In patients with nonbulging lesions, EUS-guided transmural drainage seems to be helpful and was reported to provide a high success rate in one recent series [46,47].

Endoscopic debridement/necrosectomy has been recently reported [44,45]. A larger balloon dilation of the enteric-cyst stoma is required to allow passage of the end-viewing endoscope for debridement under direct vision. Alternatively, the cavity can be trolled with stone retrieval balloons or baskets to remove debris [46]. Seewald and colleagues [44] reported on a small series of 13 patients who had infected pancreatic necrosis/abscess and were unfit for surgery. With aggressive daily endoscopic debridement and lavage providing successful drainage, surgery could be completely avoided in 9 patients. Three of 4 patients with bleeding required endoscopic therapy. A recent series that included a proportion of patients undergoing endoscopic debridement (22 procedures) reported an overall success rate at 81%. Concomitant percutaneous drainage was required in 40% of patients, however, and subsequent surgery was eventually required in 23% of patients [45].

In summary, endoscopic therapy for pancreatic necrosis and abscess is technically feasible, but experience remains limited. Larger scaled studies are required to define its use fully. Such therapy should be considered as part of the team (interventional radiology, surgery, and endoscopy) approach.

Endoscopic treatment of chronic pancreatitis

CP is characterized by progressive and irreversible pancreatic injury. Alcohol abuse is the most common cause of CP in the Western world. In patients who have CP, the aims of endoscopic therapy are to alleviate outflow obstruction of the pancreatic duct to decrease ductal hypertension, drain fluid collections, and relieve pain. Available endoscopic modalities include ERCP, which is used to treat pancreatic strictures, pancreatic ductal stones, bile duct strictures, and pseudocysts. EUS can be used to perform celiac plexus neurolysis or blockade to improve pain. Jejunal tube placement for enteral feeding may be sometimes used for gut rest and to decrease pancreas stimulation.

Pancreatic endotherapy should be considered in patients with a failed response to medical treatment or a dilated MPD. Although most studies suggest that endotherapy does not improve pancreatic function, one MRCP-based secretin study suggests that pancreatic exocrine function can improve after endoscopic therapy [48].

Endoscopic diagnosis of chronic pancreatitis

ERCP (Fig. 3) and EUS can confirm the diagnosis of CP. ERCP detects PD changes, including ductal dilation, strictures, abnormal side branches, communicating pseudocysts, PD stones, and PD leaks. ERCP is effective at visualizing these ductal and duct-related findings, with a sensitivity for the diagnosis of CP of 73% to 94% and a specificity of 90% to 100% [49]. ERCP may not detect changes of less advanced CP, but functional

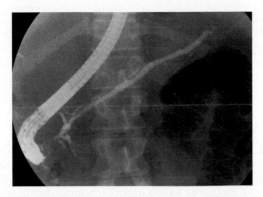

Fig. 3. Dorsal pancreatogram shows irregularity of main duct with dilated/irregular side branches indicating chronic pancreatitis in the PD.

assessment of the pancreas can be achieved during ERCP by performing an intraductal secretin stimulation test.

EUS allows visualization of ductal and parenchymal changes, such as lobularity, hyperechogenic foci and strands, focal areas of hypoechogenic tissue, and the presence of cysts. Ductal changes seen at EUS include hyperechogenic duct walls, dilation or irregularity of the main PD, PD stones, and visible side branches.

Endoscopic therapy in chronic pancreatitis

Pancreatic sphincterotomy

Pancreatic sphincterotomy can be done with a needle-knife incision over a guiding pancreatic stent or with a pull-type sphincterotome passed over a guidewire. This can be used to treat manometrically documented or suspected pancreatic SOD. Most pancreatic sphincterotomies are done as a part of pancreatic stone, stricture, or pseudocyst management or as part of a combined pancreatobiliary sphincterotomy for SOD, however. After such a sphincterotomy, a 3-French single-pigtail plastic stent 4 to 6 cm in length is used to prevent postprocedure pancreatitis unless a larger diameter stent is required for treatment of a simultaneous stricture. The small diameter single-pigtail stent in the duodenal lumen generally passes into the gastrointestinal tract within 7 to 14 days without the need for a second endoscopic procedure for stent retrieval. Risks for pancreatic sphincterotomy include early complications of pancreatitis (2%–7%), bleeding (0%–3%), perforations (< 1%), and late complication of sphincter stenosis (up to 10%) [50].

Dilation and stenting of pancreatic strictures

Benign strictures of the main PD are generally attributable to inflammation or fibrosis around the main PD. Focal strictures of the pancreatic head or body can be approached by endoscopic dilation or stent placement. If the narrowing involves the sphincter per se, this is classified as SOD and is best diagnosed by manometry. In most patients, pancreatic sphincterotomy (with or without biliary sphincterotomy) by way of the major or minor papilla is performed to facilitate placement of accessories. A guidewire must be maneuvered upstream to the narrowing. High-grade strictures require dilation before insertion of the endoprosthesis. This may be performed with graduated dilating catheters or hydrostatic balloon-dilating catheters. Pancreatic duct strictures from CP are often densely fibrotic; therefore, simple balloon dilation alone does not generally result in satisfactory long-term responses. Therefore, one or more polyethylene pancreatic duct stents are placed through the strictures to expand the lumen chronically. The goal is to expand the narrowing adequately, such that it allows good flow long after the stent is removed. In general, the diameter of the stent should not exceed the downstream duct diameter. Stent calibers range from 3 to 10 French. For pancreatitis prophylaxis 3- to 5-French stents are usually used, whereas stricture therapy usually requires single or multiple 7-, 8.5-, or 10-French stents.

Weber and colleagues [51] investigated in a prospective study the clinical success in 19 patients after initial ERCP and relapse rates during a 2-year follow-up period. The overall patient assessment of the stent therapy revealed complete satisfaction in 17 of 19 patients. A relapse rate of approximately 30% was seen within 2 years after stent extraction and was treated by repeated stent therapy. At 5 years of follow-up, another series [52] reported pain relief in 65% of the patients with ductal outflow obstruction attributable to dominant pancreatic duct stricture and were treated by stent drainage. Costamagna and colleagues [53] studied 19 patients who had severe CP and a single pancreatic stent through a refractory dominant stricture in the pancreatic head with the following protocol: (1) removal of the single pancreatic stent, (2) balloon dilation of the stricture, (3) insertion of the maximum number of stents allowed by the stricture tightness and the pancreatic duct diameter, and (4) removal of stents after 6 to 12 months. They reported that the median number of stents placed through the major or minor papilla was three, with diameters ranging from 8.5 to 11.5 French and length from 4 to 7 cm. Only 1 patient (5.5%) had persistent stricture after multiple stenting. During a mean follow-up of 38 months after removal, 84% of patients were asymptomatic and 10.5 % had symptomatic stricture recurrence. A recent randomized trial [54] comparing the endoscopic transampullary drainage of the pancreatic duct with operative pancreaticojejunostomy showed that complete or partial pain relief was achieved in 32% of patients assigned to endoscopic drainage as compared with 75% of patients assigned to surgical drainage ($P = .007$), however. Rates of complications, length of hospital stay, and changes in pancreatic function were similar in the two treatment groups, but patients receiving endoscopic treatment required more procedures than did patients in the surgical group (median of eight versus three; $P < .001$). The investigators concluded that surgical drainage of the pancreatic duct is more effective than endoscopic treatment in patients with obstruction of the pancreatic duct attributable to CP.

Occasionally, the pancreatic duct strictures are extremely tight or angulated and may not be traversable with conventional dilators and catheters. A case report by Familiari and colleagues [55] described the use of a guidewire placed across these types of strictures for 24 hours (used as a dilator). They hypothesized that the guidewire left in place across the stricture, in combination with its slight movements caused by breathing, facilitated a noninvasive dilation of the stenosis and allowed subsequent mechanical dilations and stent insertion.

The optimum duration of stent placement, stent number and diameter, and degree of balloon dilation are not well known. The early complications of stent placement are similar to those of sphincterotomy (eg, bleeding, pancreatitis). Late complications are mainly related to migration (10%) and occlusion (20%), which present with pain, pancreatitis, or infection [56]. In addition, PD stents may produce ductal changes, including strictures or focal areas of CP. These changes may improve with time, however.

Removal of pancreatic duct stones

Patients with obstructing stones of the head or body with main duct dilation are candidates for stone extraction (Fig. 4). Simple stone extraction can be achieved by various techniques, including balloon or basket sweep. Larger stones usually require lithotripsy by means of extracorporeal shock wave lithotripsy (ESWL), followed by balloon or basket sweep. Patients frequently require several ESWL sessions to achieve stone clearance from the duct [57]. Intraductal lithotripsy guided by pancreatoscopy has also been used to fragment PD stones, although experience is limited. Large series [58] showed pain relief in 70% to 80% of patients after stone removal. There is a pain relapse rate of approximately 30% in patients over 2 years.

Surgical removal of the pancreatic duct stones can also be achieved. In one randomized trial of endoscopic and surgical therapy, surgery was superior for long-term pain reduction in patients who have painful obstructive CP [59]. Endotherapy without conjunctive ESWL, as performed in this study, seems to be suboptimal for pancreatic duct stone therapy, however. Generally, endotherapy may be preferable, given its less invasiveness, and surgery may be considered as the second-line therapy for patients in whom endoscopic therapy fails or is ineffective. Some short-term and long-term follow-up data to 5 years showing improvements in pain (77%–100% and 54%–86%, respectively) have been reported [60,61]. It is the authors' observation that approximately 50% of patients have pain relapse within a 5-year follow-up period. This may be caused by new stone formation or underlying ongoing pancreatitis.

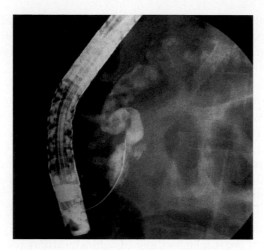

Fig. 4. Numerous pancreatic duct stones in the head of the pancreas.

Biliary obstruction in chronic pancreatitis

Distal common bile duct strictures have been reported to occur in at least 35% of patients who have CP. Such strictures are a result of a fibrotic inflammatory restriction or compression by a pseudocyst. No treatment is recommended unless the alkaline phosphatase level is two times normal or greater with ductal dilation. Most studies showed that cholestasis can be effectively resolved by ERCP plastic biliary stenting in the short-term setting. In the authors' experience, these strictures uncommonly resolve and long-term stenting, or preferably surgical bypass, is needed. Preliminary experience with placement of 4- to 8-cm 10-French plastic stents may indicate better long-term patency. Fully coated metal stents placed at ERCP are being evaluated for these strictures. To be successful, it is essential that these stents be removable after 6 to 24 months in situ and cause no ductal injury. Van Berkel and colleagues [62] reported that long-term stenting of benign biliary strictures attributable to CP using self-expanding metal was safe and provided successful and prolonged biliary drainage in a selected group of patients in whom surgical intervention was not possible or desirable. Larger prospective, randomized, long-term studies are awaited, however.

Pancreatic duct leaks

Pancreatic duct disruptions or leaks can occur as a result of CP from a blow-out upstream to obstructing strictures or stones. Disruption of the MPD may be partial or complete. At ERCP, partial disruption appears as a fluid collection communicating directly with the MPD. Complete disruption consists of MPD transection, leading to pancreatic ascites, pleural effusions, pseudocyst formation, and internal and external pancreatic fistulas. PD leaks can often be treated with endoscopic placement of transpapillary stents. Endoscopic therapy is successful in closing the leak in approximately 60% of patients [63]. Factors associated with a better outcome in duct disruption include a partial disruption, successfully bridging the disruption with a stent, and longer duration of stent placement (approximately 6 weeks). There are no comparative studies of surgical, medical, and endoscopic therapy for treatment of PD leaks.

Treatment of chronic pancreatitis attributable to pancreas divisum

Opening the minor papilla by sphincterotomy and a combined sphincterotomy/stenting technique has been shown to eliminate recurrent pancreatitis in three quarters of patients who have CP and to improve pain in approximately 50% of patients who have pain syndrome. Vitale and colleagues [64] evaluated the long-term efficacy of endoscopic stenting in 24 patients who had CP attributable to PD and underwent endoscopic stenting over a 12-year period (mean follow-up period was 59.6 months). Every patient had more than one ERCP performed for stent exchange or removal (mean number was 3.6 ERCPs per patient during the study period). Stents used for the endoscopic therapy varied between 5, 7, and 10 French. Patients had a stent placed in the minor papilla for a mean period of 5.9 months, with exchanges every 6 to 8 weeks. The mean pain score and number of hospital admissions decreased significantly after stent placement ($P < .05$). Pain medication use decreased in 58% of patients, remained the same in 21%, and increased in 13%. The authors concluded that endoscopic stenting of the pancreatic duct is a safe and effective first-line treatment for patients who have pancreatitis secondary to PD.

Endoscopic jejunal tube placement for enteral feeding

In patients with unrelenting pain attributable to CP, gut rest is recommended by enteral feeding (preferred) or parenteral nutrition. Enteral nutrition by means of a jejunal tube is replacing parenteral nutrition. By feeding the gut beyond the ligament of Treitz, enteral feeding causes negligible stimulation of the pancreas and is associated with improved immune function, reduced infections, and lower pain scores.

Celiac nerve block and neurolysis

In patients who have CP, celiac plexus blockade or neurolysis can be performed to improve their pain. Celiac plexus blockade involves injection of a steroid (triamcinolone) and an anesthetic agent (bupivacaine) into the celiac plexus. Celiac plexus neurolysis involves injection of a neurolytic agent (absolute alcohol) into the celiac plexus to ablate or destroy the ganglia, thereby interrupting pain transmission. An EUS procedure can be used in patients who have a suboptimal response to medical management. In general, EUS-guided celiac plexus blockade improves pain in approximately 50% of patients for a period of 3 to 6 months. Younger patients (<45 years of age) and those who have had previous pancreatic surgery are less likely to respond to EUS-guided celiac plexus blockade [65].

Complications of celiac plexus blockade or neurolysis are infrequent and mostly self-limited. The most common side effects are transient diarrhea and hypotension; these can be seen in up to 30% to 40% of patients. Sympathetic blockade can manifest as diarrhea and hypotension as the result of relatively unopposed visceral parasympathetic activity. In most patients, the diarrhea is mild and self-limiting and lasts less than 48 hours. Infrequent major complications have been reported, including retroperitoneal bleeding and peripancreatic abscess. It is advisable to give antibiotic prophylaxis (against mouth flora) to patients undergoing celiac plexus blockade. Antibiotics may not be necessary when alcohol is used, because alcohol has inherent bactericidal properties. In addition, ethanol causes a dense desmoplastic reaction, making any future pancreatic surgery more difficult. Therefore, the authors avoid alcohol neurolysis for CP, because these patients may require future surgery. Realizing that, celiac blockade is of clinical benefit in only half of patients. The authors use EUS-guided blockade when EUS is being done for diagnostic reasons and CP is confirmed or for patients who would benefit from a vacation from pain or pain medications.

Pancreatic pseudocysts

PPs develop in approximately 20% of patients who have CP, arising from a duct disruption in areas of inflammation or necrosis. Pseudocysts can be located within or outside the pancreas, may be single or multiple, may have persistent connection to the ductal system duct or not, and may be symptomatic or asymptomatic. Intervention is indicated for PPs that are symptomatic, in a phase of growth, or complicated (eg, infected, hemorrhage, biliary, or bowel obstruction) or in those occurring together with CP and when malignancy cannot be unequivocally excluded. Symptomatic and large pseudocysts (>7 cm) generally need drainage by an endoscopic, surgical, or percutaneous approach. Percutaneous drainage is performed for fluid collections outside the pancreas without associated necrosis (low probability of persistent ductal disruption). The endoscopic approach is performed if a significant bulge is noted against the lumen of the stomach or duodenum and the distance between the gut wall and the pseudocyst is less than 1 cm with no intervening major vascular structures (Fig. 5). This entails the creation of a fistulous tract between the PPs and the gastric lumen (cystogastrostomy) or the duodenal lumen (cystoduodenostomy). A nasocystic catheter or a stent can be placed for continuous drainage. The choice

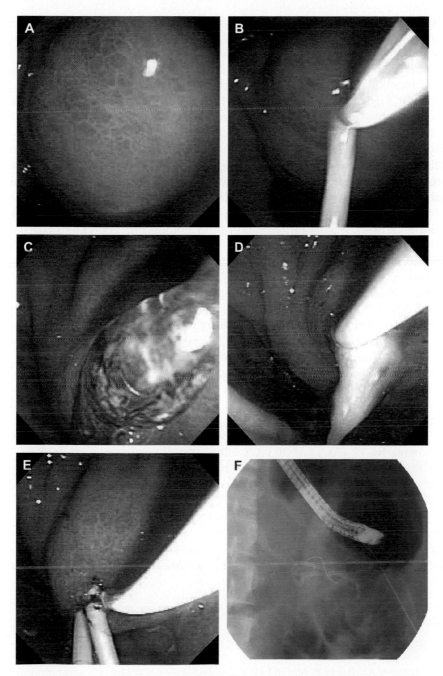

Fig. 5. (*A*) Pseudocyst bulging on gastric wall. (*B*) Cyst puncture using cystotome resulting in initial pus drainage. (*C*) Transmural (10-mm) balloon dilation. (*D*) Placement of one 7-French double-pigtail stent. (*E*) Two 7-French double-pigtail stents placed into the cyst. (*F*) Fluoroscopic view showing two double-pigtail stents in place.

between a nasocystic catheter or stent for drainage depends on the appearance of the cyst contents. A chronic cyst with clear liquid contents can be drained with one or more stents. Conversely, an infected cyst may require irrigation by means of a nasocystic catheter. Arvanitakis and colleagues [66] treated patients who had CP with apparently complete disruption of the MPD by stent placement into the PPs or peripancreatic fluid collection. Stent removal resulted in fluid reaccumulation as the duct disruption persisted. These investigators recommended long-term stenting. The authors, however, prefer definitive surgical diversion. Transpapillary drainage can also be performed if the pseudocyst connects to the MPD above the stricture. Hookey and colleagues [67] published a comparative study on transmural and transpapillary drainage for 116 patients who had PPs. The drainage technique was transpapillary in 15 patients, transmural in 60, and both in 41. Successful resolution of symptoms and collection occurred in 87.9% of cases. No significant differences were observed regarding drainage technique or site of drainage. In a summary of eight series from the literature involving 311 patients, stent placement was technically successful in 89%, with complications in 17% and death in 1%. Recurrences are seen in 10% and 20% of patients, as in surgical series, and result from persistent main duct disruption, as noted previously.

A Web-based survey was sent to US and international members of the American Society for Gastrointestinal Endoscopy [68]. Of the 3054 endoscopists to whom the survey was sent, 266 (8.7%) replied: 198 performed pseudocyst drainage. The transgastric route was the most commonly used drainage route. The number of stents placed ranged from one to five, and these remained in place for 2 to 30 weeks. A CT scan was performed before drainage by 95% of all respondents. EUS imaging was used before drainage by 72 (70%) of 103 US endoscopists compared with 56 (59%) of 95 international endoscopists. EUS-guided drainage was used by 56% of US endoscopists compared with 43% of international endoscopists.

In conclusion, endoscopic transmural drainage is the best technique for bulging PPs, whereas EUS-guided drainage is required for nonbulging pancreatic collections and in patients who have portal hypertension. For patients with complete disruption of the MPD, surgical resection or diversion is preferred.

References

[1] Draganov P, Forsmark CE. "Idiopathic" pancreatitis. Gastroenterology 2005;128(3): 756–63.
[2] Ballinger AB, Barnes E, Alstead EM, et al. Is intervention necessary after a first episode of acute pancreatitis? Gut 1996;38(2):293–5.
[3] Choudari CP, Fogel EL, Sherman S, et al. Idiopathic pancreatitis: yield of ERCP correlated with patient age. Am J Gastroenterol 1998;93(9):A1654.

[4] Fischer M, Sipe BW, Sherman S, et al. ERCP/Manometry findings based upon pre-procedure diagnosis: a sub-group analysis of 1,343 idiopathic pancreatitis patients. Gastrointest Endosc 2007;65(5):A242.

[5] Kaikaus RM, Geenen JE. Current role of ERCP in the management of benign pancreatic disease. Endoscopy 1996;28(1):131–7.

[6] Tenner S, Dubner H, Steinberg W. Predicting gallstone pancreatitis with laboratory parameters: a metaanalysis. Am J Gastroenterol 1994;89(10):1863–6.

[7] Chang L, Lo SK, Stabile BE, et al. Gallstone pancreatitis: a prospective study on the incidence of cholangitis and clinical predictors of retained common bile duct stones. Am J Gastroenterol 1998;93(4):527–31.

[8] Delhaye M, Matos C, Deviere J. Endoscopic technique for the management of pancreatitis and its complications. Best Pract Res Clin Gastroenterol 2004;18(1):155–81.

[9] Forsmark CE, Baillie J. AGA Institute technical review on acute pancreatitis. Gastroenterology 2007;132(5):2022–44.

[10] Neoptolemos JP, Carr-Locke DL, London NJ, et al. Controlled trial of urgent endoscopic cholangiopancreatography and endoscopic sphincterotomy versus conservative treatment for acute pancreatitis due to gallstones. Lancet 1988;2(8618):979–83.

[11] Fan S-T, Lai E, Mok F, et al. Early treatment of acute biliary pancreatitis by endoscopic papillotomy. N Engl J Med 1993;328(4):228–32.

[12] Nowak A, Nowakowska-Dulawa E, Marek TA, et al. Final results of the prospective, randomized, controlled study on endoscopic sphincterotomy versus conventional management in acute biliary pancreatitis. Gastroenterology 1995;108(4):A380.

[13] Fölsch UR, Nitsche R, Ludtke R, et al. Early ERCP and papillotomy compared with conservative treatment for acute biliary pancreatitis. N Engl J Med 1997;336(4):237–42.

[14] Kozarek R. Role of ERCP in acute pancreatitis. Gastrointest Endosc 2002;56(6):s231–6.

[15] Oría A, Cimmino D, Ocampo C, et al. Early endoscopic intervention versus early conservative management in patients with acute gallstone pancreatitis and biliopancreatic obstruction. A randomized clinical trial. Ann Surg 2007;245(1):10–7.

[16] Sharma VK, Howden CW. Metaanalysis of randomized controlled trials of endoscopic retrograde cholangiography and endoscopic sphincterotomy for the treatment of acute biliary pancreatitis. Am J Gastroenterol 1999;94(11):3211–4.

[17] Ayub K, Imada R, Slavin J. Endoscopic retrograde cholangiopancreatography in gallstone-associated acute pancreatitis. Cochrane Database Syst Rev 2004;CD003630.

[18] Banks P, Freeman ML, Practice Parameters Committee of the American College of Gastroenterology. Practice guideline in acute pancreatitis. Am J Gastroenterol 2006;101(10): 2379–400.

[19] Behar J, Corazziari E, Guelrud M, et al. Functional gallbladder and sphincter of Oddi disorders. Gastroenterology 2006;130(5):1498–509.

[20] Steinberg WM. Controversies in clinical pancreatology: should the sphincter of Oddi be measured in patients with idiopathic recurrent acute pancreatitis and should sphincterotomy be performed if the pressure is high? Pancreas 2003;27(2):118–21.

[21] Peterson BT. Sphincter of Oddi dysfunction, part 2: evidence-based review of the presentations, with "objective" pancreatic findings (type I and II) and of presumptive type III. Gastrointest Endosc 2004;59(6):670–87.

[22] Sgouros SN, Pereira SP. Systematic review: sphincter of Oddi dysfunction—non-invasive diagnostic methods and long-term outcome after endoscopic sphincterotomy. Aliment Pharmacol Ther 2006;24:237–46.

[23] Freeman ML, Gill M, Overby C, et al. Predictors of outcomes after biliary and pancreatic sphincterotomy for sphincter of Oddi dysfunction. J Clin Gastroenterol 2007;41(1): 94–102.

[24] Singh P, Das A, Isenberg G, et al. Does prophylactic pancreatic stent placement reduce the risk of post-ERCP acute pancreatitis? A metaanalysis of controlled trials. Gastrointest Endosc 2004;60(4):544–50.

[25] Saltzman JR. Endoscopic treatment of pancreas divisum: why, when, and how. Gastrointest Endosc 2006;64(5):712–5.

[26] Matos C, Metens T, Deviere J, et al. Pancreas divisum: evaluation with secretin-enhanced magnetic resonance cholangiopancreatography. Gastrointest Endosc 2001;53(7): 728–33.

[27] Manfredi R, Costamagna G, Brizi MG, et al. Pancreas divisum and Santorinicele: diagnosis with dynamic MR cholangiography with secretin stimulation. Radiology 2000;217:403–8.

[28] Mosler P, Fogel EL, McHenry L, et al. Accuracy of magnetic resonance cholangiopancreatography (MRCP) in the diagnosis of pancreas divisum (PD). Gastrointest Endosc 2005; 61(5):AB100.

[29] Gillams A, Pereira S, Webster G, et al. Correlation of MRCP quantification (MRCPQ) with conventional non-invasive pancreatic exocrine function tests. Abdom Imaging 2007 [e-pub ahead of print].

[30] Lans JI, Geenen JE, Johanson JF, et al. Endoscopic therapy in patients with pancreas divisum and acute pancreatitis: a prospective, randomized, controlled trial. Gastrointest Endosc 1992;38(4):430–4.

[31] Linder JD, Bukeirat FA, Geenen JE, et al. Long-term response to pancreatic duct stent placement in symptomatic patients with pancreas divisum. Gastrointest Endosc 2003; 57(5):208A.

[32] Fogel EL, Toth TG, Lehman GA, et al. Does endoscopic therapy favorably affect the outcome of patients who have recurrent acute pancreatitis and pancreas divisum? Pancreas 2007;34(1):21–45.

[33] Attwell A, Borak G, Hawes R, et al. Endoscopic pancreatic sphincterotomy for pancreas divisum using a needle-knife or standard pull-type techniques: safety and reintervention rates. Gastrointest Endosc 2006;64(5):705–11.

[34] Berkes J, Bernklau S, Halliine A, et al. Minor papillotomy in pancreas divisum: do complications and restenosis rates differ between use of the needle-knife papillotome vs ultratapered traction sphincterotome? Gastrointest Endosc 2004;59(5):A207.

[35] Samavedy R, Sherman S, Lehman GA. Endoscopic therapy in anomalous pancreatobiliary duct junction. Gastrointest Endosc 1999;50(5):623–7.

[36] Ladas SD, Katsogridakis I, Tassios P, et al. Choledochocele, an overlooked diagnosis: report of 15 cases and review of 56 published reports from 1984 to 1992. Endoscopy 1995;27(3): 233–9.

[37] Adler DG, Baron TH, Davila RE, et al. ASGE guideline: the role of ERCP in disease of the biliary tract and the pancreas. Gastrointest Endosc 2005;62(1):1–8.

[38] Harewood GC, Pochron NL, Gostout CJ. Prospective, randomized, controlled trial of prophylactic pancreatic stent placement for endoscopic snare excision of the duodenal ampulla. Gastrointest Endosc 2005;62(3):367–70.

[39] Bradley EL 3rd. A clinically based classification system for acute pancreatitis. Summary of the International Symposium on Acute Pancreatitis, Atlanta, GA, September 11 through 13, 1992. Arch Surg 1993;128(5):586–90.

[40] Baron TH, Thaggard WG, Morgan DE, et al. Endoscopic therapy for organized pancreatic necrosis. Gastroenterology 1996;111(3):755–64.

[41] Venu RP, Brown RD, Merrero JA, et al. Endoscopic transpapillary drainage of pancreatic abscess: technique and results. Gastrointest Endosc 2000;51(4):391–5.

[42] Baron TH, Harewood GC, Morgan DE, et al. Outcome differences after endoscopic drainage of pancreatic necrosis, acute pancreatic pseudocysts, and chronic pancreatic pseudocysts. Gastrointest Endosc 2002;56(1):7–17.

[43] Park JJ, Kim SS, Koo YS, et al. Definitive treatment of pancreatic abscess by endoscopic transmural drainage. Gastrointest Endosc 2002;55(2):256–62.

[44] Seewald S, Groth S, Omar S, et al. Aggressive endoscopic therapy for pancreatic necrosis and pancreatic abscess: a new safe and effective treatment algorithm. Gastrointest Endosc 2005; 62(1):92–100.

[45] Papachristou GI, Takahashi N, Chahal P, et al. Peroral endoscopic drainage/debridement of wall-off pancreatic necrosis. Ann Surg 2007;245(6):943–51.

[46] Charnley RM, Lochan R, Gray H, et al. Endoscopic necrosectomy as primary therapy in the management of infected pancreatic necrosis. Endoscopy 2006;38(9):925–8.

[47] Lopes CV, Pesenti C, Bories E, et al. Endoscopic-ultrasound-guided endoscopic transmural drainage of pancreatic pseudocysts and abscess. Scand J Gastroenterol 2007;42(4): 524–9.

[48] Bali MA, Sztantics A, Metens T, et al. Quantification of pancreatic exocrine function with secretin-enhanced magnetic resonance cholangiopancreatography: normal values and short-term effects of pancreatic duct drainage procedures in chronic pancreatitis; initial results. Eur Radiol 2005;15(10):2110–21.

[49] Enriquez WK. Diagnostic and therapeutic endoscopy of pancreas and biliary tract. Rev Gastroenterol 2006;71(1):36–8.

[50] Papachristou GI, Baron TH. Complications of therapeutic endoscopic retrograde cholangiopancreatography. Gut 2007;56(6):854–68.

[51] Weber A, Schneider J, Neu B, et al. Endoscopic stent therapy for patients with chronic pancreatitis: results from a prospective follow-up study. Pancreas 2007;34(3):287–94.

[52] Binmoeller KF, Jue P, Seifert H, et al. Endoscopic pancreatic stent drainage in chronic pancreatitis and a dominant stricture: long-term results. Endoscopy 1995;27:638–44.

[53] Costamagna G, Bulajic M, Tringali A, et al. Multiple stenting of refractory pancreatic duct strictures in severe chronic pancreatitis: long-term results. Endoscopy 2006;38(3): 254–9.

[54] Cahen DL, Gouma DJ, Nio Y, et al. Endoscopic versus surgical drainage of the pancreatic duct in chronic pancreatitis. N Engl J Med 2007;356(20):676–84.

[55] Familiari P, Spada C, Costamagna G. Dilation of a severe pancreatic stricture by using a guidewire left in place for 24 hours. Gastrointest Endosc 2007;66(3):618–20.

[56] Adler DG, Lichtenstein D, Baron TH, et al. The role of endoscopy in patients with chronic pancreatitis. Gastrointest Endosc 2006;63(7):933–7.

[57] Maydeo A, Soehendra N, Reddy N, et al. Endotherapy for chronic pancreatitis with intracanalar stones. Endoscopy 2007;39(7):653–8.

[58] Rosch T, Daniel S, Scholz M, et al. Treatment of chronic pancreatitis: a multicenter study of 1000 patients with long-term follow-up. Endoscopy 2002;34(10):765–71.

[59] Dite P, Ruzicka M, Zboril V, et al. A prospective, randomized trial comparing endoscopic and surgical therapy for chronic pancreatitis. Endoscopy 2003;35(7):553–8.

[60] Lehman GA. Role of ERCP and other endoscopic modalities in chronic pancreatitis. Gastrointest Endosc 2002;56(6):S237–40.

[61] Delhaye M, Arvanitakis M, Verset G, et al. Long-term clinical outcome after endoscopic pancreatic ductal drainage for patients with painful chronic pancreatitis. Clin Gastroenterol Hepatol 2004;2(12):1096–106.

[62] Van Berkel AM, Cahen DL, van Westerloo DJ, et al. Self-expanding metal stents in benign biliary strictures due to chronic pancreatitis. Endoscopy 2004;36(5):381–4.

[63] Varadarajulu S, Noone TC, Tutuian R, et al. Predictors of outcome in pancreatic duct disruption managed by endoscopic transpapillary stent placement. Gastrointest Endosc 2005; 61(4):568–75.

[64] Vitale GC, Vitale M, Vitale DS, et al. Long-term follow-up of endoscopic stenting in patients with chronic pancreatitis secondary to pancreas divisum. Surg Endosc 2007 [epub ahead of print].

[65] Gress F, Schmitt C, Sherman S, et al. A prospective randomized comparison of endoscopic ultrasound- and computed tomography-guided celiac plexus block for managing chronic pancreatitis pain. Am J Gastroenterol 1999;94(4):900–5.

[66] Arvanitakis M, Delhaye M, Bali MA, et al. Pancreatic fluid collections: a randomized controlled trial regarding stent removal after endoscopic transmural drainage. Gastrointest Endosc 2007;65(4):609–19.

[67] Hookey LC, Debroux S, Delhaye M, et al. Endoscopic drainage of pancreatic fluid collections in 116 patients: a comparison of etiologies, drainage techniques and outcomes. Gastrointest Endosc 2006;63(4):635–43.

[68] Yusuf TE, Baron TH. Endoscopic transmural drainage of pancreatic pseudocysts: results of a national and an international survey of ASGE members. Gastrointest Endosc 2006;63(2): 223–7.

ELSEVIER
SAUNDERS

Surg Clin N Am 87 (2007) 1403–1415

SURGICAL
CLINICS OF
NORTH AMERICA

Nutrition Support in Pancreatitis

Caitlin S. Curtis, PharmD[a],
Kenneth A. Kudsk, MD[b,c,*]

[a]Department of Pharmacy, University of Wisconsin-Madison Hospital and Clinics,
600 Highland Avenue, CSC – 1530 F6/133, Madison, WI 53792, USA
[b]Department of Surgery, Veterans Administration Surgical Services, William S. Middleton
Memorial Veterans Hospital, Madison, WI, USA
[c]Department of Surgery, University of Wisconsin-Madison Hospital and Clinics,
600 Highland Avenue, CSC H4/736, Madison, WI 53792-7375, USA

Pancreatitis poses a significant nutritional risk for various reasons, requiring that caregivers pay special attention to provision of nutrition in their treatment. First, pancreatitis increases nutritional requirements, because the disease process causes massive local and systemic inflammatory responses resulting in hypermetabolism [1] and hypercatabolism [2]. Second, the disease usually obviates the ability of patients to meet their energy needs by oral intake, as the symptoms of pancreatitis (most notably abdominal pain) prevent them from doing so. Lastly, pancreatitis impairs intestinal function, making it difficult or impossible to feed orally or enterally.

In recent years, concepts in the nutrition support of the patient with pancreatitis changed, evolving from complete bowel rest with administration of parenteral nutrition (PN) to recent recommendations for nasojejunal (NJ) and nasogastric (NG) feedings. In the past, complete bowel rest with nutrition support with PN was standard of care for pancreatitis, even though this treatment was not evidence-based. Today, multiple trials and meta-analyses [3–9] support the recommendation that enteral feeding by means of the jejunum is safe and more cost-effective than PN. In several recent trials [9–11], evidence suggested that under some conditions, nasogastric feeding may be as safe and effective as jejunal feedings. Tolerance of enteral nutrition (EN), however, varies from patient to patient in acute pancreatitis, and during the course of patient care, clinicians must make decisions regarding nutrition support that will benefit the patient most. This article explores the

_____

* Corresponding author. Department of Surgery, University of Wisconsin Hospital and Clinics, 600 Highland Avenue, CSC H4/736, Madison, WI 53792-7375.
E-mail address: kudsk@surgery.wisc.edu (K.A. Kudsk).

0039-6109/07/$ - see front matter © 2007 Elsevier Inc. All rights reserved.
doi:10.1016/j.suc.2007.08.010   *surgical.theclinics.com*

current evidence supporting nutritional supplementation in acute and chronic pancreatitis.

Mild and moderate pancreatitis

Mild and moderate pancreatitis is usually self-limiting, responds to short periods of bowel rest, and resolves before any significant malnutrition occurs. In a study by Louie and colleagues [3] comparing the route of EN to PN in acute pancreatitis, 184 patients had a Ranson's severity score of 3 or greater; of these, 120 patients tolerated oral intake within 5 days of admission. Sax and colleagues [12] reported that 80% of patients who had Ranson's criteria less than or equal to 2 tolerated an oral diet by hospital day 7. In addition, 54% of patients who had Ranson's criteria greater than or equal to 2 tolerated a diet by hospital day 7. Abou-Assi and colleagues [4] treated patients with bowel rest, intravenous fluids, and analgesics for 48 hours after establishing a diagnosis of acute pancreatitis. Seventy-five percent of these patients improved within this time period without the need for specialized nutrition support. Furthermore, 87% of patients resumed an oral diet within the next 2 days. These studies all support withholding specialized nutrition support in mild and moderate pancreatitis, since an oral diet can be instituted within a short period of time after the initial diagnosis.

Severe pancreatitis

Severe acute pancreatitis, including necrotizing pancreatitis, carries a high mortality rate and requires surgical intervention in many cases. Standard therapy for these patients includes fluid resuscitation followed by nutrition support until the patient is capable of taking an oral diet. For many years, the standard of care dictated complete bowel rest and initiation of PN, but recent trials challenge this practice and now support feeding by means of the gastrointestinal (GI) tract [3–6]. These trials show that EN in the form of NJ feeding is as safe as PN and is more cost-effective. Results of EN trials show that this treatment approach often shortens the time to initiation of oral diet, reduces complications, and shortens hospital stay. The theory is that the beneficial effects of enteral feeding are because of the maintenance of intestinal barriers and decreases in bacterial translocation. Another potential mechanism proposes that enteral feeding modulates the immune response, decreasing the systemic inflammatory response, which contributes to morbidity in acute pancreatitis. Many trials [5,6,13] have shown the benefits of jejunal feeding in pancreatitis while documenting cost savings and lower complication rates. One of the first trials by McClave and colleagues compared 32 patients admitted for acute pancreatitis; 16 patients were randomized to receive enteral nutrition by means of NJ feeding tubes, and 16 patients were randomized to receive PN. The primary goal in this study was to determine safety of EN in pancreatitis, with additional goals of determining efficacy, clinical outcomes, and cost-effectiveness of EN. The study found no difference between caloric advancement or serial pain scores between the groups but noted that Acute Physiology and Chronic Health Evaluation (APACHE) II scores, Ranson's criteria, and multiple organ failure scores decreased in the NJ group.

Every 2 to 3 days, the investigators compiled Ranson's scores. NJ-fed patients had significantly decreased Ranson's scores on the third serial measurement when compared with PN-fed patients. NJ feeding significantly reduced mean costs per patient ($3294 in the PN group and $761 in the NJ group, $P < .02$). The authors concluded that NJ feeding was as safe and effective as PN and more cost-effective [5]. Kalfarentzos and colleagues [6] studied 38 patients with acute pancreatitis, of which 18 patients received EN and 20 patients received PN. The primary aim of the study was to compare whether nutritional status could be maintained equally in each group. Secondary endpoints included the rate of complications and cost of treatment. Both groups tolerated feedings well with no significant differences in nitrogen balance between the two groups. Nitrogen balance improved through the course of the study in both groups. EN feeding significantly reduced complication rates compared with PN feeding and, specifically, lowered the mean number of infections per patient. The authors concluded that EN maintains lean tissue mass as effectively as PN and produces fewer complications. Windsor and colleagues [13] reported the feasibility of EN in patients who had severe pancreatitis and measured C-reactive protein (CRP) levels before and after treatment. They enrolled 34 patients; 16 patients were randomized to NJ feedings and 18 patients to PN. Of these patients, 13 had severe pancreatitis, and 21 had mild/moderate pancreatitis. The primary outcome of the study was the incidence of systemic inflammatory response syndrome (SIRS), with the secondary endpoints being sepsis, organ failure, hospital stay, and mortality. The authors measured CRP levels within 48 hours from time of enrollment and 7 days later. EN feeding significantly lowered CRP levels at 7 days compared with baseline, whereas PN feeding resulted in no significant change in CRP levels at day 7 compared with baseline. At baseline, 23 patients had SIRS. SIRS was present in 11 of the EN-fed patients before starting nutrition therapy, but present in only two patients after 7 days of EN, a significant decrease ($P < .05$). SIRS was present, however, in 12 of the PN-fed patients before enrollment and in 10 patients after 7 days of PN (nonsignificant). Hospital stays were not significantly different between the groups. Additionally, EN feeding was associated with significantly lower APACHE II scores from baseline, while PN feeding produced no significant effect on these scores. The authors concluded that EN is "both feasible and desirable" in patients who have acute pancreatitis, and suggested that EN stimulation attenuated the acute-phase response that improved clinical outcomes.

Several other trials testing EN versus PN support these conclusions [3]. Abou-Assi and colleagues [4] showed that pancreatitis patients randomized to NJ feeds had a significantly shorter duration of nutrition support, lower costs, and significantly fewer septic and metabolic complications when compared with patients fed with PN. Louie and colleagues showed that EN was safe and more cost-effective in pancreatitis than PN. Meta-analysis and systematic reviews [7,8] comparing methods of feeding in pancreatitis patients showed that EN is superior in cost, decreases the inflammatory response, and leads to earlier transition to oral intake when compared with PN.

One limitation to jejunal feeding remains the difficulty in obtaining access [5,14–16]. Only 5% to 15% of feeding tubes placed into the stomach migrate into the jejunum spontaneously. Thus, feeding tube advancement requires another method, usually by radiographic or endoscopic procedures [14]. These procedures are expensive and inconvenient, as they involve transporting a potentially unstable patient from the ICU setting. Additionally, they delay EN until successful placement of the tube. Bedside placement is a more popular method of placing NJ tubes; however, the procedure requires significant training with varying success rates reported [14,17].

Nasogastric feeding

Historically, the leading theory espoused that EN stimulates the release of pancreatic enzymes and worsening the pancreatitis. Therefore the belief persisted that gastric feeding was contraindicated in this condition. Animal models of acute pancreatitis, however, showed that exocrine function in the pancreas remains unresponsive to enteral feeding [18]. Several trials have shown that patients with pancreatitis tolerate nasogastric (NG) feeding well [9–11]. Preliminary work by O'Keefe and colleagues [4] showed that stimulation of exocrine function remains suppressed at basal rates in patients who have varying severity of pancreatitis. These observations provide the basis for recent trials investigating the safety and efficacy of intragastric feeding. In one trial by Eatock and colleagues [9], 50 patients who had acute pancreatitis received either NG feeding or NJ feeding after randomization. The authors compared APACHE II scores, CRP measurements, and pain patterns by visual analog scale (VAS). Twenty-two patients received NG feedings, and 27 patients received NJ feedings with no significant difference in rate of administration or target calories. Neither APACHE II scores nor CRP measurements differed significantly on any given day. VAS and analgesic requirements were not significantly different between the two groups. The authors concluded that NG feeding shows no evidence of exacerbation of disease when compared with NJ feeds, rendering NG feeding a viable option when supporting patients who have acute pancreatitis [9]. Kumar and colleagues [10] randomized 15 patients to NG feeding and 16 patients to NJ feeding, comparing tolerance and recurrence of pain between the groups. Pain recurred in only one patient in each group, with no significant rise in serum amylase or worsening of pancreatitis. The authors, however, noted requirements for partial PN in four NJ-fed patients and six NG-fed patients, because intolerance of EN limited delivery of calories. These numbers were not significant, however. Eckerwall and colleagues [11] compared patients receiving NG feeding with patients receiving PN. Outcomes measurements included serum levels of inflammatory markers (interleukin [IL]-6, IL-8, and CRP) and clinical morbidity and feasibility of the nutritional route. Baseline inflammatory markers IL-6 and CRP levels remained similar in the groups at every time point tested. Individual complications were similar between the groups, although total complications significantly increased in the NG group compared with the PN group ($P = .04$). The complications, however, included pleural effusion and atelectasis, but the authors noted that these complications were non-nutrition related. Nevertheless, the results of these three trials comparing NG feeding with another route of feeding demonstrate that NG feeding may be a safe option in patients who have acute pancreatitis. Ultimately, tolerance determines the route of feeding, but patients benefit from NG feeding because of easy accessibility, lower costs, and earlier initiation of EN. Most practitioners (including the authors of this article) remain wary of instituting NG feedings in severe pancreatitis, preferring the NJ route if no evidence of ileus or obstruction exists on abdominal imaging. Patients generally tolerate the feedings well and advance to a general diet within 10 to 14 days. For patients who have increased nausea, bloating, or abdominal pain, after initiation of NJ feeds, the authors discontinue enteral feeds and begin PN, but monitor for resolution of symptoms to reinitiate tube feedings as soon as possible. The authors do not feed by means of an NJ tube if patients require pressor support, as it is difficult to determine tolerance to jejunal feedings in this population, and they are at increased risk of bowel ischemia. Under these conditions, the authors might attempt NG feedings while following residuals closely. High gastric residual volumes (greater than 300 mL) demonstrate that tube feedings are not tolerated. The authors initiate PN if patients develop high residuals or increased pain; as these symptoms resolve, the authors attempt NJ feeding again.

Surgical jejunal access

Jejunal feedings are efficacious in pancreatitis, and some patients who have severe disease may require long-term jejunal access until they recover fully [15,19]. Surgical jejunostomy tubes or gastrostomy tubes with jejunal extension are both ways in which long-term jejunal access is achieved. In the event of pancreatitis with infection requiring surgical debridement, it is reasonable to gain enteral access by surgically placing a feeding jejunostomy tube. Kudsk and colleagues [19] described success in placing feeding jejunostomies during exploratory laparotomy for complicated pancreatitis. In this prospective study, 11 patients underwent placement of a large bore

Red Robinson or small bore needle–catheter jejunal tube at the time of celiotomy. Two of the patients died of pancreatitis-related complications, with a jejunal leak in one of the nonsurvivors. Otherwise, there were no complications. The nine survivors were supported entirely with tube EN after surgery; none required PN. Weimann and colleagues [15] reported the use of needle catheter jejunostomies in 13 patients with acute pancreatitis who underwent surgery for necrosis or an acute abdomen. They initiated EN by the tube while tapering PN off. No severe tube-related complications occurred in any of the patients. One patient required replacement of the needle catheter jejunostomy after dislodgement during a subsequent laparotomy and washout [15]. These studies verify the safety of placing a jejunostomy in acute pancreatitis patients during surgery, and the ability to feed by this route after surgery [15,19]. Yoder and colleagues [16] investigated the safety and efficacy of jejunal feedings in pancreatitis patients discharged home. Thirty-three patients went home with jejunal feedings, either by means of NJ tubes or percutaneous endoscopic gastrostomy (PEG)-jejunostomy tubes. Of these patients, 77% achieved goal tube feeding rates, and 61% maintained weight or gained weight on this regimen. The authors concluded that home jejunal nutrition is safe and efficacious.

Parenteral nutrition

Even though EN provides the optimal route when feeding patients who have acute pancreatitis, intolerance can occur because of severity of disease, including pain, prolonged ileus, or gastric outlet obstruction caused by pancreatic pseudocyst. These complications often limit the use of enteral nutrition; therefore starting PN is reasonable in these cases. Patients classified as having mild or moderate pancreatitis (eg, Ranson's scores no more than 2) should be treated with fluid resuscitation alone without nutrition support, because early PN provides no benefit (Fig. 1) [20]. Sax and colleagues [12] showed this in a randomized study comparing early PN with conventional therapy. Patients who received PN within 24 hours of diagnosis of pancreatitis experienced similar outcomes to those patients who received no early PN, with no significant differences in lengths of hospital stay, numbers of complications, or days to advancement to oral diet. Early PN was not beneficial, and in fact, the authors reported that early PN may have been harmful, as the patients randomized to this arm had a significantly higher rate of catheter-related sepsis than those patients who received conventional therapy. Therefore, a prudent approach is to wait several days before initiating PN in those who need it [17]. Patients who have severe pancreatitis requiring PN often need several days of fluid resuscitation and pain management before they tolerate any form of nutrition support [17,20]. Patients should get a NJ tube for enteral feeding after receiving adequate analgesia and correcting fluid and electrolyte abnormalities. If patients fail to tolerate enteral feeding because of pain or abdominal distention, or if other

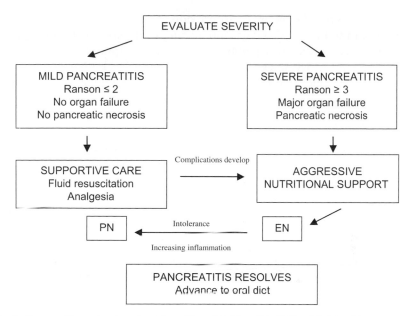

Fig. 1. Pancreatitis evaluation algorithm. (*From* McClave SA, Snider HL. Nutrition support in pancreatitis. In Kudsk KA, Pichard C, volume editors. From nutrition support to pharmacologic nutrition in the ICU. Vincent J, series editor. Updated in intensive care medicine. New York: Springer; 2002. p. 323; with kind permission of Springer Science and Business Media.)

contraindications to EN such as ileus or small bowel obstruction exist, it is appropriate to place a central line and begin PN therapy. The clinician must take special care in initiating nutrients by this route, as hyperglycemia and electrolyte abnormalities are common. The clinician should assess the patient's nutritional status at the onset of onset of pancreatitis, because approximately one-third of pancreatitis patients present with malnutrition at baseline [21]. PN requires careful monitoring when initiated in patients with pre-existing malnutrition, as they are at high risk of refeeding syndrome and the resulting fluid and electrolyte abnormalities. The initial PN should contain half or less of the calculated goal kilocalories for the patient, with increasing kilocalories in subsequent bags of PN until the patient is at goal [17]. The recommended goal kilocalories for PN are 25 to 35 kcal/kg/d, with 1.2 to 1.5 g of protein/kg. Advancing PN kilocalories requires frequent monitoring of blood glucose levels, because hyperglycemia occurs because of impaired exocrine function [22]. To prevent hyperglycemia, add insulin to the first bag of PN in a dose of 0.1 units/g of dextrose, and increase the insulin as dextrose kilocalories increase to keep blood glucose levels no more than 150 mg/dL. Guidelines for glycemic control recommend adding 0.15 units of insulin per gram of dextrose to patients who remain hyperglycemic before starting PN [23,24]. Often, adding a continuous insulin infusion helps, especially if blood glucose levels are highly variable, or very high levels of insulin are required [24]. In addition to protein and dextrose, PN should contain fat to provide 20% to 30% of nonprotein kilocalories. Initiating fat mandates monitoring triglyceride levels. If triglycerides rise to greater than or equal to 400 mg/dL, it is appropriate to withhold fat and reinitiate it when levels decrease below this level. PN should be continued until the enteral route can be accessed, or oral intake is initiated [17].

Enteral formula

An issue in feeding enterally during pancreatitis is the choice of enteral formula. Prior approaches suggested that semielemental or elemental formulas were more appropriate for use in pancreatitis, as these minimally stimulated pancreatic secretions and were absorbed without pancreatic enzymes [17,25]. Some authorities [6], however, argue that because the GI tract absorbs these formulas in the proximal gut, they may not maintain healthy intestinal flora in the distal intestine. One trial addressed this issue by comparing a semielemental versus a polymeric (ie, intact protein and long-chain triglycerides) formula in 30 patients requiring EN with a diagnosis of acute pancreatitis. This trial randomized patients to receive either a semielemental formula or a polymeric formula by means of an NJ tube and found no significant difference between the groups in terms of tolerance (measured by pain visual analog scales, presence of bloating, and days of analgesics) or absorption (measured by 24-hour stool weights, the presence of protein in the stool, presence and quantity of steatorrhea, and number of stools per day). Patients receiving the semielemental formulas (versus the polymeric diet) experienced a shorter length of hospital stay (23 days plus 2 days versus 27 days plus or minus 1 day, respectively, $P = .006$) and showed significantly less weight loss (-1.3 plus or minus 1.1 kg versus -2.4 plus or minus .0 kg, respectively, $P = .01$). Neither tolerance nor numbers of infectious complications differed significantly between the groups. The authors hypothesized that a semielemental diet led to more favorable outcomes in these patients by better maintaining gut integrity than a polymeric formula, and thus preventing bacterial translocation. The authors concluded that only a larger trial testing the rate of GI-derived infections could confirm this theory [25].

Benefits of enteral nutrition

One of the leading theories to explain the benefit of EN is that EN maintains gut integrity and decreases intestinal permeability [5,13,17]. Results from a recent study [11] refute this theory, however. Eckerwall and colleagues [11] assessed the safety and efficacy of early NG feeding compared with PN in patients who had predicted severe acute pancreatitis. They also tested intestinal permeability by measuring excretion of polyethylene glycol. Blood levels of polyethylene glycol were not significantly different between the two groups except for day 3, when patients randomized to NG feeding had higher blood levels than the patients randomized to PN. They concluded that EN does not decrease intestinal permeability and that the benefits of EN may be due to other reasons.

Another hypothesis of why EN feeding improves outcome proposes that EN feeding maintains gut mucosal immunity to decrease infectious complications [17,26]. Most of the body's immune capability resides just below the mucosa of the intestine, where T and B cells produce large amounts of IgA. IgA is the body's primary specific immune defense against bacterial antigens. Work in people and animals demonstrates that starving the gut alters T and B cell mass and function, therefore leading to a decrease in luminal levels of IgA. Also, the lack of enteral stimulation up-regulates gut endothelial adhesion marker expression and levels of inflammatory cytokines, both of which can alter immune system response to injury, resulting in more inflammatory complications [26]. When EN is used, all of these pathways for immunity are normalized and capable of normal responses to infectious challenges. When PN is used, however, lack of enteral stimulation impairs mucosal immunity. This perhaps explains why pancreatitis patients provided enteral feeding have lower complication rates than those patients fed with PN.

Potential therapies

Numerous potential nutritional therapies for acute pancreatitis exist, including supplementation of enteral feeding with probiotics and/or supplementation of formulas with omega-3 fatty acids, glutamine, and arginine. As inflammation and bacterial invasion appear to complicate acute pancreatitis, a proposed preventative treatment is through administration of prebiotics and probiotics to suppress pathogenic bacterial overgrowth and dampen the inflammatory response [27]. The few trials investigating enteral probiotic administration pancreatitis show promising results. Olah and colleagues [27,28] randomized patients who had acute pancreatitis to receive live cultures of *Lactobacillus plantarum* and substrate of oat fiber or to similar nutrients with heat-inactivated *Lactobacillus*. Forty-five patients completed the study, with 22 patients receiving active cultures and 23 patients receiving inactive cultures. The clinicians were blinded to randomization. All patients received enteral feeding via by means of NJ tube. Main outcome variables included organ failure, septic complications requiring surgery, length of hospital stay, and death. Results showed a significant reduction in the number of patients with septic complications requiring surgery with active treatment, as seven patients in the control group required surgery versus one patient in the treatment group ($P = .046$). Treatment reduced hospital length of stay compared with the control group (21.4 days versus 13.7 days), but this failed to reach statistical significance [27]. Another study by Olah and colleagues [28] randomized 62 enterally fed patients with severe acute pancreatitis to receive or not receive a mixture of lactobacilli preparation. Active treatment of patients was associated with a significantly reduced incidence of complications. The incidence of SIRS and multi-organ failure combined was lower in the treatment group (8 versus 14, $P < .05$).

No data exist to support the use of enteral supplementation with a combination of arginine, glutamine, and omega-3 fatty acids. Pearce and colleagues [29] randomized 31 patients who had pancreatitis to standard enteral feedings or an enteral diet containing glutamine, arginine, tributyrin, and omega-3 fatty acids. The primary outcome of the study was reduction of CRP by 40 mg/dL after 3 days of enteral feeding. Other clinical outcomes measured included length of stay, APACHE II scores, incidence of multi-organ failure, incidence of SIRS, and mortality. The investigators also measured carboxypeptidase activation peptide (CAPAP) levels throughout the study as an indicator of pancreatic damage. Fifteen patients received the study formula, and 16 patients received the standard formula. Results showed no significant reduction of CRP levels in the supplemented group or the control group after 72 hours of enteral feeding. In fact, when CRP levels were measured during an extension period up to a maximum of 15 days of enteral feeding, CRP levels significantly increased in the supplemented group compared with the control ($P = .028$). Mortality dropped in the treatment group versus the control (no patients versus three patients, respectively), but this difference failed to reach statistical significance., CAPAP levels dropped significantly compared with baseline in both groups, including every day in the initial 3-day period of the study. The authors concluded that the although the treatment group had higher levels of CRP and lower levels of CAPAP with no worsening in mortality, that a rise in CRP may reflect a better immune response. They suggested that immunonutrition required more trials with greater numbers of patients enrolled [29].

Two recent trials have shown promise using parenteral glutamine in acute pancreatitis [30,31]. Sahin and colleagues [30] compared 40 patients with pancreatitis with a Ranson's score between 2 and 4 randomized to glutamine-supplemented PN or standard PN. Outcomes included nutritional parameters, occurrence of complications, and length of hospital stay. Of the nutritional parameters measured, most failed to reach a statistical difference between the two groups, except for serum transferrin levels, which increased by 11.7% in the treatment group and decreased by 12.1% in the control group. Complication rates dropped significantly in the treatment group versus the control group (10% and 40%, respectively, $P < .05$). The authors concluded that parenteral glutamine supplementation provided a benefit to patients who have acute pancreatitis [30].

Ockenga and colleagues [31] showed that PN enriched with glutamine benefited patients with acute pancreatitis. This trial randomized 28 patients who had acute pancreatitis to PN-enriched glutamine or standard PN. Results showed a decrease in length of PN therapy in patients receiving the glutamine ($P < .05$) and significant increases in levels of albumin and lymphocyte count compared with those not receiving glutamine. The authors concluded that PN enriched with glutamine provided some benefit

[31], but it remains unclear why. It is unknown whether enteral glutamine alone produces the same benefits, but no trials have compared patient groups with and without enteral glutamine.

Chronic pancreatitis

Chronic pancreatitis involves progressive loss of endocrine and exocrine pancreatic function, both of which must be addressed in the treatment. Pharmacologic therapy can manage losses of both pancreatic functions [32]. Because 70% to 90% of chronic pancreatitis is alcohol-related, however, compliance with medication regimens remains a challenge, especially for blood glucose control [33]. The American Diabetes Association classifies the loss of endocrine function as diabetes mellitus type IIIc [34]. Destruction of acinar cells results in reduced pancreatic secretion of insulin and glucagon, and impaired ability to tightly regulate blood glucose. Treatment with long-acting insulin for basal control of blood glucose is best, as patients use few injections and are more compliant.

Loss of exocrine function manifests as steatorrhea (fecal fat greater than 7 g/d) and weight loss. It is appropriate to initiate pancreatic enzymes, beginning with 1000 U (USP units) of lipase per meal and with snacks, titrating upwards as needed for this problem [32]. The best form of pancreatitic enzymes are enteric-coated tablets or microspheres (Pancrease, Cotazym, and Promylin-HL16) [35]. Patients should consume smaller, more frequent meals, and not be fat-restricted when taking the pancreatic enzymes. If severe steatorrhea occurs despite adequate pancreatic enzyme supplementation, then consider restricting fat and administering medium-chain triglycerides. Patients who have severe steatorrhea risk deficiencies of fat-soluble vitamins and require these as supplements. Patients with alcoholic pancreatitis who continue to drink remain at risk of water-soluble vitamin depletion also. Clinicians should encourage abstinence, because studies show abstinence from alcohol improves outcomes [32].

Summary

Nutrition support in acute and chronic pancreatitis presents challenges related to choice of route, formula, and use of supplements. Evidence supports refraining from nutritional support during mild or moderate pancreatitis, because patients usually recover ability to take oral nutrition within 7 days. Evidence currently supports NJ or NG feeding in patients who have severe pancreatitis, with the caveat that some patients may be intolerant to feeding and develop bloating or increased pain. PN may be instituted in these patients, but only after failing a trial of EN. Enteral feeding by means of a surgically placed jejunal feeding tube is safe and effective. The optimal type of enteral feeding used remains controversial, but most literature supports the use of semielemental tube feedings. Management of chronic pancreatitis includes the use of insulin to control blood glucose levels and pancreatic enzymes to control steatorrhea. Management also includes supplementation with fat- and/or water-soluble vitamins based on the clinical situation. Research has changed the nutritional approach to this disease process dramatically.

References

[1] Dickerson RN, Vehe KL, Mullen JL, et al. Resting energy expenditure in patients with pancreatitis. Crit Care Med 1991;19:484–90.

[2] Shaw JHF, Wolfe RR. Glucose fatty acid and urea. Kinetics in patients with severe pancreatitis. Ann Surg 1986;204:665–72.

[3] Louie BE, Noseworthy T, Hailey D, et al. Enteral or parenteral nutrition for severe pancreatitis: a randomized controlled trial and health technology assessment. Can J Surg 2005;48: 298–306.

[4] O'Keefe S, Abou-Assi S, Lee R, et al. Impairment of nutrient -stimulated pancreatic trypsin and lipase secretion in patients with acute pancreatitis. Gastroenterology 2000 (abstract).

[5] McClave S, Greene L, Snider H, et al. Comparison of the safety of early enteral vs parenteral nutrition in mild acute pancreatitis. J Parenter Enter Nutr 1997;21:14–20.

[6] Kalfarentzos F, Kehagias J, Mead N, et al. Enteral nutrition is superior to parenteral nutrition in severe acute pancreatitis: results of a randomized prospective trial. Br J Surg 1997;84: 1665–9.

[7] McClave S, Chang W, Dhaliwal R, et al. Nutrition support in acute pancreatitis: a systematic review of the literature. J Parenter Enter Nutr 2006;30:143–56.

[8] Marik P, Zaloga G. Meta-analysis of parenteral nutrition versus enteral nutrition in patients with acute pancreatitis. BMJ 2004;328:1407–12.

[9] Eatock F, Chong P, Menezes N, et al. A randomized study of early nasogastric versus nasojejunal feeding in severe acute pancreatitis. Am J Gastroenterology 2005;100:432–9.

[10] Kumar A, Singh N, Prakash S, et al. Early enteral nutrition in severe acute pancreatitis: a prospective randomized controlled trial comparing nasojejunal and nasogastric routes. J Clin Gastroenterol 2006;40:431–4.

[11] Eckerwall G, Axelsson J, Andersson R. Early nasogastric feeding in predicted severe acute pancreatitis: a clinical randomized study. Ann Surg 2006;244:959–67.

[12] Sax H, Warner BW, Talamini M, et al. Early total parenteral nutrition in acute pancreatitis: lack of beneficial effects. Am J Surg 1987;153:117–24.

[13] Windsor A, Kanwar S, Li A, et al. Compared with parenteral nutrition, enteral feeding attenuates the acute-phase response and improves disease severity in acute pancreatitis. Gut 1998;42:431–5.

[14] Zaloga G. Bedside method for placing small bowel feeding tubes in critically ill patients. A prospective study. Chest 1991;100:1643–6.

[15] Weimann A, Braunert M, Muller T, et al. Feasibility and safety of needle catheter jejunostomy for enteral nutrition in surgically treated severe acute pancreatitis. J Parenter Enter Nutr 2004;28:324–7.

[16] Yoder AJ, Parrish C, Yeaton P. A retrospective review of the course of patients with pancreatitis discharged on jejunal feedings. Nutr Clin Pract 2002;17:314–20.

[17] McClave SA, Snider HL. Nutrition support in pancreatitis. In: Kudsk KA, Pichard C, volume, editors. From nutrition support to pharmacologic nutrition in the ICU. Vincent J, series editor. Update in intensive care medicine. New York: Springer; 2002. p. 317–26.

[18] Neiderau C, Niederau M, Luthen R, et al. Pancreatic exocrine secretion in acute experimental pancreatitis. Gastroenterology 1990;99:1120–7.

[19] Kudsk K, Campbell S, O'Brien T, et al. Postoperative jejunal feedings following complicated pancreatitis. Nutr Clin Pract 1990;5:14–7.

[20] Tenner S. Initial management of acute pancreatitis: critical issues during the first 72 hours. Am J Gastroenterol 2004;99:2489–94.

[21] Robin AP, Campbell R, Panlani CK. Total parenteral nutrition during acute pancreatitis: clinical experience with 156 patients. World J Surg 1990;14:572–9.

[22] Dejong CH, Greve JW, Soeters PB. Acute pancreatitis. In: Rolandelli R, editor. Clinical nutrition: enteral and tube feeding. Philadelphia: Elsevier; 2005. p. 436–44.

[23] ASPEN Board of Directors and the Clinical Guidelines Task Force. Guidelines for the use of parenteral and enteral nutrition in adult and pediatric patients. J Parenter Enteral Nutr 2002; 26SA:1SA–138SA.

[24] McMahon M, Rizza R. Nutrition support in hospitalized patients with diabetes mellitus. Mayo Clin Proc 1996;71:587–94.

[25] Tiengou LE, Gloro R, Pouzoulet J, et al. Semielemental formula or polymeric formula: is there a better choice for enteral nutrition in acute pancreatitis? Randomized comparative study. J Parenter Enteral Nutr 2006;30:1–5.

[26] Kang W, Kudsk KA. Is there evidence that the gut contributes to mucosal immunity in humans? J Parenter Enteral Nutr 2007;31:246–58.

[27] Olah A, Belagyi A, Issekutz M, et al. Randomized clinical trial of specific *Lactobacillus* and fibre supplement to early enteral nutrition in patients with acute pancreatitis. BJM 2002;89: 1103–7.

[28] Olah A, Belagyi T, Poto L, et al. Symbiotic control of inflammation and infection in severe acute pancreatitis: a prospective, randomized, double-blind study. Hepatogastoenterology 2007;54:590–4.

[29] Pearce CB, Sadek SA, Walters A, et al. A double-blind, randomized, controlled trial to study the effects of an enteral feed supplemented with glutamine, arginine, and omega-3 fatty acid in predicted acute severe pancreatitis. J Pancreas 2006;7:694-71.

[30] Sahin H, Mercanligil SM, Inanc N, et al. Effects of glutamine-enriched total parenteral nutrition on acute pancreatitis. Eur J Clin Nutr 2007 [epub ahead of print].

[31] Ockenga J, Borchert K, Rifal K, et al. Effect of glutamine-enriched total parenteral nutrition in patients with acute pancreatitis. Clin Nutr 2002;21:409–16.

[32] Witt H, Apte MV, Keim V, et al. Chronic pancreatitis: challenges and advances in pathogenesis, genetics, diagnosis, and therapy. Gastroenterology 2007;132:1557–73.

[33] Spieker MR, et al. Diseases of the pancreas. In: David AK, Johnson TA, Phillips DM, editors. Family medicine: principles and practice. 6th edition. New York: Springer-Verlag; 2003 [accessed through STAT!Ref Online Electronic Medical Library, July 2007].

[34] The Expert Committee on the Diagnosis and Classification of Diabetes Mellitus. Follow-up report on the diagnosis of diabetes mellitus. Diabetes Care 2003;26:3160-7.

[35] Thomson M, Clague A, Cleghorn G, et al. Comparative in vitro and in vivo studies of enteric-coated pancrelipase preparations for pancreatic insufficiency. J Pediatr Gastroenterol Nutr 1993;17:407–13.

SURGICAL
CLINICS OF
NORTH AMERICA

Surg Clin N Am 87 (2007) 1417–1429

Diagnosis and Management of Sphincter of Oddi Dysfunction and Pancreas Divisum

James A. Madura II, MD[a,b,]*, James A. Madura, MD[c]

[a]Department of General Surgery, Rush University Medical Center,
1725 West Harrison Street, Suite 818, Chicago, IL 60612, USA
[b]Division of General Surgery, John Stroger Hospital of Cook County,
1901 West Harrison Street, Suite 3350, Chicago, IL 60612, USA
[c]Department of Surgery, Indiana University School of Medicine,
9525 Copley Drive, Indianapolis, IN 46260, USA

Sphincter of Oddi dysfunction (SOD) and pancreas divisum (PD) are rare diagnoses, but complaints attributed to the disorders are quite similar and common: episodic abdominal pain attributed to the biliary tract or pancreas. In the face of normal ultrasounds (US), computerized tomography (CT), and normal laboratory evaluations (usually performed in between episodes), many patients are written off as difficult or histrionic and practitioners are hesitant to pursue more extensive, expensive, or invasive evaluations. Furthermore, even when the diagnoses are entertained, the quantitative findings are at times inconsistent or contradictory. Fortunately, correct diagnosis results in good response to treatment. Both disorders are the result of an abnormal sphincteric mechanism draining the biliopancreatic system. Though simple in concept, the sphincter of Oddi is really quite complex in embryonic origin, normal function, and control.

The sphincter of Oddi

The smooth muscle sphincter at the distal common bile duct that regulates the flow of bile and exocrine pancreas secretion was first described in 1887 by Rugero Oddi [1]. Subsequent investigations have defined three

* Corresponding author. Department of General Surgery, Rush University Medical Center, 1725 West Harrison Street, Suite 818, Chicago, IL 60612.
 E-mail address: jmadura@rush.edu (J.A. Madura II).

discrete zones to a sphincteric system of connective tissue, circular smooth muscle, and finally longitudinal muscle fibers, as the common bile and pancreatic ducts traverse and enter the duodenum: (1) a common bile duct sphincter (sphincter choledocus), (2) a pancreatic duct sphincter (sphincter pancreaticus), and (3) a common sphincter (sphincter papillae) (Fig. 1) [2]. Anatomic variants of the ductal anatomy exist.

The blood supply to the sphincter of Oddi (SO) typically arrives via a plexus formed by the anterior superior and posterior superior pancreaticoduodenal branches of the retroduodenal artery. The distance between the retroduodenal artery and the papillary orifice is typically greater than 3 centimeters, but may be much closer in 5% of the population. This obviously places the artery within range of sphincterotomy maneuvers.

Intrinsic innervation of the SO is complex, with many neurotransmitters and hormones appearing to have regulatory effects on an outer myenteric plexus and separate submucosal plexus. Neurons in the SO have been demonstrated to be immunoreactive to or express choline acetyltransferase, substance P, enkephalin, nitric oxide synthase, vasoactive intestinal peptide, and cholecystokinin (CCK) [3]. The major regulatory function seems to derive from neurons that originate in the duodenal mucosa [4]. Although not well understood, extrinsic innervation consists of parasympathetic vagal fibers and sympathetic nerves by way of the superior mesenteric ganglion similar to the rest of the biliary tract. The net result of known innervation

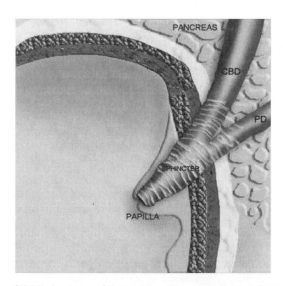

Fig. 1. Sphincter of Oddi. Anatomy of the papilla, with pancreatic duct (PD) and the common bile duct (CBD) fused as they follow a variable course through the submucosal layer of the duodenum to form the common channel. (*From* Bosch A, Pena LR. The sphincter of Oddi. Dig Dis Sci 2007;52:1212; with permission.)

seems to be the promotion of bile and pancreatic secretions into the duodenum.

In addition to the control of bile and pancreatic flow into the duodenum, the SO also prevents reflux of enteric contents from the duodenum into the pancreatic and biliary system, and in the resting state diverts bile into the gallbladder for concentration between meals. In the fasted state, myoelectric activity consists of normal basil SO pressures of 3 mm Hg to 35 mm Hg (abnormal defined as greater than 40 mm Hg), with phasic contractions thought to promote flow into the duodenum, normally 130 mm Hg above basil pressures, with an average frequency of four per minute and lasting an average of 6 seconds [5]. While there is a relationship to the migrating motor complex of the duodenum, most bile flow in humans seems to be passive between contractions of the sphincter mechanism and augmented by gallbladder contraction, antral distention, CCK, and decreased amplitude of phasic contractions of the SO in the fed state [6].

Sphincter of Oddi dysfunction

Sphincter of Oddi dysfunction may be a structural (stenosis) or functional (dyskenesia) disorder of the SO. Clinical presentations of SOD mimic biliary and pancreatic pain as recurrent episodic abdominal pain. The pain may be associated with common bile duct and pancreatic duct dilatation, transient elevations in liver or pancreatic enzymes, and delayed emptying of contrast after biliary imaging. The entity has also been referred to as postcholecystectomy syndrome, papillary stenosis, biliary dyskenesia, and biliary spasm. Up to 20 % of patients with persistent pain after cholecystectomy, and 10% to 20 % of patients with idiopathic recurrent pancreatitis may suffer from SOD. Box 1 lists a number of factors thought to contribute to the incidence of papillary stenosis. Biliary type SOD pain is commonly epigastric or right upper quadrant, lasts for more than 45 minutes but not more than several hours, and is similar to that attributed to biliary stone disease. Pancreatic type SOD pain is typically episodic, postprandial,

---

Box 1. Factors implicated in sphincter of Oddi stenosis

Choledocholithiasis
Endoscopic retrograde cholangiopancreatography or surgical
  instrumentation
Cholesterolosis
Pancreatitis
Peptic ulcer disease
Ascaris
Malignancy

prolonged, and located in the mid-upper abdomen or back. Some remain unconvinced that primary motor disturbances of the sphincter of Oddi cause severe episodic abdominal pain [7]. Nevertheless, acalculus biliopancreatic pain is a real and challenging entity for the clinician.

A rational and well-planned approach investigating a cause for these often difficult and problematic patients should include a methodical evaluation. Early referral to centers with advanced endoscopic and radiologic capabilities and expertise should be considered. Initial evaluation should include transabdominal ultrasound, CT, or magnetic resonance cholangiopancreatography (MRCP) of the abdomen, with serum liver and pancreatic enzyme determination. Bile sampling has determined that the frequency of biliary sludge or microlithiasis in patients with recurrent pancreatitis may be as high as 75% and is uncommon after cholecystectomy, leading to a recommendation that patients with an intact gallbladder be considered for cholecystectomy as an initial therapeutic modality [8].

Other noninvasive tests have been used to investigate the diagnosis of SOD. The morphine neostigmine provocative test (Nardi test) [9] consists of the intramuscular injection of 10-mg morphine sulfate and 1-mg neostigmine with venous blood samples obtained before injection and at 30-minute intervals after injection. The samples are analyzed for amylase, lipase, alanine aminotransferase (ALT), and aspartate aminotransferase (AST) levels. Patients are monitored for the reproduction of pain or symptoms of nausea or vomiting. A positive result of enzyme elevation to greater than four times normal, or reproduction of symptoms, has been documented in over 90% of patients so tested [10]. MRCP and secretin stimulated MRCP can demonstrate or exclude structural abnormalities, but lack sensitivity and accuracy in predicting success of sphincterotomy in patients with SOD [11,12]. Endoscopic ultrasound (EUS) can also delineate anatomic abnormalities but with very poor sensitivity or specificity in diagnosing SOD [13]. Hepatobiliary scintigraphy can provide evidence of SOD manifested as delayed biliary emptying, but negative studies do not reliably correlate with sphincter of Oddi manometry (SOM) [14].

Endoscopic retrograde cholangiopancreatography (ERCP) with SOM is the gold standard for the diagnosis of SOD. Elevation of resting SO pressure greater than 40 mm Hg is diagnostic for SOD and an excellent predictor of successful relief of symptoms after sphincterotomy [15]. The drawback to ERCP with SOM is clearly the finite complication rate of pancreatitis; the highest rate of post ERCP pancreatitis occurs in young females being investigated for SOD (up to 20%). Because of the potential complications of ERCP with SOM, patients can first be classified according to evidenced based schemata designed to predict the need for additional testing, indications for intervention, and therapeutic response (Table 1) [15,16].

Management of type I SOD is the most straight forward. After exclusion of structural lesions with noninvasive imaging (US, CT, MRCP, or EUS), patients with biliary type SOD should undergo cholecystectomy if the

Table 1
Contemporary classification of sphincter of Oddi dysfunction

Type	Biliary SOD	Pancreatic SOD
Type I	1. Biliary type pain (lasting 30 min and occurring at least once per year) 2. Elevated AST/ALT on two occasions 3. Dilated CBD (>12 mm), or delayed biliary drainage (>45 min)	1. Recurrent pancreatitis or pain suspected of pancreatic origin 2. Elevated amylase or lipase 3. Dilated pancreatic duct or delayed emptying of the pancreatic duct
Type II	Biliary type pain and at least one additional factor above	Presumed pancreatic pain and at least one additional factor above
Type III	Biliary type pain alone	Pancreatic type pain alone

gallbladder is present. If the gallbladder has been removed, biliary sphincterotomy should be performed without SOM because all patients are felt to benefit from sphincterotomy and manometry may be normal in as many as 65% [10,17–20]. Presenting pain can be expected to resolve in most and be improved in the remainder of patients treated with surgical or endoscopic sphincterotomy. Type I pancreatic SOD requires biliary sphincteroplasty with pancreatic septectomy (biliary and pancreatic sphincterotomies). In the current era of endoscopic evaluation and treatment, few patients are referred for surgical treatment unless endoscopic therapy has failed or is technically unsuccessful. However, long term follow-up after surgical intervention is documented to be quite good, while endoscopic treatment studies are limited in follow-up and have a disappointing rate of pancreatic duct restenosis. Several proposed advantages to surgical intervention that may explain better long-term results with less restenosis include the ability to create longer ductotomies, suture control of the opening (sphincteroplasty), and avoidance of cautery and the attendant proximity thermal injury.

Type II and III biliary and pancreatic SOD probably represent a heterogeneous group of disorders with longstanding controversy and lack of consensus on pathophysiology, natural history, and treatment. Noninvasive imaging to exclude structural lesions should be performed as above. Biliary scintigraphy should be performed to rule out gallbladder dysfunction, and cholecystectomy considered if the gallbladder is present. Manometry of both the biliary and pancreatic ducts is proposed for Type II SOD, but not without detractors, as summarized in a review by Sherman [20]. Alternative treatment algorithms recommend sphincterotomy without manometry because of the relative success of sphincterotomy, lack of correlation between manometry and results of intervention, and complications of SOM. Results of SOM are less predictive of response to therapy but basal SO pressure greater than 40 mm Hg best predicts resolution of symptoms after sphincterotomy. Most studies of Type II and III SOD report results in mixed groups of patients, but response to sphincterotomy is as high as

90%, again best correlating with elevated sphincter pressures [21,22]. It seems logical that SOM pressures should guide intervention in a diverse group of patients, and in the case of pancreatic SOD, biliary sphinctero-plasty with pancreatic septectomy (or endoscopic biliary and pancreatic sphincterotomies) should be performed. The authors' experience with surgical intervention has demonstrated good and long lasting results, particularly in the patients who were operated on as a primary intervention, compared with reintervention after failed endoscopic procedures. Long-term results after endoscopic therapy for this group of patients are elusive.

Type III SOD, the largest group of SOD patients, are the most difficult to diagnose and the most likely not to benefit from therapy [22]. In the absence of laboratory and imaging abnormalities, trials of calcium channel blockers, anticholinergics, and antidepressants are recommended before invasive diagnostic and therapeutic procedures. A single randomized controlled trial evaluated the outcomes of therapy for Type III SOD [23]. Symptom improvement was only modestly better in patients undergoing surgical and endoscopic intervention (sphincteroplasty or sphincterotomy) compared with sham endoscopic sphincterotomy. Other, uncontrolled studies, have demonstrated lasting results leading to recommendations for routine endoscopic evaluation and therapy for presumptive Type III SOD [24]. Diagnostic ERCP has no role in the assessment according to the National Institutes of Health Conference Statement [14]. However, ERCP with SOM and dual sphincterotomy should be considered at specific referral centers and in randomized controlled trials for this group of patients.

Pancreas divisum

Failure of the dorsal and ventral pancreatic ducts to fuse during the 7th week of embryologic development results in an anatomic variant of pancreatic ductal drainage, referred to as pancreas divisum. As a result, the dorsal duct drains the body and tail of the pancreas via the accessory ampulla, known as the duct of Santorini. This results in an almost vestigal duct of Wirsung draining the ventral portion (2%–20% by mass) of the pancreas. Three variants of ductal abnormalities have been proposed: type I, classical PD with total failure of fusion; type II with dorsal duct dominant drainage; and type III, incomplete divisum where a small communicating branch is present (Fig. 2). Both autopsy and ERCP reports suggest an incidence of approximately 7% (range 1%–14%) [25]. The clinical significance of PD has been debated for years. The vast majority of patients with this alternative pancreatic drainage are unaffected by the condition. Less than 5% of PD patients ever develop pancreatic symptoms, yet a disproportionate number of acute, recurrent, idiopathic pancreatitis and postcholecystectomy syndrome patients are discovered to have PD (8%–50%), suggesting the anomaly is a risk factor in their complaints [26–28]. In addition to the implication

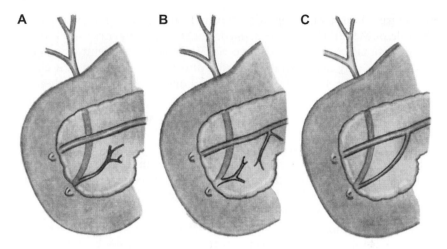

Fig. 2. Duct variations in pancreas divisum. Three variants of ductal abnormalities: (*A*) Type I, classical PD with total failure of fusion; (*B*) Type II with dorsal duct dominant drainage; and (*C*) Type III, incomplete divisum where a small communicating branch is present.

of PD in idiopathic pancreatitis, the small ventral duct must be differentiated at ERCP from the main pancreatic duct cutoff of pancreas cancer, as well as the identification and cannulation of the minor papilla, for a complete pancreatogram to evaluate the entire main pancreatic duct [25].

Inadequate drainage of the dorsal pancreatic duct results in high intraductal pressure, duct distension, pain, and pancreatitis. This is not a result of PD per se, but rather a relative stenosis of the minor papilla, referred to as the dominant dorsal duct syndrome [29,30]. Another variant of PD describes a normal dorsal duct with abnormal drainage of the ventral pancreatic duct, resulting in recurrent pancreatitis of the ventral pancreas [31].

The clinical management of coincidentally discovered PD in patients being evaluated for, or discovered to have common bile duct stones, sclerosing cholangitis, or liver disease is expectant. The diagnosis of PD in the setting of a patient with no clinical history of pancreatitis and normal imaging studies is purely coincidental. Patients with mild or infrequent episodes of acute pancreatitis should be managed with supportive medical therapy to include pain control, low fat diet, and abstinence from alcohol. Clinically significant disability related to recurrent acute pancreatitis or severe episodes should trigger evaluation of the minor papilla, with serious consideration for intervention.

Computed tomography of the pancreas may suggest PD when selective dilation of the dorsal duct or changes of chronic pancreatitis confined to the body and tail of the pancreas are identified. Prolonged secretin stimulated pancreatic duct dilation, as observed by ultrasound, correlates with pancreatic outflow obstruction and response to therapy [30,32]. Precise criteria for abnormal findings and confirmation of these findings are needed. The role of MRCP is yet to be defined, but is increasingly reported to identify the anomalous drainage. Diagnostic ERCP with both ventral and dorsal ductography may demonstrate a dilated dorsal duct or changes of chronic pancreatitis in the distribution of the dorsal duct, suggesting pathologic minor papilla stenosis or a cystic dilation of the distal dorsal duct ("Santorinicele"), but these are not common findings [33,34]. ERCP with SOM has demonstrated elevated basal minor papilla pressures (greater than 40 mm Hg) in the rare reports in which it has been performed [35,36].

Surgical intervention for PD has historically been in the setting of recurrent idiopathic pancreatitis, and has typically consisted of a cholecystectomy, if not already performed, and dual sphincteroplasty of the major and minor papillae, to include a septoplasty at the major papilla (Fig. 3). Results of surgical intervention for PD are summarized by Fogel, Toth and Lehman [25]. In general, patients with acute recurrent pancreatitis have a high rate of symptomatic relief after surgical intervention, whereas chronic pancreatitis and continuous pain are less reliably addressed with surgical drainage of the sphincter mechanism. Endoscopic therapy has been less reliable in long term pain relief but is improving with better patient selection.

Endoscopic address of the minor papilla has been approached with dilatation, stenting, and sphincterotomy [37,38]. Balloon dilatation should be

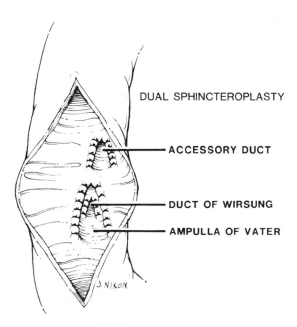

Fig. 3. Surgical sphincteroplasty of the ampulla of Vater, pancreatic septum, and minor papilla. (*From* Madura JA. Pancreas divisum: stenosis of the dorsally dominant pancreatic duct, a surgically correctable lesion. Am J Surg 1986;151:744; with permission).

discouraged because of the risk of severe pancreatitis. Endoscopically placed pancreatic stents have been effective as a trial before sphincterotomy; relief of pain after stenting correlates to long term relief after sphincterotomy, as well as therapeutic benefits in over 50% of patients treated with periodic exchange stenting of the minor papilla [39]. Pancreatitis after these procedures remains a concern, as do chronic duct changes with prolonged stenting.

Considerable controversy continues to exist regarding the relative importance of PD in chronic pancreatitis. Results of intervention are universally less successful in this setting, and careful consideratioin should be taken in the proposal of therapeutic intervention.

Technique of dual surgical sphincteroplasties

The usual approach to transduodenal sphincteroplasty is through a right subcostal incision. Cholecystectomy, without ligation of the proximal cystic duct, should be performed if the gallbladder is present. A number 3 or number 4 Bakes dilator is then passed through the cystic and common ducts into the duodenum to allow for an accurately centered longitudinal duodenotomy. In the case of previous cholecystectomy, the dudenotomy is performed by best estimate of the location of the ampulla by palpation, without entering the common bile duct (Fig. 4). The ampulla of Vater is opened sharply at

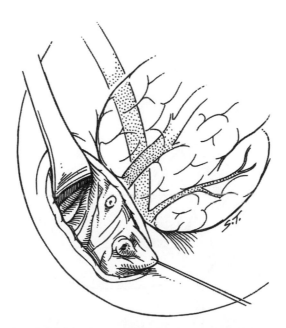

Fig. 4. Locating the major and minor papilla through a longitudinal duodenotomy. Infra-ampullary suture placed to control ampulla of Vater.

the 12 o'clock position, and controlled with an infra-ampullary silk stay suture. Adequate length of sphincterotomy may be assessed by passing a 9 or 10
French Bakes dilator in a retrograde fashion. The duct of Wirsung is then
identified and intubated with a malleable probe to protect the pancreatic
ductal orifice during choledochal sphincteroplasty. The pancreatic duct is
then opened with fine tenotomy scissors. Sphincteroplasties are completed
with interrupted, 5-0 absorbable synthetic suture. The minor papilla is
then located in its usual location, 1-cm superior and medial to the main ampulla. If not easily found, an intravenous injection of secretin (one unit
per kg) may be given to illicit a stream of pancreatic juice from the orifice
within a minute or two. Once identified, the duct is sequentially dilated
with lacrimal duct probes (Fig. 5) and then opened sharply in the 12 o'clock
position, with extension into the duct as far as possible using Potts (or tenotomy) scissors (Fig. 6). A small wedge biopsy should be taken for histopathology. The sphincteroplasty is completed with interrupted sutures, as above. A
nonabsorbable 5-0 monofilament suture is often used to mark the opening in
case future endoscopic evaluation is necessary. The duodenotomy may be
closed in either longitudinal or transverse fashion. The cystic duct, if it has
been opened, is simply ligated without t-tube drainage.

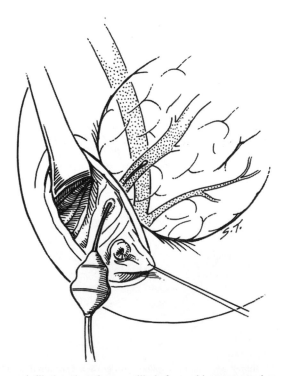

Fig. 5. Locating and dilating the minor papilla before sphincterotomy in pancreas divisum.

[6] Worthly CS, Baker RA, Iannos J, et al. Human fasting and post-prandial sphincter of Oddi motility. Br J Surg 1989;76:706–14.

[7] Moody FG, Poots JR. Dysfunction of the ampulla of Vater. In: Braasch JW, Tompkins RK, editors. Surgical Diseases of the Biliary Tract and Pancreas, multidisciplinary management. St. Louis: Mosby; 1994. p. 334–48.

[8] Kaw M, Brodmerkel G. ERCP, biliary crystal analysis, and sphincter of Oddi manometry in idiopathic recurrent pancreatitis. Gastrointest Endosc 2002;55:157–62.

[9] Nardi GL, Acosta JM. Papillitis as a cause of pancreatitis and abdominal pain: role of evocative test, operative pancreatography and histologic evaluation. Ann Surg 1966;164:611–21.

[10] Madura JA, Madura JA II, Sherman S, et al. Surgical sphincteroplasty in 446 patients. Arch Surg 2005;140:504–12.

[11] Piccinni G, Angrisano A, Testini M, et al. Diagnosing and treating sphincter of Oddi dysfunction: a critical literature review and reevaluation. J Clin Gastroenterol 2004;38:350–9.

[12] Pereira SP, Gillams A, Sgouros SN, et al. Prospective comparison of secretin-stimulated magnetic resonance cholangiopancreatography with manometry in the diagnosis of sphincter of Oddi dysfunction types II and III. Gut 2007;56:742–4.

[13] Vijayakumar V, Briscoe EG, Pehlivanov ND. Postcholecystectomy sphincter of Oddi dyskenesia—a diagnostic dilemma—role of noninvasive nuclear and invasive manometric and endoscopic aspects. Surg Laparosc Edosc Percutan Tech 2007;17:10–3.

[14] Cohen S, Bacon BR, Berlin JA, et al. National Institutes of Health State-of-the-Science Conference Statement: ERCP for diagnosis and therapy, January 14–16, 2002. Gastrointest Endosc 2002;56:803–9.

[15] Hogan WJ, Geenen JE. Biliary dyskenesia. Endoscopy 1988;20(suppl 1):179–83.

[16] Sherman S, Troiano FP, Hawes RH, et al. Frequency of abnormal sphincter of Oddi manometry compared with the clinical suspicion of sphincter of Oddi dysfunction. Am J Gastroenterol 1991;86:586–90.

[17] Cicala M, Habib FI, Vavassori P, et al. Outcome of endoscopic sphincterotomy in post cholecystectomy patients with sphincter of Oddi dysfunction as predicted by manometry and quantitative choledochoscintigraphy. Gut 2002;50:665–8.

[18] Rolny P, Geenan JE, Hogan WJ. Post-cholecystectomy patients with "objective signs" of partial bile outflow obstruction: clinical characteristics, sphincter of Oddi manometry findings, and results of therapy. Gastrointest Endosc 1993;39:78–81.

[19] Thatcher BS, Sivak MV, Tedesco FJ, et al. Endoscopic sphincterotomy for suspected dysfunction of the sphincter of Oddi. Gastrointest Endosc 1987;33:91–5.

[20] Sherman S. What is the role of ERCP in the setting of abdominal pain of pancreatic or biliary origin (suspected sphincter of Oddi dysfunction)? Gastrointest Endosc 2002;56:S258–66.

[21] Geenen JE, Nash JA. The role of sphincter of Oddi manometry (SOM) and biliary microscopy in evaluating idiopathic recurrent pancreatitis. Endoscopy 1998;30:A237–41.

[22] Peterson BT. Sphincter of Oddi dysfunction, part 2: evidenced-based review of the presentations, with "objective" (types I and II) and of presumptive type III. Gastrointest Endosc 2004;59(6):670–87.

[23] Sherman S, Lehman G, Jamidar P, et al. Efficacy of endoscopic sphincterotomy and surgical sphincteroplasty for patients with sphincter of Oddi dysfunction (SOD): randomized, controlled study [abstract]. Gstrointest Endosc 1994;40:P125.

[24] Fogel EL, Toth TG, Lehman GA, et al. Does Endoscopic therapy favorably affect the outcome of patients who have recurrent acute pancreatitis and pancreas divisum? Pancreas 2007;34:21–45.

[25] Delhaye M, Engelholm L, Cremeer M. Pancreas divisum: congenital anatomic variant or anomaly? Contribution of endoscopic retrograde dorsal pancreatography. Gastroenterology 1985;89:951–8.

[26] Bernard JP, Sahel J, Giovannini M, et al. Pancreas divisum is a probable cause of acute pancreatitis: a report of 137 cases. Pancreas 1990;5:248–54.

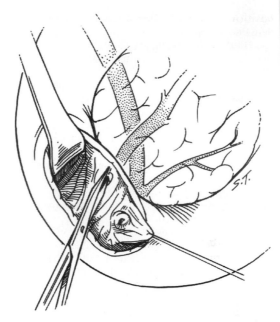

Fig. 6. Performing sphincterotomy of the minor papilla in pancreas di

Summary

Sphincter of Oddi dysfunction and pancreas divisum are unu disorders of the pancreas. They are commonly diagnosed under ical scenarios and often elude clinical diagnosis, primarily becau of consideration. However, when considered, a thoughtful evalu egy may reveal abnormalities that will respond to surgical or enc tervention. Without manometric abnormalities of the sphincter c in the face of chronic pancreatitis changes, interventions are far le ful. Acknowledging the advantages of endoscopic intervention, p favors surgical sphincteroplasty over endoscopic sphincterotom term, successful relief of symptoms. Management of these patie be a cooperative effort between surgeons and gastroenterologists

References

[1] Avisse C, Flament JB, Delattre JF. Ampulla of Vater: anatomic, embryologic aspects. Surg Clin North Am 2000;80(1):201–12.

[2] Hand BH. An anatomical study of the choledochoduodenal junction. Br J S 486–94.

[3] Bosch A, Pena LR. The Sphincter of Oddi. Dig Dis Sci 2007;52:1211–8.

[4] Kennedy AL, Mawe GM. Duodenal neurons provide nicotinic synaptic input to Oddi neurons in guinea pig. Am J Physiol 1999;277:G226–34.

[5] Guelrud M, Mendoza S, Rossiter G. Sphincter of Oddi manometry in healthy Dig Dis Sci 1990;35:38–46.

SPHINCTER OF ODDI DYSFUNCTION AND PANCREAS DIVISUM

[27] O'Connor KW, Lehman GA. An improved technique for accessory papilla cannulation in pancreas divisum. Gastrointest Endosc 1985;31:13–7.

[28] Madura JA. Pancreas divisum: stenosis of the dorsally dominant pancreatic duct—a surgically correctable lesion. Am J Surg 1986;151:742–5.

[29] Warshaw AL, Simeone JF, Shapiro RH, et al. Evaluation and treatment of the dominant dorsal duct syndrome (pancreas divisum redefined). Am J Surg 1990;159:59–66.

[30] Saltzberg DM, Schriber JB, Smith K, et al. Isolated ventral pancreatitis in a patient with pancreas divisum. Am J Gastroenterol 1990;85:1407–10.

[31] Tulassay Z, Jakab Z, Vadasz A, et al. Secretin provocation ultrasonography in the diagnosis of papillary obstruction in pancreas divisum. Gastroenterol J 1991;51:47–50.

[32] Lindstrom E, Ihse I. Dynamic CT scanning of pancreatic duct after secretin provocation and pancreas divisum. Dig Dis Sci 1990;35:1371–6.

[33] Eisen G, Schutz S, Metzler D, et al. Santorinicele: new evidence for obstruction in pancreas divisum. Gastrointest Endosc 1994;40:73–6.

[34] Fogel EL, Sherman S, Kalayci C, et al. Manometry in native minor papilla and post minor papilla therapy: experience at a tertiary referral center. Gastrointest Endosc 1999;49:187A.

[35] Staritz M, Meyer zum Buschenfelde KH. Elevated pressure in the dorsal part of pancreas divisum: the cause of chronic pancreatitis? Pancreas 1988;3:108–10.

[36] Siegel JH, Cooperman AM, Pullano W, et al. Pancreas divisum: observation, endoscopic drainage and surgical treatment results in 65 patients. Surg Laparosc Endosc 1993;3:281–5.

[37] Linder JD, Bukeirat FA, Geenen JE, et al. Minor papilla sphincterotomy in patients with symptomatic pancreas divisum: long term efficacy and complications. Gstrointest Endosc 2003;57:208A.

[38] Lehman GA, Sherman S, Nisi R, et al. Pancreas divisum: results of minor papilla sphincterotomy. Gastrointest Endosc 1993;39:1–8.

[39] Kozarek RA. Pancreatic duct stents can induce ductal changes consistent with chronic pancreatitis. Gastrointest Endosc 1990;36:93–5.

SURGICAL
CLINICS OF
NORTH AMERICA

Surg Clin N Am 87 (2007) 1431–1446

Necrotizing Pancreatitis: Diagnosis and Management

John C. Haney, MD, MPH, Theodore N. Pappas, MD*

Duke University Medical Center, Duke University School of Medicine, Durham, NC 27710, USA

Episodes of acute pancreatitis account for almost a quarter of a million hospital admissions in the United States each year [1]. Over 90% of cases are caused by either excessive alcohol consumption or gallstones, with the remainder caused by various factors, including hypertriglyceridemia, anatomic duct abnormalities such as pancreatic divisum, medications, and trauma. In most cases, acute pancreatitis represents a mild, self-limited disease, but in a minority, it confers a fulminant, progressive course associated with significant morbidity and mortality. Severe pancreatitis associated with gland necrosis occurs in 10% to 20% of patients, and despite improvements in critical care, it remains associated with mortality rates of 10% to 25% [2]. Mortality is highest when necrotizing pancreatitis becomes secondarily infected, as historically occurred in 40% to 70% of these patients [3], requiring operative debridement and prolonged, intensive medical and surgical management.

Pathophysiology

The pathogenesis of acute pancreatitis is caused initially by inappropriate conversion of the pancreatic proenzyme trypsinogen to its active form, trypsin. The precise mechanisms responsible for this activation remain unclear, but work in multiple animal models has suggested that stimuli prevent appropriate export of zymogen granules from the acinar cells, leading to fusion with intracellular lysosomes and activation of trypsin by lysosomal enzymes such as cathepsin B [4,5]. Intracellular conversion of trypsinogen to trypsin initiates a cascade of activation of other zymogens, leading to

---

* Corresponding author.

E-mail address: pappa001@mc.duke.edu (T.N. Pappas).

doi:10.1016/j.suc.2007.08.013   *surgical.theclinics.com*

cellular autodigestion. Once activated, these pancreatic enzymes are responsible for autodigestion of pancreatic and peripancreatic tissues and damage to the microvasculature supplying the gland. Necrosis of the acini, pancreatic islets, and pancreatic ducts is accompanied by interstitial fat necrosis from activated pancreatic lipase and necrotizing vasculitis with microvascular thrombosis leading to devitalization of larger areas of the pancreas [6]. The process of pancreatic necrosis occurs relatively early in the disease process, within the first 24 to 48 hours, and in at least two-thirds of patients, it remains stable throughout the course of the illness [7].

As a result of the acute pancreatic injury, a range of enzymes are released into the bloodstream, including trypsinogen, amylase, lipase, phospholipase A2, trypsinogen-activating peptide, and polymorphonuclear cell elastase. In addition, injury to the pancreatic parenchyma stimulates the production of inflammatory cytokines such as interleukin (IL)-1 and tumor necrosis factor-α (TNF α) [8]. Some of the pancreatic damage may be caused directly by the inflammatory response itself, as TNF α has been shown to cause acinar cell apoptosis [9]. The release of these cytokines triggers an inflammatory cascade, resulting in the production of additional cytokines including IL-2, IL-6, IL-8, IL-10, bradykinin, and platelet-activating factor. The end point of this cascade is often the systemic inflammatory response syndrome (SIRS), characterized by loss of vascular tone and systemic vascular resistance and increased capillary permeability with third-spacing of plasma volume, all leading to hypotension and hyperdynamic cardiovascular response. If unchecked, SIRS may produce acute respiratory distress syndrome (ARDS) or multiorgan dysfunction syndrome (MODS), both with significantly high mortality. This profound inflammatory response thus marks the early (less than 2 weeks) phase of necrotizing pancreatitis. It is the body's own inflammatory reaction to the initial injury that produces most of the early morbidity and mortality, and it is against this end that initial management is geared. The second, late-phase (greater than 2 weeks) is marked by infectious complications of gland necrosis and the sequelae of organ failure.

Diagnosis

The clinical diagnosis of acute pancreatitis is made based on the patient's history and characteristic presentation of epigastric abdominal pain combined with elevated serum levels of pancreatic enzymes amylase and lipase. Serum enzyme levels two to three times normal in the setting of an appropriate history are diagnostic. Initial evaluation should seek to identify an etiology; in the absence of alcohol use, gallstone pancreatitis should be suspected. The single most sensitive laboratory predictor of gallstone pancreatitis is a serum alanine aminotransferase (ALT) elevated to three times the normal value [1]. If biliary disease is suspected, the common bile duct should be evaluated with ultrasound and by serum bilirubin measurement to assess for obstruction, although gallstone pancreatitis is caused more frequently by smaller gallstones that infrequently impact within the common duct.

Although the diagnosis of acute pancreatitis is relatively straightforward, it is critical to attempt to identify those patients destined for severe disease, as it is these patients in whom the systemic inflammatory response can produce fulminant complications. Initial risk stratification is therefore aimed at determining which patients are likely to require more intensive levels of care and more aggressive intervention. Identifying these patients is not clear-cut, however. Initial clinical presentation may be unrevealing, as hallmark indications of severe disease such as flank (Grey Turner sign) or periumbilical eccymoses (Cullen sign) occur in less than 3% of patients [10]. Although amylase and lipase remain the standard for diagnosis, they are poor predictors of severity, as is the etiology of the pancreatitis. An acute-phase reactant and marker of inflammation, C-reactive protein (CRP) predicts severity with a sensitivity and specificity of 80%, but requires 24 to 48 hours to do so, limiting its clinical utility [11]. Efforts to find more predictive serum markers have led to the investigation of procalcitonin (PCT), polymorphonuclear leukocyte elastase, trypsinogen activation peptide, TNF α, IL-1β, ghrelin, and leptin levels as markers of severity, and while some, especially procalcitonin, hold promise, none have emerged in widespread clinical use [11–13].

In the absence of an ideal serum marker for predicting severity, most clinicians continue to use various algorithms based on clinical and laboratory measurements. First published in 1974, Ranson measured 11 criteria on admission or within 48 hours to generate a score predictive of outcome. The Ranson criteria remain commonly employed today to make clinical decisions regarding patient management (Box 1). More recently, the Acute Physiology and Chronic Health Evaluation II (APACHE II) system has been used to predict severity. Designed to predict outcomes in an intensive care setting, APACHE II measures 12 distinct variables regarding current condition and underlying health. It remains one of the best predictors of severity on initial presentation, with accuracy of up to 75% depending on the score (Table 1) [6]. At 48 hours, APACHE II, Ranson's criteria, and CRP all show equivalence. In using these measures, most clinicians seek to identify patients for whom increased levels of monitoring and intervention likely will be required, but no rigorous testing has identified specific cut-off values for step-down or ICU admission.

In predicting severity, one of the most important distinctions is the identification of pancreatic necrosis. In the absence of necrosis, mortality is 1%, while in its presence mortality increases to 10% to 23% [6]. More than 80% of deaths in acute pancreatitis occur in patients who have necrosis [14]. The extent of necrosis remains an important predictor of the risk of secondary bacterial infection, and while infection rates have decreased in more recent

---

Box 1. Ranson's criteria for the prediction of severe acute pancreatitis

At presentation:
Age older than 55 years
Blood glucose level greater than 200 mg/dL
White blood cell count greater than 16,000/mm^3
Lactate dehydrogenase level greater than 350 IU/L
Alanine aminotransferase level greater than 250 U/L

48 hours after presentation:
Hematocrit—10% decrease
Serum calcium less than 8 mg/dL
Base deficit greater than 4 mEq/L
Blood urea nitrogen increase greater than 5 mg/dL
Fluid sequestration greater than 6 L
PaO2 less than 60 mm Hg

   One point is assigned to each positive factor. Scores greater than 4 are associated with significant increases in ICU stay and mortality [1].
   From Ranson JHC, Rifkind KM, Turner JW. Prognostic signs and nonoperative peritoneal lavage in acute pancreatitis. Surg Gynecol Obstet 1976;143:209–19; with permission.

---

studies from the conventional 40% to 70% to 10% to 40%, the mortality of infected pancreatic necrosis in the absence of appropriate intervention remains nearly 100% [2]. The widespread proliferation of CT scanners has improved the ability to diagnose and stage necrotizing pancreatitis dramatically. An initial grading scale published in the mid-1980s by Balthazar and colleagues [15] graded the severity of pancreatitis by the presence of peripancreatic inflammatory changes and fluid collections, with peripancreatic fluid collections (grades D and E) conferring significantly higher mortality (Table 2). Improvements in the contrast bolus techniques now allow one to image the perfusion of the pancreatic parenchyma with accuracy. Areas of necrosis with diminished or no enhancement upon contrast bolus now are detected with an accuracy of 87%. For extended necrosis (greater than 50%), the sensitivity and specificity approach 100% [6]. These findings were incorporated into Balthazar's initial grading scale to create the more accurate CT severity index [16]. As a result of these changes, an abdominal CT scan with contrast is now standard for the diagnosis and work-up of suspected severe pancreatitis. Except in cases of initial diagnostic uncertainty, it is advisable to wait 1 to 2 days to obtain the initial scan. Before this point, pancreatic necrosis may not be apparent, and in addition, the delay allows

Table 1
The Acute Physiology and Chronic Health Evaluation II scoring system

Physiologic variable	High abnormal				Low abnormal				
	+4	+3	+2	+1	0	+1	+2	+3	+4
Temperature (oC)	≥41	39–40.9		38.5–38.9	36–38.4	34–35.9	32–33.9	30–31.9	≤29.9
Mean arterial Pressure (mm Hg)	≥160	130–159	110–129		70–109		50–69		≤49
Heart rate	≥180	140–179	110–139		70–109		55–69	40–54	≤39
Respiratory rate	≥50	35–49		25–34	12–24	10–11	6–9		≤5
Oxygenation:									
FiO2≥0.5, record A-aDO2	≥500	350–499	200–349		<200				
FiO2≤0.5, record PaO2					>70	61–70		55–60	≤55
Arterial pH	≥7.7	7.6–7.69		7.5–7.59	7.33–7.49		7.25–7.32	7.15–7.24	≤7.15
Serum sodium (mmol/L)	≥180	160–179	155–159	150–154	130–149		120–129	111–119	≤110
Serum potassium (mmol/L)	≥7	6–6.9		5.5–5.9	3.5–5.4	3–3.4	2.5–2.9		≤2.5
Serum creatinine (mg/100 mL) (double score for acute renal failure)	≥3.5	2–3.4	1.5–1.9		0.6–1.4		≤0.6		
Hematocrit (%)	≥60		50–59.9	46–49.9	30–45.9		20–29.9		≤20
White blood cell count (total/mm3)	≥40		20–39.9	15–19.9	3–14.9		1–2.9		≤1
15 - (Glasgow coma scale)									
Total acute physiology score (APS):									
Age points:									

Age points:
<44   0
45–54   2
55–64   3
65–74   5
≥75   6

Chronic health points:
If the patient has a history of severe organ system insufficiency or is immunocompromised, assign points as follows:
For nonoperative or emergency postoperative patients, 5 points
For elective postoperative patients, 2 points

APACHE II score (sum of APS + age points + chronic health points)

Total score is determined by the sum of points allocated for the physiologic variables and points allocated for age and chronic organ system dysfunction. Scores of at least 8 are predictive of severe acute pancreatitis [1].

From Knaus WA, Draper EA, Wagner DP, et al. APACHE II: a severity of disease classification system. Crit Care Med 1985;13(10):818–29; with permission.

Table 2
CT severity index

CT grade	Points	Necrosis %	Extra points	Severity index
A (normal pancreas)	0	0	0	0
B (pancreatic enlargement)	1	0	0	1
C (Pancreatic/peripancreatic fat inflammation)	2	<30	2	4
D (single peripancreatic fluid collection)	3	30–50	4	7
E (two or more fluid collections/ retroperitoneal air)	4	>50	6	10

Points are allocated for grade (A–E) of inflammation and for percentage of gland necrosis. A severity index score of 7–10 yields a 17% mortality and 92% complication rate [16].

From Balthazar EJ, Robinson DL, Megibow AJ, et al. Acute pancreatitis: value of CT in establishing prognosis. Radiology 1990;174:331–6; with permission.

the patient to receive initial aggressive fluid resuscitation, thus reducing the risk of contrast-induced nephropathy. Once an initial CT scan has been obtained, it is uncommon to require a follow-up study for 3 to 4 weeks, as pancreatic necrosis typically remains stable in appearance [7].

Early management

Initial management of necrotizing pancreatitis is geared toward maintenance of adequate intravascular volume and end-organ perfusion in the face of the systemic inflammatory response caused by the injury. The capillary leak and peripancreatic inflammation can cause substantial third-spacing of fluid; thus initial management should be geared toward aggressive crystalloid resuscitation. All patients should be monitored closely for assessment of intravascular volume and adequacy of organ perfusion. This includes frequent physical examination and evaluation of vital signs for signs of tachycardia or hypotension, monitoring of hourly urine output, and frequent analysis of serum acid–base status and oxygenation by arterial blood gas. It is during this initial resuscitation period that the clinician must diagnose those patients who have severe pancreatitis from the majority who have a more benign course by fluid requirements and signs of organ dysfunction. Clinical evaluation is aided by the predictive measures discussed previously, such as Ranson's criteria or APACHE II score, but ultimately it is the patient's early clinical course that will be most informative. Patients in whom there are early signs of severe fluid requirements or end-organ dysfunction, or in whom baseline chronic conditions leave little physiologic margin for error, should be monitored in a step-down or even ICU setting. In rare patients in whom concomitant cardiovascular disease makes accurate assessments of volume status or cardiac function difficult, ICU admission will allow for invasive monitoring of central venous and pulmonary wedge pressures with a Swann-Ganz catheter.

In addition to crystalloid resuscitation, patients who have necrotizing pancreatitis should be made nulla per os (NPO) to reduce pancreatic stimulation. If there are signs of gastric ileus and distension, a nasogastric tube should be placed for gastric decompression. The patient's abdominal pain should be managed with intravenous narcotics. Most patients should receive stress ulcer prophylaxis and deep vein thrombosis prophylaxis with subcutaneous low molecular weight or unfractionated heparin unless contraindicated. Numerous additional pancreatitis-specific therapies have been investigated, including the use of pharmacologic agents targeting various components of the inflammatory cascade [17,18]. These have included the trypsin inhibitor aprotinin, a platelet-activating factor inhibitor lexipafant, the protease inhibitor gabexate mesilate, and octreotide for pancreatic suppression. Various trials were undertaken to investigate these therapies with mixed results, although a recent meta-analysis from Switzerland found no evidence for benefits of any of these agents [19].

An additional area that has merited thorough investigation is the optimal delivery of nutritional support to these patients. Severe pancreatitis induces a highly catabolic state; thus early nutritional support is essential if malnutrition is to be avoided. Oral intake is prohibited to avoid pancreatic exocrine stimulation; additionally, pancreatitis often produces gastric ileus or outright obstruction from perigastric inflammation. As a result, there was initial enthusiasm for total parenteral nutrition (TPN). Studies in healthy volunteers demonstrated that enteral feedings administered in the jejunum by means of nasojejunal tube do not stimulate pancreatic exocrine function as previously suspected [20]. In addition, enteral feeding provides several potential benefits. In the absence of enteral nutrition, the intestinal mucosa atrophies, and the normal barrier to enteric bacterial microorganisms is compromised. The role of enteric nutrition in maintaining this healthy gut barrier has been well established [2]. Furthermore, as will be discussed, the late stage of necrotizing pancreatitis is characterized by septic complications related to infection of the necrotic gland, infection that most commonly is caused by gram-negative gut flora. This observation, in conjunction with the known infectious risks of TPN, led to more enthusiasm for enteral nutrition to reduce episodes of late infection. Numerous well-designed, prospective clinical trials have compared nasojejunal nutrition directly with TPN. In most of these studies, enteral nutrition proved equivalent or superior in outcomes of infection, end-organ failure, and mortality at lower cost. A recent meta-analysis concluded that, although mortality rates did not differ, enteric feeding was associated with lower risk of infectious complications and lower overall cost [19]. For these reasons, most treatment guidelines advocate early nasojejunal feeding in patients who have necrotizing pancreatitis, including guidelines offered by the International Association of Pancreatology (IUP) in 2002 [21] and those presented by the international consensus conference on acute pancreatitis in 2004 [20]. The nasojejunal tube is placed best under fluoroscopic guidance by gastrointestinal radiology or in the ICU as tolerated by the patient's level of critical illness.

In conjunction with nutrition, the role of hyperglycemia in the critically ill patient has been a cause of significant research within the last decade. While primarily based on two randomized, single-center trials, intensive insulin therapy achieving a mean blood glucose of less than 110 mg/dL reduces mortality by 3% to 4% [22]. Tight glucose control with intravenous insulin infusion thus is recommended. Because of ileus, which commonly occurs early in the course of severe pancreatitis, patients may need to receive a week of TPN until the ileus resolves, and nasojejunal feeding can be tolerated.

The management of early stage necrotizing pancreatitis is thus one of aggressive resuscitation and support in an attempt to avoid end organ dysfunction from hypoperfusion. Although the management in the early stages remains intensive, surgical intervention during this period is limited. Historically, there has been enthusiasm for early surgical intervention in the setting of extensive necrosis, but this has fallen out of favor after more recent data have shown increased mortality with early intervention, as will be discussed. Indications for early intervention are limited. First, in the setting of gallstone pancreatitis and evidence of common bile duct obstruction, urgent endoscopic retrograde cholangiopancreatography (ERCP) with sphincterotomy is indicated to remove the impacted stone [20,21]. Some authors caution against ERCP in the absence of clear evidence of common duct obstruction because of concerns for introducing infection [23], but most studies on the subject have suggested that urgent ERCP lowers morbidity and mortality in the setting of severe pancreatitis. Patients who have suspected gallstone pancreatitis should be evaluated by both ultrasound and serum bilirubin for evidence of biliary obstruction, and if found, they should undergo ERCP [19,20].

In the absence of biliary obstruction, early intervention in necrotizing pancreatitis is limited. It has been suggested that a subset of patients will present with a fulminant, deteriorating clinical course despite aggressive intensive care. Surgery may be indicated for these patients. It has become clear that the number of these patients is small, and that, although a large percentage of patients with significant necrosis ultimately will need an operation, early intervention is associated with worse morbidity and mortality. One suggested indication for early laparotomy is the development of acute abdominal compartment syndrome (ACS), defined as intra-abdominal pressures greater than 25 mm Hg [2]. Abdominal compartment syndrome reduces venous return and thoracic expansion, compromising renal perfusion and ventilation. Although the incidence of ACS in necrotizing pancreatitis is unclear, it is likely that fewer than 10% of patients qualify for decompressive laparotomy. When indicated, laparotomy often produces rapid improvement in hemodynamic, pulmonary, and renal function. An index of clinical suspicion should be maintained throughout the early phase of the disease, especially in patients who have worsening renal function and urine output despite active resuscitation.

Late management

In addition to supporting patients through the systemic inflammatory phase of their illness, management of severe necrotizing pancreatitis must also be geared toward reducing the incidence of late-stage complications, characterized primarily by the development of secondary bacterial infection of the necrotic gland. Infection of necrotic pancreatic parenchyma generally occurs after the second week of the acute attack, and based on experimental models, it is thought to result from the translocation of enteric flora from the small bowel and colon. Gram-negative enterics such as *Escherichia coli* traditionally have been the most common species isolated [14], but recent data have suggested that antibiotic use has altered the bacteriology in favor of gram-positive organisms such as *Enterococcus* and *Staphylococcus* species [24]. Infection has been found in up to 70% of cases of necrosis, with the most recent studies suggesting that the infection rate has dropped closer to 10% to 40%. The presence of infection is a major predictor of outcome, increasing mortality threefold [14,21]. As discussed previously, the degree of necrosis correlates with the risk for secondary infection, with extensive (greater than 50%) necrosis associated with an eightfold increase in infection rate over less substantial (30% to 50%) cases [2]. The refined CT severity index created by Balthazar and colleagues [6] combines grade of severity (A to D) with percentage of necrosis to provide an excellent early predictor of morbidity and mortality that compares favorably to either Ranson's criteria or APACHE II score.

The presence of infected necrosis also determines management strategy, as the mortality of infected necrosis approaches 100% in the absence of surgical debridement [2,3]. By contrast, multiple studies have shown that sterile necrosis is now managed best nonoperatively, demonstrating increased mortality rates in patients with sterile necrosis who have undergone debridement, with rates ranging from 12% to 21% with surgery versus 2% to 5% with nonoperative management [19,25]. As a result, most authors advocate nonoperative strategies for noninfected patients, including those recommendations from the IUP and international consensus conference, and those from major treating institutions [19–21,25,26].

Antibiotics

Because of the clinical significance of infection, there has been much interest paid to the role of early intravenous antibiotics in necrotizing pancreatitis with the goal of reducing infectious complications. Appropriate antibiotic therapy must demonstrate both penetration of pancreatic tissue and coverage of the expected infectious flora. Carbapenems, quinolones, and nitroimidazoles all fit this profile [3]. Initial enthusiasm for antibiotic prophylaxis was generated by several small prospective trials in the 1990s, which showed that early antibiotic prophylaxis in patients with severe pancreatitis could reduce both infection rates and mortality. The initial studies were performed with imipenem–cilastin (Primaxin), and this has remained the most common antibiotic studied, with ciprofloxacin (Cipro) and metronidazole (Flagyl) commonly advocated as an alternative in beta lactam-sensitive patients [2]. Although many of the initial studies suffered from various shortcomings such as small patient size and different outcome measures, meta-analysis remained suggestive of a benefit to prophylaxis [27]. Since 2004, however, two large, placebo-controlled, double-blind trials have failed to show a benefit to prophylaxis with regard to either infection rates or mortality. The first, published by Isenmann and colleagues [28] in 2004, randomized 114 patients who had severe pancreatitis to ciprofloxacin and metronidazole or placebo and showed no difference in infection or mortality. Several meta-analyses, including an updated Cochrane database review, were then published incorporating this study, and now showed a mortality benefit with the use of beta lactam prophylaxis only, but without difference in the rate of pancreatic infection or surgical intervention [19,29]. Most recently, Dellinger and colleagues [30] have published a multicenter, prospective, double-blind placebo-controlled randomized study in which 100 patients who had severe, necrotizing pancreatitis were randomized to early prophylactic meropenem (Merrem) or placebo. This study, like its predecessor, found no statistical difference between groups with regard to infection, mortality, or surgical intervention rates. Both studies have been criticized for several flaws [27]. First, while powered for a 40% expected infection rate, the actual rates observed in the control groups were significantly lower (17% and 12% respectively), resulting in underpowered studies. Second, there remained significant cross-over as a high percentage (46% and 54% respectively) of placebo patients received intravenous antibiotics of some kind. Despite these weaknesses, these studies remain the best designed investigations to date, and neither show a benefit to prophylaxis. The concern with prophylaxis, of course, is that overuse of antibiotics may promote antibiotic resistance and, perhaps more importantly, promote late fungal infection, an event shown to increase mortality fourfold independent of APACHE II status [31]. These concerns were investigated by Howard and colleagues [24], and, while antibiotic use altered the species isolated, shifting the predominance toward gram- positive species, the use of antibiotics was associated neither with increased beta lactam resistance nor with increased fungal superinfection. In light of these mixed data, the debate on prophylaxis continues [27,32].

Despite this debate, the importance of early antibiotic use in severe necrotizing pancreatitis remains unquestioned. Given the role of infection in causing morbidity and mortality, early empiric use of carbapenems in patients who have a clinical picture of infection suggested by fever, leukocytosis, and hemodynamic instability is indicated. The authors have typically continued these antibiotics to complete a 14-day course in the case of clinical improvement. In cases of persistent illness, antibiotics are continued and empiric antifungal coverage should be considered. The data do not support use of prophylaxis in all patients who have severe pancreatitis, but in those who have clinical signs of infection, early empiric use is advocated by all. Both Isenmann [28] and Dellinger [30] support this strategy as treatment on demand. The critical distinction is that the determining factor in prescribing antibiotics should be the clinically sick patient who has necrosis rather than the necrosis alone.

Fine needle aspiration

Infected pancreatic necrosis necessitates surgical debridement, while sterile necrosis is managed best nonoperatively [19–21,25,26]. This dichotomy of treatment strategies based on the presence of infection has led to the widespread advocacy for early fine needle aspiration (FNA) of the necrotic pancreas. Radiographic evidence alone is rarely conclusive, as retroperitoneal gas, the most definitive sign of infection, is a rare finding and, while the degree of necrosis does correlate with infection risk, the size of the necrosis is suggestive but not definitive. It therefore has been the practice of some authors to advocate early FNA to identify infection and determine which patients will benefit from necrosectomy. In contrast, it is the authors' contention that FNA remains unnecessary in most cases and that clinical presentation is sufficient to make an operative determination [33].

To examine the appropriate role of FNA, one must consider the timing of surgical intervention. Although early necrosectomy was once advocated, numerous more recent studies have confirmed that delayed surgical intervention is associated with better outcomes. Delaying surgery for at least 2 weeks has been associated with reduced mortality and major complications [34–36]. The rationale for this strategy includes the ebbing of the systemic inflammatory response and the clear demarcation of necrotic tissues and their organization and separation from healthy parenchyma, making dissection planes easier to identify. As a result, the current consensus is for delayed surgical intervention, even in the setting of infected necrosis. The critical argument against routine FNA, then, is that during this delay, the clinical course of the patient will readily predict who will need debridement and who will not [32,37]. Plainly stated, most patients who have sterile necrosis will improve clinically, while those who have infected necrosis will not. Examination of the data from two studies advocating FNA shows that the mean time from presentation to surgery in patients who had positive aspirates was 3 to 4 weeks (21 to 27 days), while the mean total length of hospital stay in those patients with negative aspirates, or sterile necrosis, was of similar range (23 to 34 days) [25,26]. In other words, by the time patients who had positive FNA aspirates were taken to the operating room, those patients who had sterile necrosis were nearly well enough to go home.

FNA under CT or ultrasound guidance has become a relatively safe, reliable test. It is not without risk, however, including the chance of seeding an otherwise sterile collection with bacteria. If the data from the FNA do not produce changes in clinical management, however, any risk is too much. In these studies, patients undergoing FNA were treated with prophylactic antibiotics for several weeks regardless of the aspiration data, and surgical debridement for infection was delayed appropriately for several weeks [24–26,34,36]. At this point, patients continuing to have fevers, leukocytosis, and clinical signs of sepsis after several weeks of supportive care, including intravenous antibiotics, will need surgical exploration. Most of these patients will have infection; the few who do not would meet criteria for exploration and debridement based on their lack of improvement. Patients for whom surgery is indicated typically fall into three groups:

- A rare group of patients in whom early intervention is necessary because of unrelenting deterioration despite aggressive care
- Patients who have infected necrosis
- Patients who have sterile necrosis in whom several weeks of supportive care have produced little improvement and who remain clinically unwell

Few, if any, surgeons would decline surgical intervention at this junction based on a negative FNA. Unless the results of the FNA push the clinician to intervene earlier or withhold antibiotics pending the result, it remains unnecessary. There is no evidence that use of FNA reduces mortality, and it has been the authors' practice to avoid aspiration and rely exclusively on clinical evaluation to guide surgical intervention with good results [33,38,39].

Surgical intervention

Surgical intervention is thus indicated in the patient with necrotizing pancreatitis in whom the clinical course has continued to deteriorate after 3 to 4 weeks of intensive management. Percutaneous drainage, while appealing, has a low likelihood of success in extracting the thick, liquefied pancreatic tissue, and open necrosectomy usually is required [23]. Before intervention, a repeat CT scan may guide the operation by delineating the extent of extrapancreatic disease. Operative interventions classically have come in two forms: necrosectomy followed by closed drainage, or debridement followed by open abdominal packing [3]. The latter method, with return trips to the operating room for dressing changes, has fallen out of favor, likely because the delay in surgical intervention has promoted organization of the necrotic tissue to facilitate complete debridement at the time of initial laparotomy. A recent meta-analysis of the two techniques even concluded that open packing was associated with higher morbidity and possibly higher mortality [19]. The operation typically is performed through a subcostal incision, entering the retroperitoneum through the lesser sac. Debridement is performed primarily with blunt finger dissection, stopping once bleeding tissue is encountered in an effort to spare the viable remainder of the gland. Formal pancreatic resection is associated with higher morbidity than organ-sparing debridement. Extension of the necrosis into the retroperitoneal peri colic gutters or mesentery is common, and this should be explored gingerly with blunt dissection. If feasible, cholecystectomy may be performed in cases of gallstone pancreatitis [26]. Some authors have advocated placement of a feeding jejunostomy tube. Given the high incidence of postoperative enterocutaneous fistula however, it has been the authors' practice to avoid even intentional enterotomies. Following debridement of the necrotic tissue, the cavity should be drained with several large-bore closed-suction drains. If all necrotic material is removed, the abdomen may be closed over the drains. Earlier studies of necrosectomy often employed continuous lavage through the drains as initially described by Berger [19]. In most cases in which surgical intervention has been delayed, the demarcation of necrotic tissue allows for adequate debridement, and suction with intermittent drain irrigation will be sufficient. Surgical necrosectomy is often followed by the reaccumulation of peripancreatic fluid, but recurrent collections may be drained percutaneously after the manual removal of the necrotic parenchyma. A failure in postoperative improvement after surgery should be investigated with repeat abdominal CT scan, and an aggressive percutaneous drainage strategy is advocated following initial debridement.

Current investigations into the strategy for surgical debridement include enthusiasm for minimally invasive, retroperitoneal approaches by means of a small flank incision [40]. One initial study compared favorably toward laparotomy, and currently a prospective randomized controlled multicenter trial (PANTER trial) is investigating this approach, with results due in 2008 [41].

Complications following debridement of necrotizing pancreatitis remain common; however, recent data have shown that the overall morbidity and mortality have declined [36]. These complications include pancreatic or enterocutaneous fistula, wound infection, and wound dehiscence and hernia [3]. Bleeding is a rare complication usually managed angiographically [2]. Fistulae occur in up to 30% of patients undergoing laparotomy, and initially it should be managed conservatively, with surgical repair deferred until such time as the pancreatitis has resolved completely [3,26]. Wound infection and dehiscence must be treated more aggressively. Nonoperative complications include end organ damage such as renal failure from underperfusion during the inflammatory phase. Endocrine and exocrine insufficiencies of the pancreas are also relatively common [3]. Other late complications include organized, sterile necrosis in patients in whom no surgical intervention was indicated. These patients may present with persistent abdominal pain and inability to tolerate oral feeding [26]. In these cases, delayed debridement also may be indicated. Despite the high incidence of morbidity, the long-term quality of life for patients requiring debridement approaches that of patients who have chronic pancreatitis [38].

Summary

Although most patients who have acute pancreatitis will experience a self-limited disease course, it is imperative that the clinician respect the severity of the disease in the unlucky minority. Initial diagnosis is geared toward risk stratification through a combination of clinical criteria such as Ranson's criteria and APACHE II score, although no test or analytical tool yet replaces clinical judgement in assessing disease severity. Early clinical evaluation should focus on measures of intravascular volume status and end organ perfusion, and aggressive intervention should be geared toward volume resuscitation. For patients in whom there appear clinical signs of deterioration or in whom there exists little clinical reserve, early transfer to the ICU is advised. An initial abdominal CT scan with intravenous contrast is advocated ideally after 48 hours to assess for the presence of gland necrosis, thus predicting severity of disease. In patients who have significant clinical illness within the first several days, including hemodynamic instability, leukocytosis, and/or fever, early empiric treatment with an intravenous carbapenem is indicated. If clinical stabilization does not occur, addition of empiric antifungal therapy is justifiable given its increased mortality. Intensive therapy for these sick patients includes early enteric feeding by means of a nasojejunal feeding tube, volume resuscitation, and tight glycemic control. Early intervention is indicated only for precipitous decline or for release of abdominal compartment syndrome. The most important single factor in determining long-term outcome is the presence of infection; however, even in the presence of infection, surgical intervention is best deferred several weeks. If patients who have significant illness are being treated empirically with antibiotics, then routine FNA is not needed. After several weeks, the patient's clinical status will determine the need for operative debridement. Necrosectomy is best performed as a single, definitive operative debridement using limited, blunt finger dissection. Most patients may be closed over standard suction drains. Recurrent fluid collections should be aggressively drained percutaneously. Although the postoperative complication rate remains high, the long-term quality of life compares favorably with other chronic pancreatic conditions.

References

[1] Whitcomb DC. Acute pancreatitis. N Engl J Med 2006;354(20):2141–50.
[2] Hughes SJ, Papachristou GI, Federle MP, et al. Necrotizing pancreatitis. Gastroenterol Clin North Am 2007;36(2):313–23, viii.

[3] Werner J, Ühl W, Büchler MW. Acute pancreatitis. In: Cameron JL, editor. Current surgical therapy. 8th edition. Philadelphia: Elsevier Mosby; 2004. p. 459–69.

[4] Sharp KW, Chapman WC, Potts JR III, et al. Liver, biliary tract, and pancreas. In: O'Leary JP, editor. The physiologic basis of surgery. 3rd edition. Philadelphia: Lippencott Williams & Wilkins; 2002. p. 523–4.

[5] Hirano T, Manabe T. A possible mechanism for gallstone pancreatitis: repeated short-term pancreaticobiliary duct obstruction with exocrine stimulation in rats. Proc Soc Exp Biol Med 1993;202(2):246–52.

[6] Balthazar EJ. Acute pancreatitis. assessment of severity with clinical and CT evaluation. Radiology 2002;223:603–13.

[7] Vitellas KM, Paulson EK, Enns RA, et al. Pancreatitis complicated by gland necrosis: evolution of findings on contrast-enhanced CT. J Comput Assist Tomogr 1999;23(6):898–905.

[8] Makhija R, Kingsnorth AN. Cytokine storm in acute pancreatitis. J Hepatobiliary Pancreat Surg 2002;9(4):401–10.

[9] Norman J. The role of cytokines in the pathogenesis of acute pancreatitis. Am J Surg 1998; 175(1):76–83.

[10] Meyers MA, Feldberg MAM, Oliphant M. Grey Turner's sign and Cullen's sign in acute pancreatitis. Gastrointest Radiol 1989;14:31–7.

[11] Al-Bahrani AZ, Ammori BJ. Clinical laboratory assessment of acute pancreatitis. Clin Chim Acta 2005;362(1–2):26–48.

[12] Rau BM, Kemppainen EA, Gumbs AA, et al. Early assessment of pancreatic infections and overall prognosis in severe acute pancreatitis by procalcitonin (PCT): a prospective international multicenter study. Ann Surg 2007;245(5):745–54.

[13] Kerem M, Bedirli A, Pasaoglu H, et al. Role of ghrelin and leptin in predicting the severity of acute pancreatitis. Dig Dis Sci 2007;52(4):950–5.

[14] Beger HG, Rau B, Mayer J, et al. Natural course of acute pancreatitis. World J Surg 1997;21: 130–5.

[15] Balthazar EJ, Ranson JHC, Naidich DP, et al. Acute pancreatitis: prognostic value of CT. Radiology 1985;156(3):767–72.

[16] Balthazar EJ, Robinson DL, Megibow AJ, et al. Acute pancreatitis: value of CT in establishing prognosis. Radiology 1990;174:331–6.

[17] Turkyilmaz S, Alhan F, Ercin C, et al. Effects of enalaprilat on acute necrotizing pancreatitis in rats. Inflammation 2007; [Epub ahead of print].

[18] Takeda K. Antiproteases in the treatment of necrotizing pancreatitis: continuous regional arterial infusion. JOP 2007;8(4 Suppl):526–32.

[19] Heinrich S, Schäfer M, Rousson V, et al. Evidence-based treatment of acute pancreatitis: a look at established paradigms. Ann Surg 2006;243(2):154–68.

[20] Nathens AB, Curtis JR, Beale RJ, et al. Management of the critically ill patient with severe acute pancreatitis. Crit Care Med 2004;32(12):2524–36.

[21] Ühl W, Warshaw A, Imrie C, et al. IAP guidelines for the surgical management of acute pancreatitis. Pancreatology 2002;2:565–73.

[22] Vanhorebeek I, Langouche L, Van den Berghe G. Tight blood glucose control with insulin in the ICU: facts and controversies. Chest 2007;132:268–78.

[23] Bouvet M, Moussa AR. Pancreatic abscess. In: Cameron JL, editor. Current surgical therapy. 8th edition. Philadelphia: Elsevier Mosby; 2004. p. 476–80.

[24] Howard TJ, Temple MB. Prophylactic antibiotics alter the bacteriology of infected necrosis in severe acute pancreatitis. J Am Coll Surg 2002;195:759–67.

[25] Büchler MW, Gloor B, Müller CA, et al. Acute necrotizing pancreatitis: treatment strategy according to the status of infection. Ann Surg 2000;232(5):619–26.

[26] Ashley SW, Perez A, Pierce EA, et al. Necrotizing pancreatitis: contemporary analysis of 99 consecutive cases. Ann Surg 2001;234(4):579–80.

[27] Howard TJ. As good as it gets: the study of prophylactic antibiotics in severe acute pancreatitis. Ann Surg 2007;245(5):684–5.

[28] Isenmann R, Runzi M, Kron M, et al. Prophylactic antibiotic treatment in patients with pre-dicted severe acute pancreatitis: a placebo controlled, double-blind trial. Gastroenterology 2004;126:232–9.

[29] Villatoro E, Bassi C, Larvin M. Antibiotic therapy for prophylaxis against infection of pan-creatic necrosis in acute pancreatitis. Cochrane Database Syst Rev 2006;4:CD002941. doi:10.1002/14651858.CD002941.pub2.

[30] Dellinger EP, Tellado JM, Soto NE, et al. Early antibiotic treatment for severe acute necro-tizing pancreatitis: a randomized, double-blind, placebo-controlled study. Ann Surg 2007; 245(5):674–83.

[31] Hoerauf A, Hammer S, Muller-Myhsok B, et al. Intra-abdominal *Candida* infection during acute necrotizing pancreatitis has a high prevalence and is associated with increased mortal-ity. Crit Care Med 1998;26(12):2010–5.

[32] Tenner S. Antibiotics in patients with pancreatic necrosis: the controversy continues. Am J Gastroenterol 2007;102(5):1127 [author reply: 1127–8].

[33] Pappas TN. Con: computerized tomographic aspiration of infected pancreatic necrosis. The opinion against its routine use. Am J Gastroenterol 2005;100(11):2373–4.

[34] Hungness ES, Robb BW, Seeskin C, et al. Early debridement for necrotizing pancreatitis: is it worthwhile? J Am Coll Surg 2002;194(6):740–4.

[35] Mier J, Luque-de Leon E, Castillo A, et al. Early versus late necrosectomy in severe necro-tizing pancreatitis. Am J Surg 1997;173:71–5.

[36] Howard TJ, Patel JB, Zyromski N. Declining morbidity and mortality rates in the surgical management of pancreatic necrosis. J Gastrointest Surg 2007;11:43–9.

[37] Rau B, Pralle U, Uhl W, et al. Management of sterile necrosis in instances of severe acute pancreatitis. J Am Coll Surg 1995;181(4):279–88.

[38] Broome AH, Eisen GM, Harland RC, et al. Quality of life after treatment for pancreatitis. Ann Surg 1996;223(6):665–72.

[39] Sarraf-Yazdi S, Pappas TN. European surgical survey of acute pancreatitis—union of diver-sity. Am J Gastroenterol 2004;99(4):729–30.

[40] van Santvoort HC, Besselink MG, Bollen TL, et al. Case-matched comparison of the retro-peritoneal approach with laparotomy for necrotizing pancreatitis. World J Surg 2007;31(8): 1635–42.

[41] Besselink MG, van Santvoort HC, Nieuwenhuijs VB, et al. Minimally invasive "step-up approach" versus maximal necrosectomy in patients with acute necrotising pancreatitis (PANTER trial): design and rationale of a randomised controlled multicenter trial [ISRCTN38327949]. BMC Surg 2006;6:6.

SURGICAL
CLINICS OF
NORTH AMERICA

ELSEVIER
SAUNDERS

Surg Clin N Am 87 (2007) 1447–1460

Operative and Nonoperative Management of Pancreatic Pseudocysts

Simon Bergman, MD[a], W. Scott Melvin, MD[b],*

[a]Department of Surgery, Center for Minimally Invasive Surgery,
The Ohio State University, 558 Doan Hall, 410 West 10th Avenue,
Columbus, OH 43210, USA
[b]Division of General Surgery, The Ohio State University,
N729 Doan Hall, 410 West 10th Avenue, Columbus, OH 43210, USA

Since the first description of a pancreatic pseudocyst was made in 1761 by Morgagni [1], the diagnosis, definition, and especially the management of this entity have been in constant evolution. In an effort to reduce the variability of terms used to describe pancreatitis and its complications, the Atlanta International Symposium on Acute Pancreatitis has defined pseudocysts as amylase-rich fluid collections contained within fibrotic pseudocapsules and usually occurring 4 to 6 weeks following an episode of acute pancreatitis. Any collection lacking this pseudocapsule and diagnosed earlier in the course of disease is termed an acute fluid collection and has very different management implications. When a pseudocyst is infected, it is termed a pancreatic abscess, which encompasses a spectrum ranging from infected fluid collection to infected pancreatic necrosis [2].

The principles of pancreatic pseudocyst management long have been based on a study by Bradley and colleagues [3] documenting the natural history of pancreatic pseudocysts, which were followed until resolution or development of complications. Major complications, such as rupture, abscess, jaundice, and hemorrhage, arose in 40% of patients, with resolution occurring in only 20%. They further showed that observation past 7 weeks exposed the patients to a risk greater than the mortality of elective surgery. The dogma became that pseudocysts larger than 6 cm or which persisted for longer than 6 weeks had to undergo intervention. Subsequent reports have suggested that this management algorithm may be exposing many patients to unnecessary surgery. In a retrospective study of 68 patients

---

* Corresponding author.

E-mail address: melvin-1@medctr.osu.edu (W.S. Melvin).

followed conservatively, Vitas and Sarr [4] showed that while 9% of patients developed complications, mainly pseudoaneurysm, perforation, and abscess, and one third underwent surgery because of progressing symptomatology, the remaining patients were observed safely for over 4 years. Similarly, other groups have shown that 40% to 50% of asymptomatic pancreatic pseudocysts, regardless of size, could be followed conservatively, with the expectation that complete cyst resolution would occur in 60% [5,6]. Currently, there is no clear consensus on the absolute indications for intervention, although most would agree that size and time cut-offs rarely should justify intervention. On the other hand, symptomatic pseudocysts, whether causing pain, gastric outlet or biliary obstruction, pseudocysts complicated by infection and sepsis, hemorrhage, or pseudoaneurysm, enlarging pseudocysts, and pseudocysts in which malignancy cannot be excluded, are much more valid reasons to intervene.

Surgical management is still considered the gold standard intervention in pseudocyst management. This usually is performed by internal drainage by means of a cystenteric anastomosis, either in the form of a cystgastrostomy, cystduodenostomy, or cystjejunostomy, or by excision such as distal pancreatectomy, depending on the location and size of the pseudocyst. Open external drainage largely has fallen to the wayside because of the resulting morbidity, but sometimes may be considered in more complex situations, such as in the context of a pancreatic necrosectomy [7]. The literature on open surgical internal drainage of pancreatic pseudocysts demonstrates uniformly successful results. In a cumulative review of 14 studies comprising 1032 patients, internal drainage was associated with a mortality rate of 5.8% and a complication rate of 24% [8], although in individual series, complication rates as high as 40% have been reported [9–11]. Even though complications associated with pseudocyst surgery often are thought to reflect the underlying state of pancreatitis or general health of the patient and not the surgical procedure itself, these outcomes may be improved upon [12].

The technological advances seen in medicine over the last two decades, such as the continued refinement of minimally invasive surgical technique and experience, the advent of therapeutic endoscopy, and the development of multislice CT scanners, have made open surgery a second-line therapy in managing pancreatic pseudocysts, reserved for those patients who fail less invasive forms of intervention. This article summarizes the techniques, benefits, and outcomes of laparoscopic, endoscopic, and percutaneous approaches to pseudocyst management. Their role in the armamentarium of those caring for patients with pancreatic disease will be defined.

Laparoscopic pancreatic pseudocyst drainage

The laparoscopic approach to treatment of benign pancreatic disorders was developed over 10 years ago, and while the literature contains several case reports or small case series demonstrating the feasibility of laparoscopic pancreatic pseudocyst drainage [13–16], there are only a handful of larger case series (n ≥ 10) providing data on the early and late outcomes associated with these procedures. There are no prospective comparative trials comparing the risk and benefits of these procedures versus the traditional open approach.

Transgastric (anterior) cystgastrostomy

In 1994, a laparoscopic approach to pancreatic pseudocysts involving access to the pseudocyst through an anterior wall gastrotomy, similar to the open approach, was described [17,18]. After obtaining access to the peritoneal cavity, working ports are inserted in the subxiphoid area and in the left subcostal area at the level of the midclavicular line. An assistant provides retraction through a subcostal port placed lateral to the surgeon's right hand port. The abdomen is inspected, and, using either ultrasonic sheers or electrocautery, an anterior gastrotomy is made over the area of maximal bulging, usually along the greater curvature of the body. The pseudocyst indentation is identified against the posterior wall of the stomach, and an 18- to 22-gauge needle is used to confirm proper positioning and to confirm the presence of drainable fluid. Alternatively, if available, intraoperative ultrasound may be a useful adjunct in determining the exact relationship of the pseudocyst to the stomach and other vascular structures. The pseudocyst then is entered through the posterior wall of the stomach. A biopsy of the cyst wall and pathologic confirmation for the absence of malignancy are obtained before performing the anastomosis. The cystgastrostomy is performed, either with a linear stapler, or if energy has been used to divide stomach and pseudocyst, the posterior gastric wall is sutured to the pseudocyst. The anterior gastrotomy finally is either sutured or stapled closed [7].

Around the same time, a similar anterior approach was described, but using intraluminal surgical techniques [19,20]. After gaining access to the peritoneal cavity, two to three balloon-tipped trocars are inserted into the peritoneal cavity and then guided into the gastric lumen by means of separate 10 mm gastrotomies. The balloons are then inflated and pulled up, essentially fastening the anterior gastric wall to the abdominal wall and allowing direct intraluminal access. Upper endoscopy may be used to guide trocar placement and creation of the cystgastrostomy, or a laparoscope can be inserted by means of one of the intragastric trocars. The cystgastrostomy is performed using either a linear stapler or energy and subsequent suturing of the anastomosis. Finally, anterior wall gastrotomies are sutured or stapled closed [7]. The minilaparoscopic technique is a recent refinement of this procedure and involves insertion of 2 mm instruments directly into the gastric lumen by means of endoscopic guidance without the need for pneumoperitoneum. Because of the trocar size limitations, this technique only allows for the use of electrocautery and a minilaparoscopic suturing device for cystgastrostomy creation [7,16,21].

In one of the earliest and largest series to date, Park and Heniford [7] described their experience with various approaches to laparoscopic pancreatic pseudocyst drainage in 29 patients over a period of 5 years. Pseudocysts were approached through an anterior gastrotomy in 11, through the lesser sac in nine. Five patients underwent minilaparoscopy, three cystjejunostomy, and one external drainage. The authors reported one conversion to open due to extensive gastric varices in the minilaparoscopic group and two bleeding complications from cystgastrotomy anastomoses. There were no recurrences or septic complications. Bleeding during laparoscopic cystgastrostomy also has been reported in 11% of patients in a series by Mori and colleagues [22], in which they described outcomes in 18 patients who underwent intragastric cystgastrostomy. Bleeding complications may be avoided by performing smaller anastomoses, but often to the detriment of anastomosis patency. Early closure of the cystgastrostomy has led to recurrence and septic complications in 6% to 13% of patients undergoing anterior approaches [22–24], even when using standard stapling devices and performing 9 cm diameter anastomoses [24]. Over 10% of patients also require conversion, because the pseudocyst either could not be localized or was found to be nonadherent to the posterior gastric wall, despite appropriate preoperative imaging with CT, even when the imaging was reviewed retrospectively [22–24]. To address the technically challenging nature and associated anastomotic complications of laparoscopic transgastric cystgastrostomy, the lesser sac cystgastrostomy technique was developed.

Lesser sac (posterior) cystgastrostomy

The lesser sac, or posterior approach to laparoscopic cystgastrostomy has been described as an alternative technique to pseudocyst drainage, which requires only a single posterior gastrotomy. Furthermore, as opposed to the previously described technique, which requires the pseudocyst to be adherent and have a wide contact surface area with the posterior gastric wall, a successful lesser sac approach only requires the pseudocyst to be in contact with the greater curvature of the stomach [25]. Several authors believe that the posterior approach is technically less demanding, allows for better visualization, may cause less bleeding, and allows for a larger anastomosis, thus presumably decreasing the risk of occlusion and recurrence [7,15,26]. The decision is made based on intraoperative findings. If the lesser sac is accessible and the cyst adherent to the back wall of the stomach, then the posterior approach can be used. Otherwise, the pseudocyst can be accessed through the transverse mesocolon or through an anterior approach as described above.

Port placement is similar to that for the anterior approach. The lesser sac is accessed through the greater omentum, which is divided along the greater curvature of the stomach. Using ultrasonic energy or electrocautery, a posterior wall gastrotomy and cystotomy are created. The two limbs of a linear stapler are inserted within the two lumina, and the stapler is fired, much like a side-to-side enteric anastomosis. The resultant defect is closed with laparoscopic sutures [26,27]. In a study comparing laparoscopic cystgastrostomy performed through either the anterior approach or the lesser sac approach, Barragan and colleagues [15] demonstrated no complications in either group. One patient in the posterior group was converted to the anterior group because of dense adhesions in the lesser sac, a potential limitation to this approach. Similar results showing no complications or recurrences also have been reported by Park and Heniford [7].

Cystjejunostomy

Other alternative approaches include laparoscopic cystjejunostomy, either directly to the jejunum, or to a Roux-Y limb, as first described by Bacca and colleagues [28] and Mouiel and Crafa [29], respectively. In their series of eight patients having undergone the latter procedure, Texeira and colleagues [30] demonstrated no conversions, no septic or bleeding complications, and no residual or recurrent pseudocysts, with a mean follow-up of 2 years. Their technique involves placement of five ports: two 12 mm and three 5 mm ports positioned in an arc in the lower abdomen. Intraoperative laparoscopic ultrasound and needle aspiration are used to confirm adequate localization. Using ultrasonic sheers, the pseudocyst is entered through the transverse mesocolon, and a 3 cm window is created. Following cyst wall biopsy, the biliary is taken. The biliary limb is created by dividing the jejunum 35 cm distal to the ligament of Treitz. It then is anastomosed 50 cm distally, thus creating a 50 cm drainage limb. A 3 cm enterotomy then is created in the Roux limb. The cystjejunostomy is hand sewn as opposed to stapled to allow compensation for pseudocyst wall thickness variability.

Although cystjejunostomies are more technically demanding due to the addition of the entero–enteric anastomosis, they may be preferable in cases in which the pseudocyst is not in close proximity to the stomach. Because there is flexibility in positioning of the Roux limb in relation to the pseudocyst, drainage to the most dependant part of the cyst is made possible [7,30].

Table 1 summarizes complication rates following laparoscopic pseudocyst drainage in series reporting on 10 or more patients. Cumulatively, these studies demonstrate a conversion rate of 10.1% (9/89) of patients, bleeding complications in 6.7% (6/89) of patients, five of whom were in anterior cystgastrostomies, and septic complications in 5.6% (5/89) of patients. Furthermore, 3.4% (2/89) of patients suffered a pseudocyst recurrence, while 4.5% (4/89) required a subsequent procedure. Mortality was 1.1%. These results are very similar if not favorable to what has been reported in the open cystenterostomy literature. Despite the absence of prospective randomized trials, the benefits of laparoscopy over open surgery such as improved pain, length of stay, return to work and regular activities, wound

Table 1
Large series (n ≥ 10) of laparoscopic pancreatic pseudocyst drainage

	n	Conversions	Bleeding complications	Septic complications	Recurrence	Need for second procedure	Mortality
Park [7]	29	1	2	0	0	0	1
Mori et al [22]	18	4	2	1	1	1	0
Hauters et al [23]	17	1	0	2	0	2	0
Hindmarsh et al [24]	15	3	1	1	2	1	0
Davila-Cervantes et al [25]	10	0	1	1	0	1	0
Total	89	9 (10.1%)	6 (6.7%)	5 (5.6%)	3 (3.4%)	4 (4.5%)	1 (1.1%)

Data are presented as absolute number (percentage).

infection, and incisional hernias rates, have been stated clearly in other studies and may hold true for this procedure as well.

Percutaneous pancreatic pseudocyst drainage

With the advent of better imaging techniques and interventional radiology, percutaneous techniques have gained popularity. Although a report as early as 1865 described percutaneous drainage of a posttraumatic pseudocyst [31], it was not until the 1980s that this technique gained acceptance as a primary modality of treatment for pancreatic pseudocysts. In addition to transcutaneous external drainage of pseudocysts, percutaneous transgastric internal drainage is now also being performed.

External drainage

Under ultrasound, CT, or MRI guidance, the anterior wall of the abdomen and the stomach is pierced with a 22-gauge needle, through which a guidewire is introduced. An 8- to 10-gauge percutaneous drainage catheter then is exchanged over the guidewire and introduced into the cavity. Although there are many studies comparing percutaneous and surgical approaches to pancreatic pseudocyst, the data are somewhat difficult to interpret. First, most studies, despite reporting it as a major outcome, fail to define what constitutes treatment failure. Furthermore, and most importantly, most of these studies are retrospective and suffer greatly from selection bias. This is evident in many series that compare percutaneous and surgical outcomes, but in which the indication for percutaneous drainage was pancreatic abscess for high-risk surgical candidates. Furthermore, institutional referral patterns, both for day-to-day patient care and for the choice of treatment modality, also can introduce significant bias [32]. Although the data remain informative, they must be interpreted with caution.

This bias is illustrated in a population based study using the National Inpatient Sample administrative database, in which 8121 patients who had a diagnosis of pancreatic pseudocyst between 1997 and 2001 were drained percutaneously, while 6409 were drained surgically [9]. Patients treated percutaneously suffered more complications, in particular intra-abdominal abscesses and cardiorespiratory complications and had higher mortality rates (6% versus 3%) and longer length of stay (21 versus 15 days). In fact, the percutaneous approach increased the odds of mortality by 1.4-fold, an association that also has been demonstrated by others [33]. Despite the fact that these patients were significantly older and sicker on presentation, when correcting for comorbidity and disease severity, the differences in complications and mortality persisted.

Recent studies of external percutaneous drainage of pancreatic pseudocyst have reported failure rates ranging between 25% to 55%, caused by sepsis, bleeding, recurrence, or the need for a subsequent salvage surgical drainage [34–37]. These results are similar to the 40% to 60% failure rate quoted in earlier reports [10,38], and much higher than what has been reported in the surgical literature. In large comparative retrospective studies, complication rates are also higher, ranging from 50% to 75% with percutaneous treatment and from 19% to 24% with surgery [33,34]. On the other hand, in studies in which both groups of patients were similar in terms of comorbidities and severity of disease, morbidity and mortality were either similar or lower in the percutaneously drained groups. Nevertheless, these patients had higher recurrence rates and suffered complications such as drain tract infections and persistent pancreatico–cutaneous fistulas with drainage of up to 6 weeks, which were not seen in the open surgical groups [6,11,39].

In the only prospective study comparing percutaneous with surgical drainage of pancreatic pseudocyst, the authors found that, in patients with pancreatic abscess who underwent percutaneous drainage as the initial treatment modality, 44% were cured; 44% were palliated, meaning that their clinical condition improved, making them more suitable candidates for definitive surgical drainage, and 9% died. If initially treated surgically, 37% were cured; 44% were palliated, and 19% died. On the other hand, in patients who had noninfected pseudocysts, 93% were cured by surgery, as opposed to 75% cured by percutaneous drainage. The authors concluded that percutaneous drainage was highly effective for initial palliation of a critically ill population with pancreatic abscess, until stabilization occurred, and definitive surgical treatment could be offered [40].

The importance of proper patient selection is emphasized further by authors who believe that better outcomes for percutaneous drainage could be expected with better knowledge of underlying pancreatic pathology and ductal anatomy. In patients who had D'Egidio type 1 pseudocysts (normal duct anatomy and rare communication with the pancreatic duct) [38], 82% were treated successfully with percutaneous drainage. This fell to 60% in patients who had type 2 pseudocysts (diseased pancreatic duct without stricture, but often with a duct–pseudocyst communication). No patients who had type 3 pseudocysts (duct stricture and duct communication) were drained percutaneously because of the assumption that the failure rate would be unacceptably elevated [41]. In addition, Morton and colleagues found that the use of endoscopic retrograde cholangiopancreatography (ERCP) used in the preoperative setting was associated with better outcomes, most likely because it helped determine the most appropriate treatment modality [9,34]. Finally, other studies have demonstrated that 77% to 91% of patients with treatment failures following percutaneous drainage had pancreatic duct strictures or obstruction [34,42].

Internal drainage

Despite the reported success of this technique, internal drainage of pancreatic pseudocysts by percutaneous approaches has been much more popular in Europe than in North America. The technique involves ultrasound or CT-guided puncture of the anterior abdominal wall and anterior gastric wall. Under fluoroscopic or endoscopic guidance, the needle is advanced into the pseudocyst through the posterior gastric wall, then exchanged over a guidewire to a catheter delivery system that allows for the placement of double-J or double-mushroom catheter, usually 5 to 10 French in size, that lies within pseudocyst and gastric lumen. These catheters usually require an additional endoscopic procedure for removal, although some may pass spontaneously. The largest study to date describes this approach in 74 patients with chronic pancreatic pseudocysts. The authors report successful catheter placement in 92% of patients, with an immediate complication rate of only 6%, abscess formation in 11%, and a mortality rate of 1%. Pain resolved or improved in 90% of patients, and weight gain was seen in 80% [43]. Smaller studies have shown equally impressive results, with rates of successful resolution following internal catheter placement between 88% and 100% and septic complications in 12% to 18% of patients [44–47]. Although studies are few, these results seem to compare very favorably with those of surgery.

In conclusion, given the limitations of the literature in this field, the data seem to favor operative over percutaneous approaches when managing pancreatic pseudocyst. With the latter approach, overall morbidity seems to be higher, as are treatment failure rates, with persistent pancreatico–cutaneous fistulas and secondary drain tract or pseudocyst infections commonly seen. Furthermore, this technique does not allow cyst wall biopsy. Nevertheless, there seems to be a role for percutaneous external drainage in patients who have a prohibitive surgical risk and perhaps in patients who have a pancreatic abscess as a temporizing method to allow medical optimization before the definitive procedure. Nevertheless, adequate drainage of a viscous infected peripancreatic tissue is almost always inadequate. Finally, there may be promise for percutaneous internal drainage procedures, although additional studies of this technique are needed. Percutaneous drainage rarely is used in the authors' institution as a primary treatment modality for pseudocysts.

Endoscopic pancreatic pseudocyst drainage

Transenteric

Endoscopic transenteric drainage of pancreatic pseudocysts is performed either as a cystgastrostomy or cystduodenostomy. For this technique to succeed, the pseudocyst must be in close approximation to the enteric wall, so that it causes a visible intraluminal bulge. When the cyst is not found to bulge, which is the case in almost 50% of patients, but is known to be adherent to the organ to which it will be drained, endoscopic ultrasound (EUS) may be used for localization and evaluation of the distance between the two structures, and identification of interposed vessels. Furthermore, the information it provides on cyst wall thickness and presence of necrosis may change the proposed modality of treatment in up to 20% of patients. Fine needle aspiration is used to puncture the pseudocyst at the optimal site, after which contrast is injected to confirm entry into the cyst and further identify its anatomy. An enterotomy and cystotomy then are performed with a diathermy needle knife in that location, and a guidewire is passed into the pseudocyst. A sphincterotome or a 6 to 8 mm balloon can be used to enlarge the opening over the guidewire. One or two 7 to 10 French stents, straight or double pigtail, are inserted into the cyst. These can be left in place for several months or until radiological resolution of the pseudocyst, at which point most must be removed endoscopically [48]. Like percutaneous drainage, cyst wall biopsy is usually not possible using this technique.

In one of the earliest studies with long-term follow-up of endoscopic cystduodenostomy and cystgastrostomy for chronic pancreatitis, Cremer and colleagues [49] reported 97% initial successful drainage, with bleeding or perforation observed in only 6%. Overall recurrence rates were 12%, with 18% of patients eventually requiring some other form of therapy. In a review of series published in the following decade, results were just as good. Successful pseudocyst resolution was seen in 82% to 90% of patients, with recurrences observed in 6% to 18% of patients. Complications were seen on average in 20% of patients, with most being bleeding in 4% to 8% of patients or perforation in up to 8%. Mortality was less than 1%. Additional therapy, most often surgical, for recurrences or complications, was required in an average of 17% of patients [50,51].

In more recent series, despite growing experience with these procedures, outcomes have remained similar. Long-term successful drainage has been reported in 88% to 97% of patients, with recurrence rates varying between 5% and 18%. Presence of necrosis is associated with failure rates of 50% and higher recurrences and more complications [52,53]. The presence of necrotic debris usually can be predicted using EUS, and, given these data, should prompt surgical rather than endoscopic management. Successful endoscopic drainage also seems to depend on pseudocyst location. One study suggests that the more distal a pseudocyst is, the worst the outcome: 94% success when the pseudocyst arose from the head of the pancreas, as opposed to 84% in the body and 77% in the tail [54]. Complications have been reported in 10% to 34% of patients (hemorrhage, perforation, stent migration, and infectious complications), with a mortality of 1%. Finally, 9% to 14% of patients require further surgery because of treatment failure or complications [52,54–56].

Transpapillary

Transpapillary pseudocyst drainage is indicated only when there is a clearly established communication between duct and pseudocyst. This occurs in 60% of cases and is seen most often in the context of chronic rather than acute pancreatitis. The advantages of this technique are that pseudocysts need not be in close proximity or show bulging in the stomach or duodenum, that pseudocyst wall thickness is irrelevant, and that it avoids enterotomies and the associated risk of enteric perforations and vascular injury. The disadvantages are that only one stent may be left in place and that this stent has a reduced diameter compared with the transmural approach. Therefore, for successful transpapillary drainage, the pseudocyst must be minimally loculated, and its contents must be fairly nonviscous and contain little necrotic debris.

With ERCP, the communication between the pancreatic duct and the pseudocyst is confirmed. A guidewire then can be threaded into the pancreatic duct into the pseudocyst or as close to the disruption as possible. Biliary and pancreatic sphincterotomies then are performed and a 5 or 7 French stent is passed over the wire. In the presence of pancreatic duct strictures, these should be dilated before passage of the stent. The stent is usually left in place for 3 months, or until resolution is confirmed on follow-up imaging [57,58].

In recent studies of transpapillary drainage, successful drainage has been reported in 84% to 93% of patients, with recurrence seen in 9% to 20%, and complications, most notably pancreatitis and secondary infection of pseudocyst, reported in 0% to 12% [50,52,54,59].

Overall, endoscopic pancreatic pseudocyst drainage, either by means of the transmural or the transpapillary approach, is associated with excellent outcomes similar to those seen in the surgical literature, but with an improved morbidity profile, which make it an excellent option as a first-line treatment modality.

Proposed approach

Because there exist no randomized trials comparing the different management options for pancreatic pseudocysts, the decision to choose one type of intervention over another often is based on institutional expertise and the treating team's experience and preference. Assuming institutional experience in advanced interventional radiology and endoscopy, and a surgical team facile with laparoscopic pancreatic surgery, the authors propose the following management algorithm based on the data that have been presented.

Faced with a patient who has a pancreatic pseudocyst, initial efforts should be directed toward excluding the possibility of a cystic neoplasm, by history, biochemical, and radiological means. Once done, the decision to drain the pseudocyst must be made based on the patient's symptoms or progression of pseudocyst size. An asymptomatic patient probably should be observed and followed with serial imaging. Symptomatic patients, or patients who have enlarging pseudocysts, should undergo an intervention. Those presenting with sepsis or with evidence of a pancreatic abscess probably should undergo external drainage and debridement by means of an open surgical approach. Alternatively, percutaneous drainage has been reported as an acute intervention, but this usually would not be the authors' first choice.

Patients who have a history or CT suspicious for chronic pancreatitis should undergo ERCP to further characterize the anatomy of the pancreatic duct. Those who have normal ducts and no communication with the pseudocyst (D'Egidio type 1) should be treated similarly to those who have pseudocysts secondary to acute pancreatitis and presumed normal ductal anatomy. In this population, endoscopic cystgastrostomy or cystduodenostomy should be performed with or without EUS guidance. Patients who have D'Egidio type 2 or 3 ducts should undergo endoscopic transpapillary stenting of the duct and pseudocyst. Finally, those patients who have a clear history of chronic pancreatitis and very diseased, dilated ducts may be served better with a longitudinal pancreaticojejunostomy or proximal pancreatectomy/Whipple's resection, especially in the setting of biliary obstruction. Similarly, patients who have proximal pancreatic duct strictures and pseudocysts in the tail of the pancreas should undergo distal pancreatectomy.

Immediate treatment failures or recurrences should be treated surgically. A laparoscopic cystgastrostomy, through the lesser sac approach, should be performed if the lesser sac is accessible, and the pseudocyst is near the greater curvature of the stomach. Otherwise, a laparoscopic anterior approach should be undertaken if the pseudocyst is located more cephalad in a hostile lesser sac. Pseudocysts that bulge into the transverse mesocolon can be accessed from beneath the transverse colon; however, care must be taken to avoid mesenteric vessels. Finally, a distally located pseudocyst should be drained by means of a laparoscopic cystjejunostomy.

The operative management and nonoperative management of pancreatic pseudocyst are evolving, as surgery continues to favor less invasive approaches to disease. Laparoscopic internal pseudocyst drainage has shown equivalent outcomes to open surgery, with probable improved morbidity.

Percutaneous external drainage of pseudocysts is clearly a less effective therapy with a higher risk of recurrence, and this should be reserved for postoperative situations and unusual cases. Finally, endoscopic therapies may be the best overall treatment modality and probably should be considered first-line therapy. Until randomized clinical trials, so far lacking in this field, are published, the optimal management of pancreatic pseudocyst remains debatable, and should remain individualized based on institutional expertise and experience. The authors believe that their suggested approach, based on the currently available data, is safe and most likely to benefit patients suffering from pancreatic pseudocyst.

References

[1] Morgagni JB. De sedibuset causis morborum per anatomen indagatis, vol. 4. Paris; 1821. p. 86–123.
[2] Bradley EL. A clinically based classification system for acute pancreatitis. Summary of the International Symposium on Acute Pancreatitis. Arch Surg 1993;128:586–90.
[3] Bradley EL, Clements JL, Gonzalez AC. The natural history of pancreatic pseudocysts: a unified concept of management. Am J Surg 1979;137(1):135–41.
[4] Vitas GJ, Sarr MG. Selected management of pancreatic pseudocysts: operative versus expectant management. Surgery 1992;111(2):123–30.
[5] Yeo CJ, Bastidas JA, Lynch-Nyhan A, et al. The natural history of pancreatic pseudocysts documented by computed tomography. Surg Gynecol Obstet 1990;170(5):411–7.
[6] Cheruvu CV, Clarke MG, Prentice M, et al. Conservative treatment as an option in the management of pancreatic pseudocyst. Ann R Coll Surg Engl 2003;85(5):313–6.
[7] Park AE, Heniford BT. Therapeutic laparoscopy of the pancreas. Ann Surg 2002;236(2): 149–58.
[8] Gumaste VV, Pitchumoni CS. Pancreatic pseudocyst. Gastroenterologist 1996;4(1):33–43.
[9] Morton JM, Brown A, Galanko JA, et al. A national comparison of surgical versus percutaneous drainage of pancreatic pseudocysts: 1997–2001. J Gastrointest Surg 2005;9(1): 15–20.
[10] Heider R, Meyer AA, Galanko JA, et al. Percutaneous drainage of pancreatic pseudocysts is associated with a higher failure rate than surgical treatment in unselected patients. Ann Surg 1999;229(6):781–7.
[11] Spivak H, Galloway JR, Amerson JR, et al. Management of pancreatic pseudocysts. J Am Coll Surg 1998;186(5):507–11.
[12] Cooperman AM. An overview of pancreatic pseudocysts: the emperor's new clothes revisited. Surg Clin North Am 2001;81(2):391–7.
[13] Obermeyer RJ, Fisher WE, Salameh JR, et al. Laparoscopic pancreatic cystgastrostomy. Surg Laparosc Endosc Percutan Tech 2003;13(4):250–3.
[14] Ramachandran CS, Goel D, Arora V, et al. Gastroscopic-assisted laparoscopic cystgastrostomy in the management of pseudocysts of the pancreas. Surg Laparosc Endosc Percutan Tech 2002;12(6):433–6.
[15] Barragan B, Love L, Wachtel M, et al. A comparison of anterior and posterior approaches for the surgical treatment of pancreatic pseudocyst using laparoscopic cystgastrostomy. J Laparoendosc Adv Surg Tech A 2005;15(6):596–600.
[16] Heniford BT, Iannitti DA, Paton BL, et al. Minilaparoscopic transgastric cystgastrostomy. Am J Surg 2006;192(2):248–51.
[17] Petelin JB, Renner P. Laparoscopic pancreatic pseudocyst gastrostomy. Surg Endosc 1994; 8:448.

[18] Frantzides CT, Ludwig KA, Redlich PN. Laparoscopic management of a pancreatic pseudocyst. J Laparoendosc Surg 1994;4:55–9.

[19] Way LW, Legha P, Mori T. Laparoscopic pancreatic cystgastrostomy: the first operation in the new field of intraluminal laparoscopic surgery. Surg Endosc 1994;8:235.

[20] Gagner M. Laparoscopic transgastric cystgastrostomy for pancreatic pseudocyst. Surg Endosc 1994;8:239.

[21] Libby ED, Taylor J, Mysh D, et al. Combined laparoendoscopic cystgastrostomy. Gastrointest Endosc 1999;50(3):416–9.

[22] Mori I, Abe N, Sugiyama M, et al. Laparoscopic pancreatic cystgastrostomy. J Hepatobiliary Pancreat Surg 2002;9(5):548–54.

[23] Hauters P, Weerts J, Navez B, et al. Laparoscopic treatment of pancreatic pseudocysts. Surg Endosc 2004;18:1645–8.

[24] Hindmarsh A, Lewis MP, Rhodes M. Stapled laparoscopic cystgastrostomy. Surg Endosc 2005;19(1):143–7.

[25] Dávila-Cervantes A, Gómez F, Chan C, et al. Laparoscopic drainage of pancreatic pseudocysts. Surg Endosc 2004;18:1420–6.

[26] Park AE, Schwartz R. Laparoscopic pancreatic surgery. Am J Surg 1999;177:158–63.

[27] Roth JS, Park AE. Laparoscopic pancreatic cystgastrostomy: the lesser sac technique. Surg Laparosc Endosc Percutan Tech 2001;11(3):201–3.

[28] Baca I, Klempa I, Gotzen V. Laparoscopic pancreato–cystojejunostomy without entero–entero anastomosis. Chirurg 1994;65:378–81.

[29] Mouiel J, Crafa F. Pancreatic cyst treated by laparoscopic cysto–jejunal anastomosis on a Roux-en-Y loop. Surg Endosc 1995;9:625.

[30] Texeira J, Gibbs KE, Vaimakis S, et al. Laparoscopic Roux-en-Y pancreatic cyst–jejunostomy. Surg Endosc 2003;17(12):1910–3.

[31] LeDentu M. Rapport sur l'observation précédente. Bulletins de la Société Anatomique de Paris 1865;10:197–213.

[32] Nealon WH, Walser E. Surgical management of complications associated with percutaneous and/or endoscopic management of pseudocyst of the pancreas. Ann Surg 2005;241(6): 948–57.

[33] Soliani P, Franzini C, Ziegler S, et al. Pancreatic pseudocysts following acute pancreatitis: risk factors influencing therapeutic outcomes. Journal of the Pancreas 2004;5(5):338–47.

[34] Nealon WH, Walser E. Main pancreatic ductal anatomy can direct choice of modality for treating pancreatic pseudocysts (surgery versus percutaneous drainage). Ann Surg 2002; 235(6):751–8.

[35] Will U, Wegener C, Graf KI, et al. Differential treatment and early outcome in the interventional endoscopic management of pancreatic pseudocysts in 27 patients. World J Gastroenterol 2006;12(26):4175–8.

[36] Kariniemi J, Sequeiros RB, Ojala R, et al. Feasibility of MR imaging—guided percutaneous drainage of pancreatic fluid collections. J Vasc Interv Radiol 2006;17:1321–6.

[37] Andersson B, Nilsson E, Willner J, et al. Treatment and outcome in pancreatic pseudocysts. Scand J Gastroenterol 2006;41(6):751–6.

[38] D'Egidio A, Schein M. Pancreatic pseudocysts: a proposed classification and its management implications. Br J Surg 1991;78(8):981–4.

[39] Adams DB, Anderson MC. Percutaneous catheter drainage compared with internal drainage in the management of pancreatic pseudocyst. Ann Surg 1992;215(6):571–6.

[40] Lang EK, Paolini RM, Pottmeyer A. The efficacy of palliative and definitive percutaneous versus surgical drainage of pancreatic abscesses and pseudocysts: a prospective study of 85 patients. South Med J 1991;84(1):55–64.

[41] Zhang A-B, Zheng S-S. Treatment of pancreatic pseudocysts in line with D'Egidio's classification. World J Gastroenterol 2005;11(5):729–32.

[42] Adams DB, Srinivasan A. Failure of percutaneous catheter drainage of pancreatic pseudocyst. Am Surg 2000;66(3):256–61.

[43] Henriksen FW, Hancke S. Percutaneous cystogastrostomy for chronic pancreatic pseudo-cyst. Br J Surg 1994;81(10):1525–8.

[44] Cox MR, Davies RP, Bowyer RC, et al. Percutaneous cystogastrostomy for treatment of pancreatic pseudocysts. Aust N Z J Surg 1993;63(9):693–8.

[45] Davies RP, Cox MR, Wilson TG, et al. Percutaneous cystogastrostomy with a new catheter for drainage of pancreatic pseudocysts and fluid collections. Cardiovasc Intervent Radiol 1996;19(2):128–31.

[46] Sacks D, Robinson ML. Transgastric percutaneous drainage of pancreatic pseudocysts. AJR Am J Roentgenol 1988;151(2):303–6.

[47] Sacks BA, Greenberg JJ, Porter DH, et al. An internalized double-J catheter for percutane-ous transgastric cystogastrostomy. AJR Am J Roentgenol 1989;152(3):523–6.

[48] Giovanni M. Endoscopic ultrasound-guided pancreatic pseudocyst drainage. Gastrointest Endosc Clin N Am 2006;15:179–88.

[49] Cremer M, Deviere J, Engelholm L. Endoscopic management of cysts and pseudocysts in chronic pancreatitis: long-term follow-up after 7 years of experience. Gastrointest Endosc 1989;35(1):1–9.

[50] Beckingham IJ, Krige JE, Bornman PC, et al. Endoscopic management of pancreatic pseu-docysts. Br J Surg 1997;84:1638–45.

[51] Lo SK, Rowe A. Endoscopic management of pancreatic pseudocysts. Gastroenterologist 1997;5(1):10–25.

[52] Hookey LC, Debroux S, Delhaye M, et al. Endoscopic drainage of pancreatic fluid collec-tions in 116 patients: a comparison of etiologies, drainage techniques, and outcomes. Gastro-intest Endosc 2006;63(4):635–43.

[53] Baron TH, Harewood GC, Morgan DE, et al. Outcome differences after endoscopic drain-age of pancreatic necrosis, acute pancreatic pseudocysts, and chronic pancreatic pseudo-cysts. Gastrointest Endosc 2002;56(1):7–17.

[54] Weckman L, Kylänpää M-L, Puolakkainen P, et al. Endoscopic treatment of pancreatic pseudocysts. Surg Endosc 2006;20:603–7.

[55] Lopes CV, Pesenti C, Bories E, et al. Endoscopic ultrasound-guided endoscopic transmural drainage of pancreatic pseudocysts and abscesses. Scand J Gastroenterol 2007;42(4):524–9.

[56] Kahaleh M, Shami VM, Conaway MR, et al. Endoscopic ultrasound drainage of pancreatic pseudocyst: a prospective comparison with conventional endoscopic drainage. Endoscopy 2006;38(4):355–9.

[57] Pitchumoni CS, Agarwal N. Pancreatic pseudocysts. When and how should drainage be per-formed? Gastroenterol Clin North Am 1999;28(3):615–39.

[58] Vidyarthi G, Steinberg SE. Endoscopic management of pancreatic pseudocysts. Surg Clin North Am 2001;81(2):405–10.

[59] De Palma GD, Galloro G, Puzziello A, et al. Endoscopic drainage of pancreatic pseudocysts: a long-term follow-up study of 49 patients. Hepatogastroenterology 2002;49(46):1113–5.

ELSEVIER
SAUNDERS

SURGICAL
CLINICS OF
NORTH AMERICA

Surg Clin N Am 87 (2007) 1461–1475

Resectional Therapy for Chronic Pancreatitis

Ronald F. Martin, MD[a,b,*], Michael D. Marion, MD[a]

[a]*Department of Surgery, Marshfield Clinic and Saint Joseph's Hospital,
1000 North Oak Avenue, Marshfield, WI 54449, USA*
[b]*Department of Surgery, H4/785 Clinical Science Center, University of Wisconsin School
of Medicine and Public Health, 600 Highland Avenue, Madison, WI 53792, USA*

Eat when you can, sleep when you can and don't operate on the pancreas. That was the advice often repeated when the senior author of this manuscript was in early medical training. Since then we have developed a national obesity epidemic, the 80-hour work week has been established for residency training (although not yet for staff work weeks), and a large number of preeminent surgeons have made their careers by mainly operating on the pancreas. This article describes the current state of affairs for resectional therapy for chronic inflammatory conditions of the pancreas.

To understand which operation might benefit the patient who has chronic pancreatitis we must first consider the problems that such a patient might encounter. The pancreas, nestled in its retroperitoneal location, is an organ that when functioning properly, as is the case for most of us, goes about its business without fanfare or attention. The properly functioning pancreas secretes digestive enzymes by way of a ductal system and produces and secretes hormones that predominantly regulate metabolism. Anatomically the pancreas is intimately associated with the duodenum, the extrahepatic bile duct, and the major splanchnic vessels. When the pancreas is acutely inflamed patients can experience anything form mild viral-like symptoms to life-threatening illness complicated by profound metabolic disturbance and major organ failure. Patients who have chronic inflammation of the pancreas can also suffer life-ending complications, yet most present with less imminently threatening problems along the course of their disease.

The main indication for operation in the management of chronic pancreatitis is medically intractable pain. Other indications include biliary or

---

* Corresponding author. Department of Surgery, Marshfield Clinic and Saint Joseph's Hospital, 1000 North Oak Avenue, Marshfield, WI 54449.
E-mail address: martin.ronald@marshfieldclinic.org (R.F. Martin).

pancreatic ductal obstruction (with or without pseudocyst formation), mass effect impinging on other organs or adversely affecting their function, or diagnostic insecurity regarding the possibility of periampullary or pancreatic neoplasms.

Pathogenesis of chronic pancreatitis

The pathogenesis and genetic predispositions to chronic pancreatitis are well described elsewhere in this issue. Some fundamental review is essential here, however.

The hallmark of chronic pancreatitis is the replacement of normal pancreatic tissue with fibrotic tissue. This change leads to mass formation, ductal obstruction, encasement of other structures, or some combination of the above [1]. The mechanism by which fibrosis takes place is incompletely understood but several advances have been made in the last several years.

Ethanol is believed to largely contribute to the development of chronic pancreatitis [2], although many people over-consume ethanol and do not develop chronic pancreatitis and a sizable percentage of patients who develop chronic pancreatitis have not over-consumed ethanol. There seems to be a direct toxic effect on the pancreas by ethanol or perhaps its metabolites. Ethanol seems to stimulate pancreatic stellate cells (PSCs) through its metabolite acetaldehyde. PSCs are the cells that regulate extracellular matrix proteins within the pancreas and are also primarily responsible for collagen deposition within the gland. PSCs also respond to and produce various cytokines that can result in a self-sustaining cycle of inflammation and fibrosis [3]. Pancreatic stone protein (PSP), or lithostathine, is also affected by ethanol and may be over- or underproduced in patients who have chronic pancreatitis. The role of PSP is to stabilize inorganic ion complexes and to prevent precipitation of calcium carbonate [4]. Alterations in PSP production can lead to protein plugs or pancreatic duct stones, which in turn can lead to ductal obstruction, intraductal and parenchymal hypertension, and subsequent continued cellular and organ damage.

The most likely explanation for why some patients develop pancreatitis and others do not with similar exposure risk is that some patients are born with or develop a genetic predisposition and fall ill to a multi-hit–type process. Several genetic aberrancies have been well implicated in chronic pancreatitis; PRSS1, SPINK1, and CFTR are most notable among them. PRSS1 is involved in trypsin metabolism and regulation of the conversion of pro-pancreatic enzymes to their active form [5]. SPINK1 inhibits intrapancreatic trypsin function to help prevent autodigestion [6]. The cystic fibrosis transcription repair (CFTR) gene is an essential gene for the proper regulation of pancreatic fluid, calcium, and bicarbonate secretion [5]. Regulation of bicarbonate also affects the inactive versus active form of trypsin. The net effect of all these processes is chronic injury to the parenchyma of the pancreas with subsequent fibrosis and collagen deposition. Although this accounts, at least in part, for the mass effect in found in some patients and for intraductal and glandular hypertension, it may not completely explain why some patients have pain syndromes and others do not.

The pathogenesis of pain is almost certainly linked in some degree to the above-mentioned processes, yet some patients who have chronic pancreatitis have no demonstrable mass effect and no evidence of ductal obstruction. Bockman and colleagues [7] have shown that in patients who have undergone resection histologic changes are seen in the nerves within the pancreas. There is an increased mean diameter of the nerves and altered structure to the nerve sheath. Neurotransmitters, including substance P, neuropeptide YY, and calcitonin gene-related peptide (CGRP), are also shown to be overexpressed [8]. This overexpression creates an environment for overstimulation of the local pain-sensing apparatus and a potential humoral component for pain sensation in the setting of chronic pancreatitis.

Based on review of the above data one could construct a series of mechanical solutions that could possibly alleviate pain or other symptoms in these patients. Operations that remove mass, decrease intraductal pressure, denervate the pancreas, or combine some of the above features while trying to maintain as much normal pancreatic endocrine and exocrine function as possible would be perfectly rational to consider. The remainder of this article addresses the successes and failures of these operations.

The operations

The types of operations that one would consider to offer a patient who has symptomatic chronic pancreatitis fall into three broad categories: cytoreduction, ductal decompression, and denervation. The operations that yield cytoreduction include pancreatic head resection with or without concomitant resection of the duodenum, distal pancreatectomy of varying amounts up to and including total pancreatectomy, and segmental central pancreatectomy. Operations designed for ductal decompression include pancreaticoenteric anastomosis (longitudinal pancreaticojejunostomy, end-to-side pancreaticojejunostomy, pancreaticogastrostomy), sphincteroplasty, and various internalized pseudocyst drainage procedures. Denervation procedures include chemical or mechanical splanchnicectomy and total pancreatic resection with autotransplantation. The autotransplantation group is further subdivided into those patients who undergo whole or partial intact organ autotransplantation or islet cell–only autotransplantation. Although this last group undergoes denervation by default, it is inaccurate to say that the sole strategy in this operation is denervation.

As practice patterns have evolved and clinical proficiency has increased with pancreatic resection, there has been a trend away from decompressive procedures alone toward resections or operations that combine resection with decompression [9]. For the purposes of this article we concentrate the discussion on operations that include resection as a major part of their procedure. Operations designed for decompression or denervation only are covered less extensively.

Choice of operation

In surgery if one expects good results from operations one must choose the right operation for the patient and perform it correctly. Dr. Kenneth Warren reported in 1959 [10] that operations for chronic pancreatitis failed when they were not chosen on the basis of pathology observed at the time of operation. He also stated that not all operations were successful all the time. These statements hold true today. The statements of Dr. Warren are even more remarkable if one takes into consideration that at the time of his report there were no CT scanners, MRI scanners, flexible fiberoptic endoscopes, or laparoscopes. All one really had to work with was laparotomy and intraoperative cholangiopancreatography.

The trends in choice of operation for chronic pancreatitis have not solely been based on better capacity to match the operation with the pathology discovered in the patient but also with the global level of comfort with the operations being offered. Despite a fairly consistent pattern of glandular involvement with inflammatory changes, the pattern of operative choice over time has been, roughly: decompressive procedures, distal resections, pancreaticoduodenectomy with or without pylorus preservation, duodenum-sparing pancreas resection with or without associated drainage procedures, total or completion pancreatectomy associated with autotransplantation or islet cell transplantation, and laparoscopic pancreatic resection. The common theme in this progression is that each step generally requires greater technical sophistication on the part of the surgical team (one could argue that about pancreatic head resection with or without duodenal preservation—they are both fairly technically demanding). Furthermore, if one looks at the time frame over which these operations were developed there was a general decrease in the mortality of the more complicated procedures. Also during that period a decrease in the number of surgeons performing these procedures with an increase in volume of cases per surgeon was noted [11]. Our discussion of these operations begins with the distal pancreatic resections and progress along the historical timeline.

Distal pancreatectomy

Distal pancreatectomy became the early mainstay of resective therapy for chronic pancreatitis, yet it is probably the operative procedure for complications of chronic pancreatitis that is most difficult to evaluate because of reporting trends and evolution of clinical knowledge during its period of highest use. Many of the reports that describe distal pancreatectomy predate or overlap with the availability of axial imaging and endoscopic retrograde cholangiopancreatography. Consequently, comparing series of patients can be extremely difficult because preoperative conditions or indications are widely variable. Which operations constitute a distal pancreatectomy also varies. In a report by Sawyer and Frey, distal pancreatectomy is defined as a resection of 50% to 90% of the pancreas [12].

The basic premise of distal pancreatectomy follows Warren's suggestion that the resection should match the findings at operation. This premise is confirmed in a review by Schoenberg and colleagues [13]. In their series they report that distal pancreatectomy had favorable results when compared with conservative treatment. The main indications for operation in this group of patients included pain (97.2%), corpus/cauda tumor (56.8%), pseudocysts (54.1%), suspicion of malignoma (sic) (24.3%), main pancreatic ductal stenosis (25.7%), and a collection of less frequently observed indications. The results of their series showed that 80% of patients in the late postoperative phase had little or no pain. Endocrine insufficiency was believed to be hastened or overtly caused in 20% of patients who underwent resection. Despite a nearly 45% postoperative complication rate, the conclusions they reached support the use of distal pancreatectomy while espousing the caveat of Sawyer and Frey that the procedure "is only indicated if the inflammatory disease and complications resulting from inflammation in this region are localized on the left side of the gland" [12].

Rattner and colleagues [14] reported in their series from Massachusetts General Hospital that even when preoperative imaging suggested disease confined to the tail of the pancreas and evidence of a midpancreatic ductal stricture that distal pancreatectomy seldom provided sustained relief. Fifteen percent of their patients were found to have unsuspected pancreatic carcinoma and 35% of their patients experienced significant perioperative complications. In 14 of their 20 patients there were clearly identified transition zones between normal- and abnormal-appearing pancreas at time of laparotomy. Despite this only 9 of these 14 patients had sustained pain relief postoperatively. They were able to identify a subset of patients who uniformly did well with distal resection: those who had pseudocysts confined to the tail. Whether this group of patients represented those who had commonly found pseudocysts or disconnected pancreatic tail syndrome (DPTS) is not speculated on by the authors. Our experience with patients who have DPTS confirms their observations that distal resection generally produces good outcomes in this subset of patients [15].

Splenic preservation

The spleen is rarely directly involved in patients who have chronic pancreatitis. In one large series of patients followed prospectively splenic complications secondary to chronic pancreatitis were reported to in 2.2% of nearly 500 patients [16]. These complications were more likely to be associated with splenic vein thrombosis and significant pancreatic tail pathology, such as necrosis or pseudocyst. The role of splenic preservation at the time of pancreatic resection is widely favored by most authors [13,16,17]. The reasons generally given are the usual, in that immune protection against encapsulated bacterial organisms is preserved along with the spleen's hematologic functions. One report By Govil and Imrie [18] suggests that splenic preservation while performing pancreatectomy may delay the subsequent onset of diabetes mellitus. This assertion has met with some criticism and it has been suggested that a more likely explanation for this observation may be a lesser resection of pancreatic mass or that patients in whom splenic preservation is technically feasible may have a less severe form of inflammatory disease [19].

Although the phenomenon of post-splenectomy infection syndrome is well recognized it has been a rare occurrence in the experience of the authors. In patients in whom there is evidence of splenic vein thrombosis or compromise, sinistral portal hypertension, or technical inability to preserve the splenic vasculature, we would agree with others in recommending the concomitant removal of the spleen without hesitation [12,14].

Pancreaticoduodenectomy

Traverso and Longmire reported their technique of pylorus-preserving pancreaticoduodenectomy (PPPD) in 1978 [20]. Of note is that they issued a caveat that this procedure should not be used for malignancy. Interestingly, since then it has become the most widely accepted form of treatment of periampullary neoplasm also. The intellectual basis for the shift in resection of the distal pancreas to that of the pancreatic head was the concept of the "pain pacemaker" being located in the head of the pancreas promulgated by Dr Longmire. The other root event that may have helped shift the emphasis in type of resection was the growing number of reports of large series of pancreatic head resections without mortality beginning with Dr John Howard's report of 41 consecutive patients undergoing pancreaticoduodenectomy without mortality in 1968 [21]. Other events, such as improved intensive care, the ability to use mechanical ventilation outside of an operating suite, and total parenteral nutrition, all provided a better safety net with which to try out more challenging operations, although alone they certainly did not account for the greater successes encountered.

The senior author of this paper and colleagues presented a report on 45 patients who underwent pancreaticoduodenectomy for chronic pancreatitis with a mean follow-up of more than 5 years and as long as 15 years [22]. In our series a substantial reduction in patient-reported pain scores was identified within 6 months. At 1 year following operation no patient required daily narcotic. Also, in our series those patients who had undergone pylorus preservation (some had undergone previous antrectomy for unrelated reasons) had regained more of their lost preoperative weight than those who had associated hemigastrectomy. This finding of improved weight gain in patients who had preservation of the pylorus compared with those who had antrectomy was also found in a prospective series reported by Kozuschek and colleagues [23].

Concerns raised by those who favor standard Whipple (pancreaticoduodenectomy with hemigastrectomy or Kausch-Whipple) include delayed gastric emptying and marginal ulceration. In one report from Traverso, 14% of patients undergoing PPPD had evidence of delayed gastric emptying [24]. These identified patients all had associated perigastric fluid collections and responded to drainage of these collections. In the Lahey Clinic series we did not find delayed gastric emptying to be a significant problem.

Serum gastrin and gastric acid secretion have been shown to be reduced in patients undergoing standard Whipple operations but remain normal in patients who undergo PPPD compared with non-operated control patients, thus making PPPD a relatively more ulcerogenic operation [25]. In the Lahey Clinic series we reported an 11% occurrence of marginal ulceration for which one patient required operation for hemorrhage. Since then we have modified our technique from one of predominantly external drainage of the pancreaticojejunal anastomosis to one of internalized drainage with a significant reduction in marginal ulceration to about 4% with no need for reoperation (R.F. Martin, unpublished data). This change would correlate with the presumed benefit of maintaining intraluminal bicarbonate flow to neutralize the normal gastric acid secretion at the duodenojejunostomy. Proponents of PPPD also cite the benefits of preserving the antropyloric mechanism in controlled emptying from the stomach of solids and liquids, which may improve fat absorption [26] and glucose tolerance [27].

For pain relief, preservation of endocrine and exocrine function, and global complications PPPD and standard Whipple resection are generally regarded as fairly equivalent procedures. For reconstruction, pancreaticojejunostomies of various types and pancreaticogastrostomy have all been shown to be effective. The best choice of operation in the authors' opinion is whichever procedure and reconstruction the surgeon is most comfortable with. Our preference is PPPD with end-to-side two-layered duct-to-mucosa pancreaticojejunostomy.

Duodenum-preserving resection of the head of the pancreas

Kümmerle opined that when resecting the pancreas one should resect "as much as necessary—and as little as possible" [28]. The duodenum-preserving resection of the head of the pancreas (DPRHP), or Beger procedure, was introduced in 1972, well before Kümmerle's admonition, yet it fairly well typifies the concept [29]. Based in part on the concept of Long-mire's pain pacemaker being located within the head of the pancreas the operation is designed to remove the inflammatory mass in the pancreatic head without requiring the interruption in continuity of the alimentary tract at the level of the duodenum or disrupting the biliary tract. The operation has gained traction throughout the world but certainly has been largely championed by Dr. Beger and Dr. Büchler.

Büchler and colleagues [30] reported a randomized series of patients in two groups of 20 who underwent either DPRHP or PPPD. The groups were compared for mortality, serum glucose, insulin production, glucagon production, postoperative pain, and quality of life. Mortality was found to be equal (zero) in each group. Glucose tolerance and insulin production were significantly better preserved in the DPRHP group compared with the PPPD group and glucagon production was not significantly different between the groups. Of particular interest was that the 6-month data for recurrent pain showed that 33% of the PPPD group had recurrent pain compared with only 6% of the DPRHP group. Although fascinating, this is somewhat hard to explain based on theory, because one would not expect that a lesser resection of the pancreas should yield improved pain result unless the pain were caused by some other postoperative event, such as an unrecognized complication of altered gut motility or perhaps impaired biliary flow.

In an excellent review of trials reported by Schäefer and colleagues [11], the evidence-based ranking of reports of pancreaticoduodenectomy has been listed. As one can gather from a brief review of the data there is a scarcity of true "head-to-head" trials of one operation versus the next, although there are some. The two prospective comparative studies of pancreaticoduodenectomy versus DPRHP are the above-mentioned study by Büchler and colleagues [30] and one by Evans in which the group undergoing the DPRHP operation had twice as many patients, 60% versus 30%, developing new-onset diabetes [31]. Numerous other studies comparing DPRHP versus the Frey operation (DPRHP plus longitudinal pancreaticojejunostomy, see later discussion) are also listed. In general, one could conclude that each series in which the authors focus on the operation with which they are most comfortable their best results are achieved—and for that matter results are comparable between best series from different authors. In those series in which a group of authors adopts a comparative operation with which they are perhaps less familiar, the adopted operation tends to come up short in the comparison. It is a hard point to prove scientifically, but even harder not to read between the lines.

The Frey procedure

Frey and Smith reported in 1987 the description and rationale for a new operation for chronic pancreatitis [32]. Technically the operation was a combination of two older operations and incorporated the concepts of the DPRHP with an extended longitudinal pancreaticojejunostomy (ELPJ) for complete main pancreatic ductal decompression. Conceptually this operation would address two of our above-mentioned culprits in generating ongoing pain and glandular injury: cytoreduction for the inflammatory mass and ductal decompression to address intraductal and intraglandular hypertension. One might also predict that this operation would be unlikely to perform significantly better than Beger DPRHP unless there was coexistent segmental structuring of the main pancreatic duct or unless the patient developed an anastomotic stricture postoperatively as a mechanism for recurrence of pain.

In one large randomized trial of DPRHP versus the Frey procedure, Izbicki and colleagues [33] reported a nearly 9-year follow-up of 74 patients. There was no significant difference demonstrated in short- or long-term mortality, quality of life, pain scores, or endocrine or exocrine insufficiency. Di Izbicki concluded that the choice of operation should be left to the choice of the surgeon doing the procedure.

Pancreatectomy with autotransplantation

The presence of pan-pancreatic chronic inflammatory involvement without significant ductal dilatation presents a challenging situation in which consideration of total pancreatectomy may be reasonable. Total or near-total pancreatectomy would achieve the goal of denervation but would create an apancreatic state that may be difficult to control. Two solutions present themselves for this dilemma: segmental organ pancreatic autotransplantation and pancreatectomy with islet cell autotransplantation. The respective operations introduced in the late 1970s each have benefits and drawbacks.

In segmental organ transplantation the organ is implanted with its own blood supply and cellular support system obviating the need for complex islet cell preparation. The obvious drawback of this approach is that the technical challenges of successfully restoring blood flow and drainage to the organ are daunting and the inflammatory process for which we are operating in the first place can continue and progressively destroy the remaining islet cell mass. Rossi, who has reported a significant fraction of the known cases, has outlined the technical evolution of the operation and its benefits and risk [34]. Over the years there has been a progression to internal enteric drainage, and there is now early consideration of this technique before stepwise pancreatic resection removes potentially viable islet cell mass. His group further recommends careful patient selection for this type of operation.

Since the early 1970s, work in the laboratory showed transplanting islet cells was safe and often effective in preventing insulin dependence. Using the canine model described by Mirkovich and Campiche, the group at the University of Minnesota demonstrated technical feasibility in performing the first human intraportal autotransplant [35]. Current models for digestion and isolation of pancreatic islets share basic principles based on techniques put forth by Ricordi and colleagues [36,37]: The whole excised pancreatic tissue is distended by way of intraductal instillation of a solution containing collagenase; afterward mechanical mincing of the material occurs and the islets cells are separated by centrifugation. Finally, the islet cells are grafted by way of direct injection into the portal system with the hope of implantation and viability in hepatic venous sinusoids.

Successful autotransplantation of islet cells, which is variably defined, has been less than anticipated to this point. Although the initial patient in the University of Minnesota report was rendered insulin-independent for the remainder of her life (6 years), complete insulin independence in patients who have total or near-total pancreatectomy and autologous islet cell transplantation for chronic pancreatitis currently ranges from 13% to 60% with a follow-up of up to 10 years [38–43]. More consistently, patients who have surgically induced diabetes and islet cell autotransplantation have shown, at least initially, lower daily insulin requirements, lower serum HbA1c levels, and fewer episodes of hypoglycemia or ketoacidosis, and their diabetes is generally considered easier to manage [40,44–46].

Greater insulin independence coincides with increasing the yield of islets available at the end of excising, digesting, and purifying the pancreatic tissue. The ideal ratio of insulin equivalents transfused to kilograms body weight (IEQ/kg) has yet to be determined, although recent studies suggest more than 2500 to 6635 IEQ/kg may be required [38,39,47,48]. These data suggest patients who have increased BMI are less likely to benefit from islet transplantation [38]. In addition, it has been shown that islet isolation was compromised in pancreata with extensive calcification and fibrosis, lowering the IEQ [39,41–44,49–51]. Ahmad and colleagues [38] and others [47] showed that when patients had undergone a Peustow-type procedure, there was a negative impact on islet yield because they were unable to distend the pancreatic duct with collagenase material at processing. Rodriguez and colleagues [39] found that patients who underwent total pancreatectomy as the initial procedure had higher IEQ/kg compared with patients who had completion pancreatectomy. Earlier intervention (resection when the pancreas is less diseased or fibrosed and before any number of resective/drainage procedures are done) has thus been proposed to increase the IEQ.

Preoperative pancreatic endocrine function has also been shown to affect the durability of transplant results. The likelihood of successful islet cell autotransplantation is decreased in patients who have diabetes mellitus or even impaired glucose tolerance before surgery. Assuming a less-diseased pancreas would have nearer normal endocrine function, assaying its function may well be predictive of those patients who have higher likelihood of successful transplantation [37,43,44,48,50,51].

Other developments that have been recommended for greater success in islet cell autotransplant include reducing cold ischemia time with efficient islet cell processing at experienced centers, reducing warm ischemia time by technically preserving blood supply to the pancreas as long as possible, using improved collagenase solutions, purifying islet cells before transplantation, and immediate postoperative tight insulin control to avoid toxic affects of glucose to islet cells [37,38,42,43].

Early attempts at autologous islet transplantation were plagued with life-threatening complications, such as portal hypertension, portal vein thrombosis, hepatic infarction, disseminated intravascular coagulopathy, and systemic hypotension [44,46,51]. Through technical advances, current literature argues the procedure adds little to the peri- and postoperative morbidity or mortality of patients undergoing pancreatic resection for benign disease [39–41,49].

The balance of pain relief and difficult-to-control diabetes remains delicate in patients undergoing extensive pancreatectomy for chronic pancreatitis. Although no guarantee of insulin independence can be given at this time, some centers are showing clear advantages in islet cell autotransplantation with little, if any, addition to morbidity. The decision to attempt autotransplantation should occur only after a thorough discussion of realistic outcomes with the patient.

Laparoscopic pancreatic resection

Minimally invasive techniques deserve some mention, although their adoption has been limited. Gagner and Pomp [52] reported in 1993 a successfully completed laparoscopic PPPD. The operation, performed on a cachectic 45-kg woman who had pancreas divisum, was reported to have taken 10 hours and was completed successfully. The patient's postoperative course was complicated by delayed gastric emptying and a marginal anastomotic ulcer; both complications are well documented in the open experience. The authors concluded that although the operation was technically feasible, the benefit of the laparoscopic approach "may not be as apparent as that of a less-complex laparoscopic procedure" [52]. Other studies have certainly described minimally invasive success with operation for benign and neoplastic pancreatic diseases [53]. Although there may be a slight benefit in highly selected patients for left-sided or limited pancreatic resection there does not seem to be a demonstrable benefit for patients who have disease in the pancreatic head.

Other considerations

There are several considerations that are not particular to one specific type of operation. Significantly increased perioperative mortality and morbidity is seen in patients who have major vascular involvement who undergo resections of all types, including pancreaticoduodenectomy, DPRHP, distal pancreatectomy, and total pancreatectomy [54]. Arterial and venous major vascular involvement are noted in this series. These authors recommend following patients closely preoperatively who are at risk for developing major vascular involvement.

The role of preoperative biliary stenting remains contentious with varying views expressed. We personally have not had adverse outcomes that we can attribute to preoperative biliary stenting. In a review of preoperative pancreatic ductal stenting Schellendorfer and colleagues [55] describe a threefold increase in perioperative complications, which they attribute to possible stent failure, stent-related perforation, or colonization of the stent.

The role of perioperative somatostatin analog in preventing complications following pancreatic resection has been assessed. In one multicenter trial from Europe there was a demonstrated significant reduction in complication rates in the somatostatin analog–treated group compared with the placebo group [56]. The study was criticized for its high complication rates in treatment and control arms and its results have not been reliably reproduced.

Summary

Chronic pancreatitis is a disease process that most likely results from a combination of inherited or acquired genetic predispositions coupled with glandular injury secondary to ingested compounds such as ethanol, prior mechanical injury, or injury secondary to other significant illness. The disease process creates fibrosis, which yields mass effect and obstructs ductal drainage. Chronic inflammatory changes results in pain syndromes caused by directly injuring nerves and through humoral release of pain neurotransmitters. Ductal obstruction causes conditions to persist that provide a positive feedback loop for continued glandular injury.

Despite early observations that operative management should be targeted to match the pathology found, it has taken decades for a slow but indisputable shift in management. Recognition that the inflammatory consequences throughout the gland are rarely homogenous and that the degree of ductal obstruction is variable have led to differing strategies for resection that maintain the similar goals of removing as much abnormal pancreas as possible while retaining as much normal pancreas, at least endocrine pancreas, as possible. Advances in technical capability and patient care, partially derived from operations designed to approach pancreatic and periampullary malignancies, gradually gave surgeons the confidence to progress from decompressive procedures to progressively larger distal resections to pancreatic head resection. Higher-than-desired morbidity with pancreatic head resection led to the development of DPRHP and the Frey procedure, both of which tried to focus on the removal of the pain pacemaker without unnecessary resection of associated innocent organs. The alternative strategy of larger distal pancreatic resection with either segmental or islet transplantation developed along a similar time course as a means to preserve islet cell mass while mitigating the deleterious effect of the inflamed gland on its surrounding structures. While these alternatives to pancreatic head resection were being developed, success in pancreatic head resection was growing rapidly and mortality and morbidity from these procedures was declining.

To a large extent all of the above-mentioned operations work well in many cases and rarely, if ever, work well in all cases, which, in the authors' opinion, is exactly what one would predict based on our knowledge of the structural and physiologic characteristics of the disease. Any approach the surgeon chooses to use requires an appropriate evaluation of the patient, proper selection of procedure, and excellent technical execution of the operation. For most patients the correct procedure to choose is the one with which the surgeon is most comfortable and proficient. The trick is to realize when a patient is not like "most patients" and, consequently, to avoid trying to make that patient fit your operation.

References

[1] Ammann RW, Akovbiantz A, Largiader F, et al. Course and outcome of chronic pancreatitis. Longitudinal study of a mixed medical-surgical series of 245 patients. Gastroenterology 1984;86(5 Pt 1):820–8.

[2] Levy P, Mathurin P, Roqueplo A, et al. A multidimensional case-control study of dietary, alcohol, and tobacco habits in alcoholic men with chronic pancreatitits. Pancreas 1995;10:231–8.

[3] Apte MV, Wilson JS. Stellate cell activation in alcoholic pancreatitis. Pancreas 2003;27:316–20.

[4] Bernard JP, Adrich Z, Montalto G, et al. Inhibition of nucleation and crystal growth of calcium carbonate by human lithostathine. Gastroenterology 1992;103:1277–84.

[5] Witt H, Apte MV, Keim V, et al. Chronic pancreatitis: Challenges and advances in pathogenesis, genetics, diagnosis and therapy. Gastroenterology 2007;132:1557–73.

[6] Chandak GR, Idris MM, Reddy DN, et al. Absence of PRSS1 mutations and association of SPINK1 trypsin inhibitor mutations in hereditary and non-hereditary chronic pancreatitis. Gut 2004;53(5):723–8.

[7] Bockman DE, Buchler M, Malfertheiner P, et al. Analysis of nerves in chronic pancreatitis. Gastroenterology 1988;94:1459–69.

[8] Buchler M, Weihe E, Friess H, et al. Changes in peptidergic innervation in chronic pancreatitis. Pancreas 1992;7:183–92.

[9] Sakorafas GH, Sarr MG. Changing trends in operations for chronic pancreatitis: a 22-year experience. Eur J Surg 2000;166(8):633–7.

[10] Warren KW. Pathological considerations as a guide to the choice of surgical procedures in the management of chronic relapsing pancreatitis. Gastroenterolgy 1959;36:224–31.

[11] Schafer M, Mullhaupt B, Clavien PA. Evidence-based pancreatic head resection for pancreatic cancer and chronic pancreatitis. Ann Surg 2002;236(2):137–48.

[12] Sawyer R, Frey CF. Is there still a role for distal pancreatectomy in surgery for chronic pancreatitis? Am J Surg 1994;168(1):6–9.

[13] Schoenberg MH, Schlosser W, Ruck W, et al. Distal pancreatectomy in chronic pancreatitis. Dig Surg 1999;16(2):130–6.

[14] Rattner DW, Fernandez-del Castillo C, Warshaw AL. Pitfalls of distal pancreatectomy for relief of pain in chronic pancreatitis. Am J Surg 1996;171(1):142–5 [discussion 145–6].

[15] Lawrence C, Howell DA, Stefan AM, et al. Disconnected pancreatic tail syndrome: potential for endoscopic therapy and results of long-term follow-up. Gastrointest Endosc 2007;63(6): 804–7.

[16] Malka D, Hammel P, Levy P, et al. Splenic complications in chronic pancreatitis: prevalence and risk factors in a medical-surgical series of 500 patients. Br J Surg 1998;85(12):1645–9.

[17] Beger HG, Buchler M. Duodenum-preserving resection of the head of the pancreas in chronic pancreatitis with inflammatory mass in the head. World J Surg 1990;14(1):83–7.

[18] Govil S, Imrie CW. Value of splenic preservation during distal pancreatectomy for chronic pancreatitis. Br J Surg 1999;86:895–8.

[19] White SA, Sutton CD, Berry DP, et al. Value of splenic preservation during distal pancreatectomy for chronic pancreatitis. Br J Surg 2000;87(1):124.

[20] Traverso LW, Longmire WP. Preservation of the pylorus during pancreatectomy. Surg Gynecol Obstet 1978;146:959–62.

[21] Howard JM. Pancreaticoduodenectomy: forty-one consecutive Whipple resections without an operative mortality. Ann Surg 1968;168:629–40.

[22] Martin RF, Rossi RL, Leslie KA. Long-term results of pylorus-preserving pancreatoduodenectomy for chronic pancreatitis. Arch Surg 1996;131(3):247–52.

[23] Kozuschek W, Reith HB, Waleczek H, et al. A comparison of long term results of the standard Whipple procedure and the pylorus-preserving pancreatoduodenectomy. J Am Coll Surg 1994;178:443–58.

[24] Traverso LW, Kozarek RA. The Whipple procedure for severe complications of chronic pancreatitis. Arch Surg 1993;128:1047–53.

[25] Pearlman NW, Steigman GV, Ahnen DJ, et al. Acid and gastrin levels following pyloric-preserving pancreaticoduodenectomy. Arch Surg 1986;121:661–4.

[26] Doty JE, Meyer JH. Vagotomy and antrectomy impairs absorption of fat from solid, but not liquid dietary sources (abstract). Gastroenterolgy 1987;97(5 pt 2):1374.

[27] Hongo M, Satake K, Sanoyama K, et al. Regulation of insulin demand by gastric emptying in diabetics (abstract). Gastroenterolgy 1987;97(5 pt 2):1440.

[28] Kümmerle F. Chronische pankreatitis. Dtsch Med Wochenschr 1977;102:543–7.

[29] Beger HG, Krautzberger W, Bittner R, et al. Duodenum-preserving resection of the head of the pancreas in patients with severe chronic pancreatitis. Surgery 1985;97(4):467–73.

[30] Buchler MW, Friess H, Muller MW, et al. Randomized trial of duodenum-preserving pancreatic head resection versus pylorus-preserving Whipple in chronic pancreatitis. Am J Surg 1995;169(1):65–9 [discussion 69–70].

[31] Evans JD, Wilson PG, Carver C, et al. Outcome of surgery for chronic pancreatitis. Br J Surg 1997;84:624–9.

[32] Frey CF, Smith G. Description and rationale of a new operation for chronic pancreatitis. Pancreas 1987;2:701–7.

[33] Strate T, Taherpour Z, Bloechle C, et al. Long-term follow-up of a randomized trial comparing the Beger and Frey procedures for patients suffering from chronic pancreatitis. Ann Surg 2005;241(4):591–8.

[34] Watkins JG, Krebs A, Rossi RL. Pancreatic autotransplantation in chronic pancreatitis. World J Surg 2003;27(11):1235–40.

[35] Sutherland DER, Matas AJ, Najarian JS. Pancreatic islet cell transplantation. Surg Clin North Am 1978;58:365–82.

[36] Ricordi C, Lacy PE, Scharp DW. Automated islet isolation from human pancreas. Diabetes 1989;38:140–2.

[37] Morrison CP, Wemyss-Holden SA, Dennison AR, et al. Islet yield remains a problem in islet autotransplantation. Arch Surg 2002;137(1):80–3.

[38] Ahmad SA, Lowy AM, Wray CJ, et al. Factors associated with insulin and narcotic independence after islet autotransplantation in patients with severe chronic pancreatitis. J Am Coll Surg 2005;201(5):680–7.

[39] Rodriguez Rilo HL, Ahmad SA, D'Alessio D, et al. Total pancreatectomy and autologous islet cell transplantation as a means to treat severe chronic pancreatitis. J Gastrointest Surg 2003;7(8):978–89.

[40] White SA, Davies JE, Pollard C, et al. Pancreas resection and islet autotransplantation for end-stage chronic pancreatitis. Ann Surg 2001;233(3):423–31.

[41] Berney T, Rudisuhli T, Oberholzer J, et al. Long-term metabolic results after pancreatic resection for severe chronic pancreatitis. Arch Surg 2000;135(9):1106–11.

[42] Rabkin JM, Olyaei AJ, Orloff SL, et al. Distant processing of pancreas islets for autotransplantation following total pancreatectomy. Am J Surg 1999;177(5):423–7.

[43] Wahoff DC, Papalois BE, Najarian JS, et al. Autologous islet transplantation to prevent diabetes after pancreatic resection. Ann Surg 1995;222(4):562–75 [discussion 575–9].

[44] Morrow CE, Cohen JI, Sutherland DE, et al. Chronic pancreatitis: long-term surgical results of pancreatic duct drainage, pancreatic resection, and near-total pancreatectomy and islet autotransplantation. Surgery 1984;96(4):608–16.

[45] Toledo-Pereyra LH. Islet cell autotransplantation after subtotal pancreatectomy. Arch Surg 1983;118(7).851–8.

[46] Najarian JS, Sutherland DE, Baumgartner D, et al. Total or near total pancreatectomy and islet autotransplantation for treatment of chronic pancreatitis. Ann Surg 1980;192(4): 526–42.

[47] Gruessner RW, Sutherland DE, Dunn DL, et al. Transplant options for patients undergoing total pancreatectomy for chronic pancreatitis. J Am Coll Surg 2004;198(4):559–67 [discussion 568–9].

[48] Panaro F, Testa G, Bogetti D, et al. Auto-islet transplantation after pancreatectomy. Expert Opin Biol Ther 2003;3:207–14.

[49] Farney AC, Najarian JS, Nakhleh RE, et al. Autotransplantation of dispersed pancreatic islet tissue combined with total or near-total pancreatectomy for treatment of chronic pancreatitis. Surgery 1991;110(2):427–37 [discussion 437–9].

[50] Traverso LW, Abou-Zamzam AM, Longmire WP Jr. Human pancreatic cell autotransplantation following total pancreatectomy. Ann Surg 1981;193(2):191 5.

[51] Cameron JL, Mehigan DG, Harrington DP, et al. Metabolic studies following intrahepatic autotransplantation of pancreatic islet grafts. Surgery 1980;87(4):397–400.

[52] Gagner M, Pomp A. Laparoscopic pylorus-preserving pancreatoduodenectomy. Surg Endosc 1994;8(5):408–10.

[53] Cuschieri A, Jakimowicz JJ, van Spreeuwel J. Laparoscopic distal 70% pancreatectomy and splenectomy for chronic pancreatitis. Ann Surg 1996;223(3):280–5.

[54] Alexakis N, Sutton R, Raraty M, et al. Major resection for chronic pancreatitis in patients with vascular involvement is associated with increased postoperative mortality. Br J Surg 2004;91(8):1020–6.

[55] Schnelldorfer T, Lewin DN, Adams DB. Do preoperative pancreatic stents increase operative morbidity for chronic pancreatitis? Hepatogastroenterology 2005;52(66):1878–82.

[56] Buchler M, Friess H, Klempa I, et al. Role of octreotide in the prevention of postoperative complications following pancreatic resection. Am J Surg 1992;163(1):125–30 [discussion 130–1].

ELSEVIER
SAUNDERS

SURGICAL
CLINICS OF
NORTH AMERICA

Surg Clin N Am 87 (2007) 1477–1501

The Role of Total Pancreatectomy and Islet Autotransplantation for Chronic Pancreatitis

Juan J. Blondet, MD[a], Annelisa M. Carlson, MD[b],
Takashi Kobayashi, MD[b], Tun Jie, MD[b],
Melena Bellin, MD[c], Bernhard J. Hering, MD[b],
Martin L. Freeman, MD[d], Greg J. Beilman, MD[a],
David E.R. Sutherland, MD, PhD[b],*

[a]Division of Surgical Critical Care/Trauma, Department of Surgery, University of Minnesota,
MMC 11, 420 Delaware Street Southeast, Minneapolis, MN 55455, USA
[b]Division of Transplantation, Department of Surgery, University of Minnesota, MMC 280,
420 Delaware Street Southeast, Minneapolis, MN 55455, USA
[c]Division of Pediatric Endocrinology, Department of Pediatrics, University of Minnesota,
MMC 404, 420 Delaware Street Southeast, Minneapolis, MN 55455, USA
[d]Department of Medicine, University of Minnesota, MMC 36, 420 Delaware Street,
Minneapolis, MN 55455, USA

Total pancreatectomy (TP) or near-total pancreatectomy with islet auto-transplantation (IAT) to treat chronic pancreatitis (CP) first was done in 1977 at the University of Minnesota (UMN) and described in *Surgical Clinics of North America* [1]. The idea evolved from a desire to compare metabolic outcomes between islet autografts in pancreatectomized individuals, who could not reject their graft, and islet allografts done to treat type 1 diabetes, to understand why the latter failed (was it for technical or immunologic reasons?) [2]. The main rationale from the beginning, however, was to relieve the pain of CP in patients in whom other measures had failed and, to preserve beta (β)-cell mass and insulin secretory capacity, to prevent or minimize the otherwise inevitable surgical diabetes [3].

Although IATs have been done with pancreatic resections for premalignant neoplasias, and for acute relapsing pancreatitis (ARP) before evolution to CP occurs, the major application of TP-IAT has been in patients who

* Corresponding author.
E-mail address: dsuther@umn.edu (D.E.R. Sutherland).

0039-6109/07/$ - see front matter. Published by Elsevier Inc.
doi:10.1016/j.suc.2007.08.014   *surgical.theclinics.com*

have CP and intractable pain [4]. TP, even with IAT, may appear to be a radical treatment, but for the CP patients in whom it is done, the alternative is even more radical: persistent pain and/or lifetime narcotic use. Thus, an appreciation of the spectrum of the disease, the possible lack of correlation between imaging or gross pathology results and the degree of pain, and the various mechanisms by which CP causes pain are relevant for patient selection and interpretation of outcomes in the TP-IAT series reviewed here.

Brief review of chronic pancreatitis and treatment options

CP is characterized by progressive, irreversible damage to the pancreas, with varying degrees of inflammation, fibrosis, ductal alteration, exocrine atrophy, and secondary involvement of the islets of Langerhans. The clinical manifestations also vary as to the degree of pain, maldigestion from loss of exocrine function, and occurrence of diabetes. Although lost exocrine function can be managed with oral pancreatic enzyme supplements, and diabetes, if it occurs, with insulin, the hallmark of CP is pain, often intractable and debilitating. Pain is the main symptom toward which therapies are directed, all with significant failure rates.

The acute and chronic forms of pancreatitis are not totally distinguishable. They have overlapping risk factors and share a common pathogenetic origin as a pancreatic autodigestive process. Additionally, they each may manifest as an initial episode of abdominal pain, with elevation of serum amylase and lipase, and with similar nonspecific inflammatory changes. CP is likely the result of progressive pancreatic damage after recurrent episodes of pancreatic necroinflammation. The sentinel acute pancreatitis event (SAPE) hypothesis, introduced by Schneider and Whitcomb [5], postulates that the sentinel event is a pancreatic injury that makes the gland particularly vulnerable, in the recovery phase, to additional insults such as alcohol, metabolic, and oxidative stresses. ARP may evolve to CP; patients who are initially pain free between episodes may begin to have underlying interval pain and may cease having episodes altogether. Even one episode of acute pancreatitis may be followed by evolution to CP, or CP may occur without a history of an identifiable episode of acute pancreatitis. Whatever the trigger, progression of CP to end-stage fibrosis occurs at different rates in different people, and can be caused by different mechanisms [6].

Traditionally, alcohol abuse has been thought to be the cause of most cases of CP, but this perception may not be correct. Indeed, in the TP-IAT group at UMN, only 16% of the cases of CP were attributed to alcohol, and 60% were idiopathic [7]; in the series at the University of Cincinnati, only 4% of the cases of CP were attributed to alcohol [8]. Cigarette smoking is also a major risk factor for CP [9,10]. Well-defined inherited germline mutations also can cause CP in families [11]. Hereditary pancreatitis once was thought to be rare, diagnosed only when other family members are affected. The identification of PRSS1, SPINK1, and CFTR mutations in patients with so-called idiopathic CP, however, indicates that genetic risk factors are much more common than originally envisioned [12]. These mutations have both autosomal-dominant and recessive patterns of inheritance with variable penetration and may be influenced by certain modifier genes and environmental factors. The discovery of SPINK1 mutations in various types of CP, such as tropical calcific, alcoholic, and autoimmune pancreatitis, blurs the borders between the particular CP subtypes [12–14]. Other risk factors for CP include biliary lithiasis, anatomical variants like annular pancreas or divisum, hypertriglyceridemia, hypercalcemia, sphincter of Oddi dysfunction, and trauma [7,8,12]. The key histopathologic features of CP, regardless of the etiology, are varying degrees and combinations of pancreatic fibrosis, acinar atrophy, acute and chronic inflammation, and distorted or blocked ducts.

The diagnosis of CP is based mainly on symptoms, imaging studies, and supporting laboratory tests. In certain patients, the diagnosis can be surprisingly difficult, especially in those who have early or mild small-duct or minimal-change variants [15,16]. Serum amylase and lipase levels typically are elevated during attacks early on but might be normal in later phases with progressive destruction of the gland. Imaging studies include CT, endoscopic retrograde cholangiopancreatography (ERCP) (which is associated with a risk of precipitating pancreatitis), magnetic resonance cholangiopancreatography (MRCP), and endoscopic ultrasound (EUS) [17]. Although all of the studies can detect ductal and textural abnormalities, the specificity and sensitivity of each in diagnosing CP are not defined well, given the difficulty of obtaining histopathologic correlation.

The treatment of patients who have CP is focused on mitigating their unrelenting or recurring abdominal pain. Patients who imbibe alcohol or smoke should stop. Pancreatic enzyme supplementation may help. Nonnarcotic analgesics should be tried first, but many need narcotic analgesics; patient comfort takes precedence over concerns of addiction [18–20]. Some patients need escalating doses, with the addition of fentanyl patches or even parenteral administration. Celiac ganglion blocks, percutaneous or endoscopic, can be tried but rarely give permanent pain relief, if any at all, and transient responses often cannot be repeated [21]. Patients who require narcotic analgesics, with or without complete relief, are candidates for invasive procedures in an attempt to remove or modify the root cause of the pain. The general progression is from the least to the most invasive procedure, depending on the response.

Pain in CP occurs with or without ductal obstruction. When obstruction, increased intraductal pressure, or a dilated duct can be demonstrated, efforts should be made to relieve the obstruction. If pain persists or recurs, then the next step is pancreatic resection. Because previous surgical drainage procedures (Puestow or Berger) compromise islet yield if a subsequent TP-IAT is done [7], the current UMN paradigm is to do any indicated drainage procedures endoscopically only. Then, if the endoscopic drainage is unsuccessful, the authors proceed to resection rather than surgical drainage. Although two randomized trials of highly selected subgroups of patients who had severe CP cases showed that primary surgical drainage had a better chance of relieving pain than endoscopic drainage [22,23], most gastroenterologists, because it is minimally invasive, advocate an initial trial of endoscopic therapy in an attempt to relieve pain in patients who have a dilated duct, stricture, or pancreatic stones [24]. If endoscopic drainage fails, there is little evidence that surgical drainage will be successful in relieving pain. As primary therapy, each approach has a relatively high failure rate; pain persisted in 68% of patients who had endoscopic and 25% who had surgical drainage in the study by Cahen and colleagues [23]. Even in those who have initial relief following either endoscopic or surgical drainage, it may not be sustained longer than 5 years.

The ideal CP candidates for endoscopic drainage procedures have a focal proximal stricture associated with upstream dilation of the pancreatic duct, or relatively small burden of main pancreatic duct stones that is amenable to extraction with or without extracorporeal shock wave lithotripsy, or a pseudocyst. Endoscopic therapy most often is successful in patients who have moderate disease. Successful treatment of strictures requires aggressive therapy, with repeated dilations and stenting in hope that the stricture resolves. There is wide variability in expertise, aggressiveness, and conceptual approaches to endoscopic therapy, which may influence outcomes [19,24]. Although the complication rate of endoscopic therapy is relatively low, acute episodes of pancreatitis can occur after sphincterotomy and stent placement, and in some patients, the underlying pain becomes worse; such patients are prime candidates for resection, including TP-IAT.

Pancreas resection is indicated in CP patients who have small-duct disease or those in whom endoscopic drainage fail. A TP is the most likely operation to relieve pain, and for CP patients who are already diabetic, there is little reason not to do it. For nondiabetic CP patients, a TP-IAT reduces but does not eliminate the risk of surgical diabetes. Thus, a case can be made for partial resection (usually a Whipple operation, but a distal pancreatectomy for the rare case with a mid-duct stricture and CP of the body and tail only). If pain is not relieved by a partial resection, a completion pancreatectomy with IAT can be done subsequently.

Patients tend to be referred for resection late in the course of CP, often with a pain history of years, and many opt for TP rather than a partial resection, wanting the best chance at pain relief without the risk of reoperation. TP-IAT done early in the course of CP avoids the complications of chronic narcotic use and gives the best chance at a high islet yield to prevent or minimize postpancreatectomy diabetes.

The authors' experience indicates that TP with preservation of β-cell mass by immediate isolation and intraportal transplantation of islets from the excised pancreas should be considered as a primary surgical option for patients who have painful CP refractory to less invasive procedures. The main criterion for success of the islet autograft per se is whether insulin independence is maintained or surgical diabetes made milder. The overall outcome, however, depends as much on the clinical response as on the metabolic results, specifically whether the patient's pain is reduced or eliminated, narcotic analgesics withdrawn, and the quality of life (QOL) improved.

Historical context

The first patient in the UMN series (and the world) to undergo an IAT after pancreatectomy [1], in 1977, remained insulin-independent and pain-free until she died 6 years later [25]. This case proved that a viable islet preparation could be made from a freshly excised human pancreas. It also showed that the previous failures with islet allografts were caused either by low viability or poor preservation of deceased donor pancreases, or rejection [26].

As of early 2007, the UMN IAT experience includes more than 200 cases, and the outcomes of the first two thirds have been published [1–3,7,25–35]. Shortly after the initial reports on IATs from the UMN nearly 30 years ago [1], several other centers worldwide began to do the same. To date, at least 20 centers are known to have done IAT, nearly all by embolization of the isolated islets to the liver by means of the portal vein (Fig. 1). The world

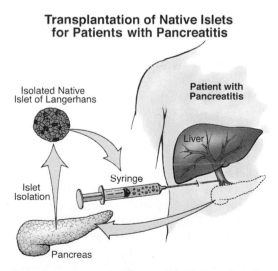

**Transplantation of Native Islets
for Patients with Pancreatitis**

Isolated Native
Islet of Langerhans

Patient with
Pancreatitis

Liver

Islet
Isolation

Syringe

Pancreas

Fig. 1. Sequence of events to preserve β-cell mass in patients undergoing a total pancreatectomy for benign disease. The resected pancreas is dispersed by collagenase digestion followed by islet isolation. Autologous islets then are embolized to the patient's liver by means of the portal vein.

literature as of 2006 contains reports of about 300 IATs, including the UMN cases cited previously and those done elsewhere [8,36–45]. After UMN, the next largest series are at the University of Cincinnati (nearly 100), the University of Leicester (more than 40), and the University of Geneva (more than 20).

For historical completeness, segmental pancreatic autotransplantation is mentioned as another method for preserving β-cell mass after pancreatic resection [46–48]. The first such case was done around the time of the first IAT [46]. This approach appears to have been used less frequently than IAT; indeed, no reports have appeared in the literature on segmental pancreas autotransplants for the past decade.

Patient selection and pain syndrome

The severity of the gross morphologic changes associated with pancreatitis, as detected by imaging studies, do not correlate necessarily with the degree of pain the patient is experiencing [49,50]. Minimal change CP was first described by Walsh and colleagues [15] in patients who had severe abdominal pain with minimal gross morphologic changes but clear histopathologic changes in the gland, with resolution of pain in most patients following pancreatectomy. Layer and colleagues [16] also described two forms of CP: early-onset CP, where pain precedes by years the development of gross pathologic changes, and late-onset CP, where gross changes are already detectable by the time the patient has pain. These two articles were published before the EUS era.

Ideally, EUS should allow minimal change CP to be detected, but because it is standard to require that five of the nine features tested for on EUS (hyperechoic parenchymal foci, strands, hypoechoic lobules, cysts, main duct irregularity, ductal dilation, hyperechoic duct walls, visible side branches, and calcifications or stones) be present for a diagnosis of CP to be made to avoid overcalling [50], the minimal change variety may be present but not diagnosed. In 15 patients of the authors' series in which recent EUS findings could be correlated with pancreatic histopathology following resection (CP confirmed in all), seven had minimal change CP with only mild fibrosis. Five had fewer than EUS criteria for CP, yet all had inflammation present (including one with no features of CP detected on EUS) [51]. Further support for the contention that the current criteria, designed to prevent overdiagnosing CP on EUS [50], may underdiagnose comes from Chong and colleagues [52] at the Medical University of South Carolina. They found that a threshold of three criteria gave the best balance between sensitivity (83%) and specificity (80%) for correlation of EUS findings with histological CP. Thus, patients who have an abdominal pain syndrome who have any one of the nine features consistent with CP on EUS may indeed have the disease, probably in the minimal change category. The authors know of no report in the literature that correlates the severity of pain and the morphologic findings of radiologic or pathologic studies.

The pain of pancreatitis is multifactorial [53–55]. Even when there is increased ductal pressure, it is not necessarily the cause of the pain [56], and pain in patients who have CP exists in the absence of increased ductal pressure. Indeed microscopic pathology with intrinsic neuritis had the best correlation in at least one study [53]. Some patients have increased sensitivity to pain of central origin, perhaps explaining the symptoms in minimal-change CP [57].

Thus, at UMN, the authors do TP-IAT in CP patients who have intractable pain, whether the gross morphologic changes detected in the pancreas are minimal or severe. It is almost always worth an attempt at islet isolation, because having even a small β-cell mass is better than having none. Occasionally, and especially in CP patients who already have impaired glucose tolerance, the pancreas is such a small atrophic rock that the authors make a decision not to go to the expense and effort of an islet isolation that is almost certain to be ultra-low.

Patients who have ARP are also candidates for TP-IAT if their episodes are frequent, disruptive, and persist over time, even if they are pain-free between episodes. Evolution of ARP into CP, where elevated levels of serum amylase and lipase cease but pain persists, is common and often misunderstood as meaning the pain is other than pancreatic. In nondiabetic patients requiring narcotics for their pain who have a history of ARP associated with even minimal criteria for CP on imaging studies, the authors recommend TP-IAT [32].

Some patients who have CP have diabetes when referred for surgical consultation. In such patients, the decision for resection is easy, especially when exocrine deficiency also exists. Most patients, however, are seen when diabetes does not exist, and thus a TP must be undertaken with the acceptance of diabetes as a tradeoff for pain relief and for the chance to discontinue narcotics. If an IAT prevents diabetes, it is a bonus. When a TP is done for CP in a nondiabetic patient, however, an IAT to preserve β-cell mass should be done whenever possible.

Surgical resection considerations

During TP, the blood supply to the pancreas should be preserved as long as possible to minimize the detrimental effects of warm ischemia on the islets [27,58,59]. To do so, never separate the distal pancreas from the splenic vessels. If the splenic vessels are ligated in the hilum, the spleen may survive on its collateral vessels, but usually it has to be taken. When the spleen is spared, there is a risk of variceal formation in the gastric veins draining the spleen leading to late intestinal bleeding, or splenomegaly that can be painful, so the authors leave it only if retains an absolutely normal appearance after hilar ligation.

At UMN, early IAT series included cases with the entire duodenum preserved (95% pancreatectomy), but the complication rate was actually lower in patients who had part of the duodenum or the entire duodenum resected [25]. For the past 15 years, the authors have done a pylorus- and fourth portion-sparing partial duodenectomy when possible, with orthotopic reconstruction by means of duodenostomy and choledochoduodenostomy (Fig. 2).

Metabolic considerations

In patients who have painful CP referred for resection, baseline metabolic studies to assess β-cell function include fasting and postprandial glucose, baseline and stimulated C-peptide, and glycosylated hemoglobin levels. Patients who have CP often have symptoms of exocrine insufficiency (steatorrhea), but formal evaluation usually is not done. IAT candidates are counseled that exocrine deficiency may be made worse or induced by TP.

Although the authors sometimes try to spare the proximal and distal duodenum during TP, data from the bariatric literature suggest that there may be a metabolic benefit of duodenectomy. GLP-1, produced by L cells in the distal intestinal tract is a powerful incretin. Patients who have a Roux-en-Y gastric bypass have increased levels of GLP-1 with improvement in diabetes, results not seen after restrictive bariatric procedures [60,61]. It is possible that complete duodenectomy at the time of TP would increase GLP-1 levels and mirror the positive impact on insulin sensitivity seen in the bariatric duodenal bypass patients, allowing a reduced islet mass to sustain insulin independence.

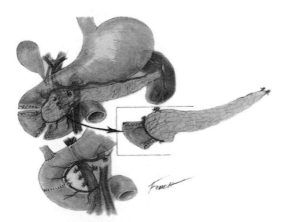

Fig. 2. Surgical technique for total pancreatectomy. Total pancreatectomy and pylorus- and distal-sparing duodenectomy with orthotopic reconstruction by means of duodenostomy and choledochoduodenostomy. (*Adapted from* Farney AC, Najarian JS, Nakhleh RE, et al. Auto-transplantation of dispersed pancreatic islet tissue combined with total or near-total pancreatectomy for treatment of chronic pancreatitis. Surgery 1991;110(2):427–37 [discussion: 437–9]; with permission. Copyright © 1991, Elsevier.)

Islet isolation and infusion considerations

In the United States, islet isolation must be done in a laboratory that meets all of the US Food and Drug Administration (FDA) criteria for processed tissue. Only a few medical centers currently have such a laboratory.

After resection, the pancreatic duct is cannulated, and the pancreas is dispersed by collagenase digestion, using the modified Ricordi technique [34,35]. At UMN, the authors do not purify preparations with a low tissue volume to maximize the islet yield [62]. If the crude tissue digest exceeds 15 mL, the authors usually reduce the volume by purifying all or part of the islet preparation, so that embolization to the liver occurs without any undue rise in portal pressure [63,64]. If portal pressure reaches 20 to 30 cm of water, the residual preparation can be dispersed freely in the peritoneal cavity or transplanted beneath the kidney capsule, or submucosal layer of the stomach, in the hope that the islets engraft [28,65]. The authors' current preference is to purify islets so that the tissue volume is reduced to an amount tolerated by the portal vein, without any undue rise in pressure, but not to the degree that a large number of islets have to be discarded or placed in alternative sites. Sometimes the authors do not purify a high-volume digest, because a high percentage of the islets are mantled by, or not cleaved from, a surrounding rim of exocrine tissue, and we will lose most by purification.

Clinical observations and animal studies indicate that the liver (by means of the portal vein) is the most efficient site for islet engraftment [28,66,67]. Other sites used, such as the renal capsule [68–71], spleen [67,72], omentum [73], and peritoneal cavity [74,75] rarely have been associated with function of islet autografts in people [76,77]. At any site, the islets initially survive by nutrient diffusion; during this period, they have reduced functional capacity, with function improving once neovascularization occurs [78,79].

To prevent intraportal clotting from the tissue thromboplastin (present in the islet preparation) [80], the authors have administered heparin since their first cases in the 1970s [2,28]. Nearly all of the reports of complications related to portal infusion of islets [80–83] were published before the standardized semiautomated pancreas dispersion techniques and before the routine use of heparinization at all centers.

In islet allograft recipients, one study by Doppler ultrasound showed a 4% incidence of radiologically detected but clinically insignificant portal vein thrombosis [63]. In the authors' IAT series, portal vein thrombosis occasionally is detected on ultrasound, but not as a clinical entity. The authors always administer heparin before islet infusion and continue the infusion for a few days if the closing portal pressures are high. Liver function tests typically show a transient rise in serum enzyme levels during the early postoperative period [35], with no implication for future hepatic dysfunction.

Intra- and postoperative considerations

The authors maintain euglycemia by an insulin drip during and after the pancreatectomy and IAT [84]. Animal studies have shown a decrease in islet engraftment with hyperglycemia; furthermore, glucose toxicity may cause dysfunction and structural lesions in the transplanted islets [85–88]. The authors promote islet engraftment by an exogenous insulin drip to maintain euglycemia, minimizing insulin secretory demand from the freshly infused islets. A transition to subcutaneous insulin is made when the patient begins to eat, with the dose again adjusted to maintain euglycemia; insulin gradually is withdrawn in patients who can achieve euglycemia without it.

Expanding application

IATs have been done after resection for benign pancreatic processes, including pancreatic pseudocysts [43], cystic neoplasms [89,90], insulinomas [90,91], and a neuroendocrine tumor [90]. In each case, pathologic evaluation was completed before the IAT to confirm that the lesions were benign.

In the UMN series, IATs have been done at the time of distal pancreatectomy for benign cystic tumors in five patients (unpublished observation). In these cases, the authors are uncertain how well the intrahepatic islets are functioning, because those in the native pancreatic remnant also are functioning. The authors' series also includes a few CP patients whose IATs were done after only a distal pancreatectomy, with the head remaining. When a completion pancreatectomy was later done, diabetes was prevented, indicating good engraftment at the initial IAT (unpublished observation).

An IAT also has been reported in a patient with pancreatic adenocarcinoma who had a Whipple operation complicated by an anastomotic leak at the pancreaticojejunostomy. The leak was treated by an urgent completion pancreatectomy with an IAT [92]. The risk of doing an IAT when a completion pancreatectomy is done because of a technical complication of a Whipple procedure cannot be calculated from one case, but conceptually the procedure is valid, because the judgment must be that the distal pancreas was tumor-free by leaving it in (otherwise a Whipple operation would not have been done). A case also could be made for doing a TP-IAT, even in situations where a Whipple otherwise would suffice, but where a TP would be safer by avoiding an enteric anastomosis to a soft pancreas that has a higher than average leakage or breakdown probability.

Transplants of islets isolated from pancreas allografts excised for technical problems or allograft pancreatitis (islet auto-allografts) also have been performed, with one case published by the authors [93]. This patient remained insulin-independent for more than 1 year while on immunosuppression, but ultimately needed exogenous insulin from decline or loss of islet function for immunologic or nonimmunologic reasons. Additionally, most of the other islet auto-allografts have had limited duration of function (unpublished observation).

Islet autotransplantation in children

CP is less common in children than in adults, but should be treated with the same aim: to relieve pain, eliminate the need for narcotics, and preserve β-cell mass. As of December 2006, the authors performed 25 IATs in children; the youngest was 5 years old. The authors reported their first pediatric case in detail [94]. In a subsequent report of their initial cases, the authors had a 50% rate of insulin independence [32]. In the authors' most recent long-term follow-up of 18 pediatric patients, more than 60% had discontinued narcotics, with a 78% rate of full or partial islet function and a 54% rate of insulin independence at 1 year [95].

Literature review

The largest series published to date on patients undergoing pancreatectomy and IAT have come from UMN [1–3,7,25,27,28,32,34,35], the University of Cincinnati [8,37], and the University of Leicester [43–45]. Reports have focused on metabolic outcomes, QOL, and pain reduction.

Insulin independence

The ability to achieve insulin independence after IATs appears to correlate directly with the islet equivalents (IEs) infused. IEs serve as an indirect measurement of β-cell mass, but there is much overlap, in that a small percentage of patients receiving less than 2000 IE/kg will become insulin-independent, while some receiving more than 5000 IE/kg will not [7,8]. The authors have shown that islet yields are poorest in patients who have prior pancreatic resections (distal pancreatectomies or surgical drainage procedures such as the Puestow procedure) [34,96]. In addition, fewer islets are recovered as pathologic fibrosis increases [28,34]. The timing of the procedure has a direct impact on islet yield. Maximal islet yield and insulin independence may be attained more easily if the IAT is performed earlier in the disease course, as recently reported by the Cincinnati group [18,37].

University of Minnesota series

In the authors' 1995 report [28], the lowest islet yields were in patients who had a prior Puestow procedure, with only an 18% rate of insulin independence in this group, in contrast to 71% in patients without a prior resection or drainage procedure. In a later update of the UMN series, at a time when the authors were much more likely to treat even mild hyperglycemia, and nearly all patients underwent a TP, insulin independence was achieved in only 16% of patients with prior resections versus 40% in those without prior resections [34]. A prior Whipple operation had less effect on the islet yield than a distal pancreatectomy [32].

As of December 2006, 198 IATs had been done at the UMN, more than half of them since 2000 (Fig. 3). A recent analysis involving 188 patients (unpublished data), whose TP-IATs were done between February 1977 and September 2006, showed a patient survival rate of 98% at 1 year and 73% at 10 years, with complete pain relief or reduction in over 90% of patients and discontinuation of narcotics in half. In addition, 55% of adult patients had full islet graft function and were insulin-independent at 1 year after transplant. A third of the patients were insulin-independent at 10 years, and another third had partial islet function with minimal insulin requirements.

The authors' latest published outcome analysis included 136 patients cared for from 1977 through 2004; of those, 120 had sufficient follow-up for analysis [7]. The age range was 5 to 70 years old (Fig. 4); duration of disease was 1 to 30 years (Fig. 5). The etiology of CP was idiopathic in 43% of the patients (Box 1). Most had had previous operations, 33% directly on the pancreas. Previous operations included:

- Abdominal operations—126 (93%)
- Cholecystectomy—57 (42%)
- Pancreatic operations—45 (33%)
- Puestow—17
- Duval—1

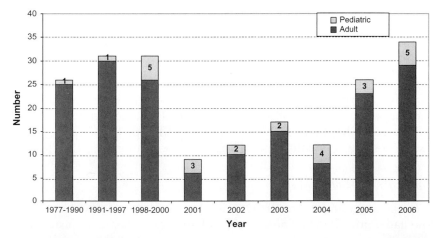

Fig. 3. Islet autograft experience at the University of Minnesota by era/year, including 198 patients (172 adults, 26 children younger than 18 years) from February 1977 to December 2006.

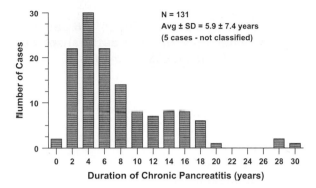

Fig. 4. Best estimated duration (in years) of chronic pancreatitis in 136 patients undergoing pancreatectomy and islet autotransplantation at the University of Minnesota from 1977 through 2004.

- Whipple—9
- Distal—12
- Combined (partial resection plus Puestow)—6

More than 75% underwent a TP or completion pancreatectomy at the time of their IAT (Box 2). This analysis [7] confirmed the correlation between the degree of pancreatic fibrosis and a prior Puestow procedure with attainment of low islet yields (Fig. 6). Again, we found a strong correlation between islet yield and insulin independence. Of patients receiving > 2000 IEQ/kg, 47% were completely insulin-independent while 25% required intermittent insulin.

From 2000 through 2005, the authors treated 43 TP patients whose metabolic status could be assessed relative to islet yield (Fig. 7). One third had

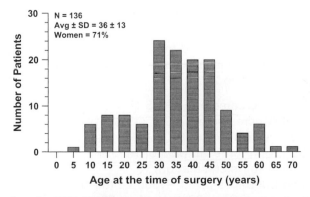

Fig. 5. Age and gender (71% female) distribution of 136 patients undergoing islet autotransplantation at the University of Minnesota from 1977 through 2004.

Box 1. Etiology of chronic pancreatitis in 136 patients undergoing pancreatectomy and islet autotransplantation at the University of Minnesota 1977 to 2004

Idiopathic—59 patients (43%)
Alcohol—21 patients (15%)
Divisum—17 patients (13%)
Familial—15 patients (11%)
Biliary—14 patients (10%)
Iatrogenic—four patients (3%)
Cystic fibrosis—three patients (1%)
Trauma—two patients
Congenital cyst—one patient

---

little or no islet function and were fully insulin-dependent. Another third had mild diabetes and needed insulin only intermittently or long-acting insulin once daily. The other third were insulin-independent. The mean islet yield was lowest in the completely insulin-dependent group and highest in the completely insulin-independent group, with the mean in the intermittent insulin group in between. There was much overlap between the groups, showing that factors other than simply the islet yield affect function and outcomes [7].

Cincinnati series

The most recent report from this group showed a 40% rate of insulin independence after TP/IAT, with a mean follow-up of 18 months [8,18]. Factors that correlated with postoperative insulin independence included the patient's weight, body mass index (BMI), and gender [37]. Patients who

---

Box 2. Operation performed in 136 patients undergoing pancreatectomy and islet autotransplantation at the University of Minnesota 1977 to 2004

- Complete pancreatectomy—105 (77%)
- Near total pancreatectomy—21 (15%)
- Distal pancreatectomy—10 (7%)
- Operating room time: 10 plus or minus 1.7 hours (2 to 4 hours waiting time for islet isolation)
- Estimated bood loss (EBL)—1500 cc (50 cc to 30 L)
- Length of stay (LOS)—22 days (1 to 89 days)

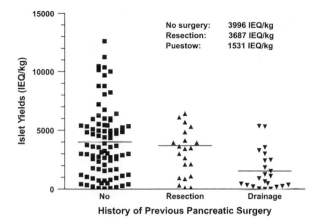

Fig. 6. Islet isolation yield by previous surgery in 136 patients undergoing pancreatectomy and islet autotransplantation at the University of Minnesota from 1977 through 2004.

had a BMI greater than 28 had a higher chance of insulin dependence [37]. Reduction to ideal body weight to minimize insulin resistance may maximize the chance for insulin independence after TP-IAT. Insulin-independent patients had lower mean insulin requirements during the first 24 hours after transplant, possibly relating to the detrimental effect of hyperglycemia on islet function [18] Recent data involving 54 CP patients who underwent a TP-IAT showed that about two thirds had discontinued narcotics, and two-thirds had full or partial islet function, with about 40% insulin-independent [18].

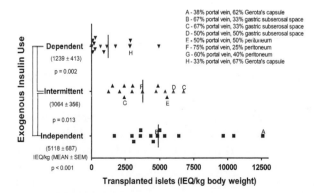

Fig. 7. Short-term metabolic outcome according to islet yield in 43 patients undergoing complete pancreatectomy and islet autotransplantation at the University of Minnesota from 2000 through 2004. The mean islet yield is higher in insulin-independent (versus -dependent) recipients, but there is considerable overlap.

Leicester series

The latest report from the Leicester series did not show any correlation between islet yield and insulin independence [43]. The results may relate to the cause of the CP (mostly alcohol) and possibly to patient compliance issues [43].

Comments

Insulin independence is only partially the goal of an IAT, because preserving any β-cell mass is beneficial. Indeed, islet allograft recipients who remain insulin dependent but have β-cell function and are C-peptide positive are metabolically more stable and less prone to hypoglycemic unawareness than those who have no β-cell function [97–99]. Furthermore, the risk of secondary complications is less in diabetics who receive or are C-peptide-positive [100–102]. By extrapolation, IAT recipients who are C-peptide positive, even with an insulin requirement, have a metabolic advantage. Although only one third of IAT recipients in the UMN series are insulin-independent long-term; another third have enough islets to achieve near normoglycemia with exogenous insulin, usually with one injection daily of the long-acting variety [7].

Although one third of the authors' IAT recipients become fully diabetic because of inadequate islet yield [7,32], as long as pain is relieved or improved, the operation is considered a success. the authors only offer IATs to patients who are fully informed about the risk of becoming diabetic, and who accept this risk in exchange for reasonable chances at both pain reduction and narcotic withdrawal. Some patients who became fully diabetic after TP-IAT because of inadequate islet yield, and who were particularly labile, have gone on to have a pancreas (allograft) transplant, and thus achieved insulin independence, but at the expense of needing immunosuppression [103]. An islet allograft also could be done in this situation, but an enteric-drained pancreas transplant is more attractive, because exocrine deficiency also can be corrected [34].

Long-term metabolic outcomes

One long-term study of metabolic outcomes in six TP-IAT recipients from the authors' center reported that diabetes mellitus was prevented for up to 13 (now 20) years (mean follow-up at study, 6.2 plus or minus 1.7 years) [33]. Normal fasting plasma glucose, intravenous glucose disappearance rate (κG), hemoglobin A_{1c}, insulin responses to intravenous glucose and arginine, and insulin secretory reserve were maintained, but insulin responses tended to decrease over time. The intravenous glucose disappearance rate correlated with the number of islets transplanted [33]. Another UMN study showed reduced functional β-cell secretory reserve in IAT recipients, as compared with healthy individuals [38]. A third UMN study showed that intrahepatic islet grafts failed to secrete glucagon in response to sustained hypoglycemia, but did in response to arginine, a peculiarity that may be site-dependent [104]. Nonetheless, intraportal autografts of as few as 265,000 islets can result in release of insulin and glucagon, at appropriate times, and thus can result in prolonged insulin independence [105].

Quality of life and pain relief

Health-related QOL is significantly worse in patients who have CP, as compared with a gender- and age-adjusted general population [106]. The authors' primary goal in performing TP-IAT is to improve QOL by alleviating pain and giving patients a chance to discontinue narcotics, while preventing or minimizing surgical diabetes. Studies evaluating health-related QOL outcomes in this population are limited. In a report from Cincinnati, QOL as measured by a standard assessment tool (SF-36) showed significant improvement a mean follow-up of 19 months [37]. Prospective studies are needed.

In the Cincinnati series, unremitting abdominal pain refractory to high-dose narcotics was the indication for surgery in all TP-IAT patients [8,37]. Narcotic independence was achieved in 58% of the most recent 26 patients, with a marked reduction in narcotic use by pre- and postoperative morphine-equivalent determinations [8].

These findings are similar to those in the 1995 UMN series of 46 patients; in 83% of them, pain resolved or improved, and 81% were able to discontinue narcotics [28]. In the authors' recent review of 120 patients through 2004, 63% showed pain resolution or improvement [7]. Furthermore, a recent UMN analysis [107], based on an ongoing retrospective survey of TP-IAT patients, showed that nearly 95% of the adult patients reached stated they had less pain after the surgery. Nearly half were able to completely discontinue narcotics, and more than 95% stated they would recommend TP-IAT. The survey reached 75 adults (71% female, 29% male) at a median of 42 months after transplant.

In a recent small series from a group in Tennessee, 100% of patients who underwent TP for CP without IAT became narcotic-independent (median follow-up, 46 months) [108].

Narcotic independence may not be obtainable in patients with opioid-induced hyperalgesia (OIH). Such patients, after receiving narcotics for chronic pain, paradoxically become more sensitive to pain, by means of mechanisms originating in afferent neurons and in the spinal cord [109–114]. Future studies are needed to identify patients at risk of OIH and to develop effective strategies for narcotic discontinuation. OIH may be highly prevalent in patients referred for TP-IAT; accordingly, an endpoint such as narcotic independence may not be ideal for assessing postoperative success.

Cancer risk of chronic pancreatitis patients

The association between longstanding CP and cancer has been established [115–118]. It is believed that pancreatic cancer develops in the setting of CP, independent of the underlying etiology, but appears to require 30 to 40 years of inflammation before manifesting in an appreciable percentage of patients [116]. This increased risk for pancreatic cancer is potentiated by cofactors such as tobacco and likely by genetic factors that are not yet entirely identified [115,116].

A TP by itself for CP completely eliminates the risk of pancreatic cancer, but even with an IAT, the risk is lowered considerably, given the marked reduction in pancreatic tissue. The autologous islets infused into the portal system are never totally pure, but the use of tissue at risk for pancreatic cancer must be minimal. Sampling the whole gland for pathologic testing is impossible in the setting of an IAT. Patients who have hereditary and tropical pancreatitis are at higher risk for developing malignant cells than the rest of CP population [116,117], but again the amount of residual pancreatic tissue after TP-IAT is very small.

In the entire series of TP-IAT patients from UMN, no patients are known to have developed cancer in the liver or in any other site where the islets were auto-grafted, so the risk of cancer appears to be extremely low.

Future directions

A basic but important limitation to more widespread clinical application of IATs is the limited number of centers with the facilities and technology to isolate and prepare human islets. Few centers, including the authors', have used distance processing for both allogenic and autologous islets successfully [119–121]. The feasibility of distance processing is enhanced by new preservation methods that extend cold ischemic times and increase islet yield and viability from suboptimal organs [112–126].

The long-term success of IATs in patients who have CP [33] contrasts with the apparently less favorable long-term results for islet allotransplants in patients who have type 1 diabetes mellitus [98]. In the Edmonton islet allograft series, only 20% of recipients who became insulin-independent remained so at 5 years, although nearly all remained C-peptide-positive [98], indicating survival of β-cells. The difference in outcomes may be because of the rejection rate of islet allografts, or if allografts are not rejected, to the diabetogenic effect of the necessary immunosuppression.

Autologous islets are as fresh as possible. They are isolated from a pancreas that, although diseased, is not under the stress of brain death (which in animal models decreases islet yield and function by the activation of proinflammatory cytokines that occurs from central nervous system (CNS) injury [127]). A native pancreas removed for IAT also is not subjected to prolonged ischemia or to hours of cold preservation that occur with deceased donor pancreases processed for allogenic islets.

Single-donor islet allografts have resulted in insulin independence in diabetic recipients at UMN [128]; yet in many cases, multiple donors are required [129]. Increasing islet viability for transplants is important; for allografts, one possibility is to use a living donor [27,130,131]. This approach should be effective, given the good outcomes in IAT recipients with an islet mass well below that required for a successful outcome with deceased donor islet allografts [132].

A secondary benefit of an IAT program is the opportunity to evaluate and compare differences in islet durability between islet autografts and allografts of the same β-cell mass. Such a comparison may allow one to make a distinction between immunologic and nonimmunologic factors that affect declines in, or sustenance of, islet graft function over time. Currently, however, it is apparent that IATs are more successful than their allogenic counterparts.

Summary

The main objective of this article was to show the benefit of IAT when combined with pancreatectomy to treat painful CP. IAT safely prevents or minimizes surgical diabetes after TP for benign disease. Pancreatic resection (even partial) with an IAT always should be considered the primary surgical option for patients who have CP and intractable pain refractory to medical or endoscopic therapy. Pain relief, enabling narcotic discontinuation, is the primary objective; the prevention of diabetes is a secondary goal. The series reviewed here, extending back 30 years, shows that both goals are achieved to a reasonable degree in a very difficult disease, CP.

References

[1] Sutherland DE, Matas AJ, Najarian JS. Pancreatic islet cell transplantation. Surg Clin North Am 1978;58(2):365–82.

[2] Najarian JS, Sutherland DE, Matas AJ, et al. Human islet autotransplantation following pancreatectomy. Transplant Proc 1979;11(1):336–40.

[3] Najarian JS, Sutherland DE, Baumgartner D, et al. Total or near total pancreatectomy and islet autotransplantation for treatment of chronic pancreatitis. Ann Surg 1980;192(4): 526–42.

[4] Carlson AM, Kobayashi T, Sutherland DER. Islet autotransplantation to prevent or minimize diabetes after pancreatectomy. Current Opinion in Organ Transplantation 2007; 12(1):82–8.

[5] Schneider A, Whitcomb DC. Hereditary pancreatitis: a model for inflammatory diseases of the pancreas. Best Pract Res Clin Gastroenterol 2002;16:347–63.

[6] Etemad B, Whitcomb DC. Chronic pancreatitis: diagnosis, classification, and new genetic developments. Gastroenterology 2001;120(3):682–707.

[7] Jie T, Hering BJ, Ansite JD, et al. Pancreatectomy and auto-islet transplant in patients with chronic pancreatitis [abstract]. J Am Coll Surg 2005;201(3 Suppl):S14.

[8] Ahmad SA, Lowy AM, Wray CJ, et al. Factors associated with insulin and narcotic independence after islet autotransplantation in patients with severe chronic pancreatitis. J Am Coll Surg 2005;201(5):680–7.

[9] Talamini G, Bassi C, Falconi M, et al. Alcohol and smoking as risk factors in chronic pancreatitis and pancreatic cancer. Dig Dis Sci 1999;44:1303–11.

[10] Maisonneuve P, Lowenfels AB, Mullhaupt B, et al. Cigarette smoking accelerates progression of alcoholic chronic pancreatitis. Gut 2005;54:510–4.

[11] Whitcomb DC. Genetic predispositions to acute and chronic pancreatitis. Med Clin North Am 2000;84:531–47.

[12] Witt H, Apte MV, Keim V, et al. Chronic pancreatitis: challenges and advances in pathogenesis, genetics, diagnosis, and therapy. Gastroenterology 2007;132:1557–73.

[13] Balakrishnan V, Nair P, Radhakrishnan L, et al. Tropical pancreatitis a distinct entity, or merely a type of chronic pancreatitis? Indian J Gastroenterol 2006;25:74–81.

[14] Ketikoglou I, Moulakakis A. Autoimmune pancreatitis. Dig Liver Dis 2005;37:211–5.

[15] Walsh TN, Rode J, Theis BA, et al. Minimal change chronic pancreatitis. Gut 1992;33(11): 1566–71.

[16] Layer P, Yamamoto H, Kalthoff L, et al. The different courses of early- and late-onset idiopathic and alcoholic chronic pancreatitis. Gastroenterology 1994;107(5):1481–7.

[17] Kahl S, Glasbrenner B, Zimmermann S, et al. Endoscopic ultrasound in pancreatic diseases. Dig Dis 2002;20:120–6.

[18] Ahmed SA, Wray C, Rilo HL, et al. Chronic pancreatitis: recent advances and ongoing challenges. Curr Probl Surg 2006;43(3):127–238.

[19] Fasanella KE, Davis B, Lyons J, et al. Pain in chronic pancreatitis and pancreatic cancer. Gastroenterol Clin North Am 2007;36:335–64.

[20] Andren-Sandberg A, Hoem D, Gislason H. Pain management in chronic pancreatitis. Eur J Gastroenterol Hepatol 2002;14(9):957–70.

[21] Warshaw AL, Banks PA, Fernandez-del Castillo C. AGA technical review: treatment of pain in chronic pancreatitis. Gastroenterology 1998;115(3):765–76.

[22] Dite P, Ruzicka M, Zboril V, et al. A prospective, randomized trial comparing endoscopic and surgical therapy for chronic pancreatitis. Endoscopy 2003;35(7):553–8.

[23] Cahen DL, Gouma DJ, Nio Y, et al. Endoscopic versus surgical drainage of the pancreatic duct in chronic pancreatitis. N Engl J Med 2007;356:676–84.

[24] Wilcox CM, Varadarajulu S. Endoscopic therapy for chronic pancreatitis: an evidence-based review. Curr Gastroenterol Rep 2006;8:104–10.

[25] Farney AC, Najarian JS, Nakhleh RE, et al. Autotransplantation of dispersed pancreatic islet tissue combined with total or near-total pancreatectomy for treatment of chronic pancreatitis. Surgery 1991;110(2):427–37 [discussion: 437–9].

[26] Najarian JS, Sutherland DER, Matas AJ, et al. Human islet transplantation: a preliminary experience. Transplant Proc 1977;9:233–6.

[27] Sutherland DE, Matas AJ, Goetz FC, et al. Transplantation of dispersed pancreatic islet tissue in humans: autografts and allografts. Diabetes 1980;29(Suppl 1):31–44.

[28] Wahoff DC, Papalois BE, Najarian JS, et al. Autologous islet transplantation to prevent diabetes after pancreatic resection. Ann Surg 1995;222(4):562–75 [discussion: 575–9].

[29] Wahoff DC, Papalois BE, Najarian JS, et al. Clinical islet autotransplantation after pancreatectomy: determinants of success and implications for allotransplantation? Transplant Proc 1995;27(6):3161.

[30] Farney AC, Hering BJ, Nelson L, et al. No late failures of intraportal human islet autografts beyond 2 years. Transplant Proc 1998;30(2):420.

[31] Hering BJ, Wijkstrom M, Eckman PM. Islet transplantation. In: Gruessner RWG, Sutherland DER, editors. Transplantation of the pancreas. New York: Splinger-Verlag; 2004. p. 583–626.

[32] Sutherland DER, Gruessner RWG, Jie T, et al. Pancreatic islet auto-transplantation for chronic pancreatitis. Clinical Transplant 2004;18(Suppl 13):17.

[33] Robertson RP, Lanz KJ, Sutherland DE, et al. Prevention of diabetes for up to 13 years by autoislet transplantation after pancreatectomy for chronic pancreatitis. Diabetes 2001; 50(1):47–50.

[34] Gruessner RW, Sutherland DE, Dunn DL, et al. Transplant options for patients undergoing total pancreatectomy for chronic pancreatitis. J Am Coll Surg 2004;198(4):559–67 [discussion: 568–9].

[35] Gores PF, Najarian JS, Sutherland DER. Islet Autotransplantation. In: Ricordi C, editor. Austin: R.G. Landers Company; 1992. p. 291–312.

[36] Watkins JG, Krebs A, Rossi RL. Pancreatic autotransplantation in chronic pancreatitis. World J Surg 2003;27(11):1235–40.

[37] Rodriguez Rilo HL, Ahmad SA, D'Alessio D, et al. Total pancreatectomy and autologous islet cell transplantation as a means to treat severe chronic pancreatitis. J Gastrointest Surg 2003;7(8):978–89.

[38] Teuscher AU, Kendall DM, Smets YF, et al. Successful islet autotransplantation in humans: functional insulin secretory reserve as an estimate of surviving islet cell mass. Diabetes 1998;47(3):324–30.

[39] Jindal RM, Fineberg SE, Sherman S, et al. Clinical experience with autologous and allogeneic pancreatic islet transplantation. Transplantation 1998;66(12):1836–41.

[40] Oberholzer J, Triponez F, Mage R, et al. Human islet transplantation: lessons from 13 autologous and 13 allogeneic transplantations. Transplantation 2000;69(6):1115–23.

[41] Farkas G, Pap A. Management of diabetes induced by nearly total (95%) pancreatectomy with autologous transplantation of Langerhans' cells. Orv Hetil 1997;138(29):1863–7.

[42] Sarbu V, Dima S, Aschie M, et al. Preliminary data on post-pancreatectomy diabetes mellitus treated by islet cell autotransplantation. Chirurgia (Bucur) 2005;100(6):587–93.

[43] Clayton HA, Davies JE, Pollard CA, et al. Pancreatectomy with islet autotransplantation for the treatment of severe chronic pancreatitis: the first 40 patients at the Leicester General Hospital. Transplantation 2003;76(1):92–8.

[44] White SA, Davies JE, Pollard C, et al. Pancreas resection and islet autotransplantation for end-stage chronic pancreatitis. Ann Surg 2001;233(3):423–31.

[45] White SA, Dennison AR, Swift SM, et al. Intraportal and splenic human islet autotransplantation combined with total pancreatectomy. Transplant Proc 1998;30(2):312–3.

[46] Hogle HH, Recemtsma K. Pancreatic autotransplantation following resection. Surgery 1978;83(3):359–60.

[47] Rossi RL, Soeldner JS, Braasch JW, et al. Segmental pancreatic autotransplantation with pancreatic ductal occlusion after near total or total pancreatic resection for chronic pancreatitis. Results at 5 to 54-month follow-up evaluation. Ann Surg 1986;203:626–36.

[48] Fukushima W, Shimizu K, Izumi R, et al. Heterotopic segmental pancreatic autotransplantation in patients undergoing total pancreatectomy. Transplant Proc 1994;26(4): 2285–7.

[49] Noh KW, Wallace MB. EUS in the diagnosis of chronic pancreatitis. Visible Human Journal of Endoscopy 2006;5(1):6–8.

[50] Sahai AV, Zimmerman M, Aabakken L, et al. Prospective assessment of the ability of endoscopic ultrasound to diagnose, exclude, or establish the severity of chronic pancreatitis found by endoscopic retrograde cholangiopancreatography. Gastrointest Endosc 1998; 48(1):18–25.

[51] Gupta K, Carlson AM, Kobayashi T, et al. EUS in early chronic pancreatitis: comparison with histopathology in patients undergoing total pancreatectomy with autologous islet cell transplantation [abstract]. Digestive Disease Week 2007. Washington, DC, May 19–24, 2007.

[52] Chong AK, Hawes RH, Hoffman BJ, et al. Diagnostic performance of EUS for chronic pancreatitis: a comparison with histopathology. Gastrointest Endosc 2007;65:808–14.

[53] Keith RG, Keshavjee SH, Kerenyi NR. Neuropathology of chronic pancreatitis in humans. Can J Surg 1985;28(3):207–11.

[54] Di Sebastiano P, Fink T, Weihe E, et al. Immune cell infiltration and growth-associated protein 43 expression correlate with pain in chronic pancreatitis. Gastroenterology 1997; 112(5):1648–55.

[55] Di Sebastiano P, di Mola FF, Buchler MW, et al. Pathogenesis of pain in chronic pancreatitis. Dig Dis 2004;22(3):267–72.

[56] Manes G, Buchler M, Pieramico O, et al. Is increased pancreatic pressure related to pain in chronic pancreatitis? Int J Pancreatol 1994;15(2):113–7.

[57] Buscher HC, Wilder-Smith OH, van Goor H. Chronic pancreatitis patients show hyperalgesia of central origin: a pilot study. Eur J Pain 2006;10(4):363–70.

[58] Corlett MP, Scharp DW. The effect of pancreatic warm ischemia on islet isolation in rats and dogs. J Surg Res 1988;45(6):531–6.

[59] White SA, Robertson GS, London NJ, et al. Human islet autotransplantation to prevent diabetes after pancreas resection. Dig Surg 2000;17(5):439–50.

[60] le Roux CW, Aylwin SJ, Batterham RL, et al. Gut hormone profiles following bariatric surgery favor an anorectic state, facilitate weight loss, and improve metabolic parameters. Ann Surg 2006;243:108–14.

[61] Greenway SE, Greenway FL 3rd, Klein S. Effects of obesity surgery on noninsulin-dependent diabetes mellitus. Arch Surg 2002;137(10):1109–17.

[62] Gores PF, Sutherland DE. Pancreatic islet transplantation: is purification necessary? Am J Surg 1993;166(5):538–42.

[63] Casey JJ, Lakey JR, Ryan EA, et al. Portal venous pressure changes after sequential clinical islet transplantation. Transplantation 2002;74(7):913–5.

[64] Robertson RP. Pancreatic islet cell transplantation: likely impact on current therapeutics for type 1 diabetes mellitus. Drugs 2001;61(14):2017–20.

[65] Cameron JL, Mehigan DG, Broe PJ, et al. Distal pancreatectomy and islet autotransplantation for chronic pancreatitis. Ann Surg 1981;193(3):312–7.

[66] Warnock GL, Rajotte RV, Procyshyn AW. Normoglycemia after reflux of islet-containing pancreatic fragments into the splenic vascular bed in dogs. Diabetes 1983;32(5): 452–9.

[67] Gray DW. Islet isolation and transplantation techniques in the primate. Surg Gynecol Obstet 1990;170(3):225–32.

[68] Gray DW, Cranston D, McShane P, et al. The effect of hyperglycaemia on pancreatic islets transplanted into rats beneath the kidney capsule. Diabetologia 1989;32(9):663–7.

[69] Gray DW, Sutton R, McShane P, et al. Exocrine contamination impairs implantation of pancreatic islets transplanted beneath the kidney capsule. J Surg Res 1988;45:432–42.

[70] Matarazzo M, Giardina MG, Guardasole V, et al. Islet transplantation under the kidney capsule corrects the defects in glycogen metabolism in both liver and muscle of streptozocin-diabetic rats. Cell Transplant 2002;11(2):103–12.

[71] Vargas F, Julian JF, Llamazares JF, et al. Engraftment of islets obtained by collagenase and liberase in diabetic rats: a comparative study. Pancreas 2001;23:406–13.

[72] Sutton R, Gray DW, Burnett M, et al. Metabolic function of intraportal and intrasplenic islet autografts in cynomolgus monkeys. Diabetes 1989;38(Suppl 1):182–4.

[73] Ao Z, Matayoshi K, Lakey JR, et al. Survival and function of purified islets in the omental pouch site of outbred dogs. Transplantation 1993;56(3):524–9.

[74] Wahoff DC, Sutherland DE, Hower CD, et al. Free intraperitoneal islet autografts in pancreatectomized dogs—impact of islet purity and post-transplantation exogenous insulin. Surgery 1994;116(4):742–8 [discussion: 748–50].

[75] Wahoff DC, Hower CD, Sutherland DE, et al. The peritoneal cavity: an alternative site for clinical islet transplantation? Transplant Proc 1994;26(6):3297–8.

[76] Fontana I, Arcuri V, Tommasi GV, et al. Long-term follow-up of human islet autotransplantation. Transplant Proc 1994;26(2):581.

[77] White SA, London NJ, Johnson PR, et al. The risks of total pancreatectomy and splenic islet autotransplantation. Cell Transplant 2000;9(1):19–24.

[78] Andersson A, Korsgren O, Jansson L. Intraportally transplanted pancreatic islets revascularized from hepatic arterial system. Diabetes 1989;38(Suppl 1):192–5.

[79] Korsgren O, Christofferson R, Jansson L. Angiogenesis and angio–architecture of transplanted fetal porcine islet-like cell clusters. Transplantation 1999;68(11):1761–6.

[80] Mehigan DG, Bell WR, Zuidema GD, et al. Disseminated intravascular coagulation and portal hypertension following pancreatic islet autotransplantation. Ann Surg 1980; 191(3):287–93.

[81] Memsic L, Busuttil RW, Traverso LW. Bleeding esophageal varices and portal vein throm bosis after pancreatic mixed-cell autotransplantation. Surgery 1984;95(2):238–42.

[82] Toledo-Pereyra LH, Rowlett AL, Cain W, et al. Hepatic infarction following intraportal islet cell autotransplantation after near-total pancreatectomy. Transplantation 1984; 38(1):88–9.

[83] Walsh TJ, Eggleston JC, Cameron JL. Portal hypertension, hepatic infarction, and liver failure complicating pancreatic islet autotransplantation. Surgery 1982;91: 485–7.

[84] Manciu N, Beebe DS, Tran P, et al. Total pancreatectomy with islet cell autotransplantation: anesthetic implications. J Clin Anesth 1999;11(7):576–82.

[85] Korsgren O, Jansson L, Andersson A. Effects of hyperglycemia on function of isolated mouse pancreatic islets transplanted under kidney capsule. Diabetes 1989;38(4): 510–5.

[86] Clark A, Bown E, King T, et al. Islet changes induced by hyperglycemia in rats. Effect of insulin or chlorpropamide therapy. Diabetes 1982;31(4 Pt 1):319–25.

[87] Dohan FC, Lukens FDW. Lesions of the pancreatic islets produced in cats by the administration of glucose. Science 1947;105:183.

[88] Makhlouf L, Duvivier-Kali VF, Bonner-Weir S, et al. Importance of hyperglycemia on the primary function of allogenic islet transplants. Transplantation 2003;76:657–64.

[89] Lee BW, Jee JH, Heo JS, et al. The favorable outcome of human islet transplantation in Korea: experiences of 10 autologous transplantations. Transplantation 2005;79(11): 1568–74.

[90] Berney T, Mathe Z, Bucher P, et al. Islet autotransplantation for the prevention of surgical diabetes after extended pancreatectomy for the resection of benign tumors of the pancreas. Transplant Proc 2004;36(4):1123–4.

[91] Oberholzer J, Mathe Z, Bucher P, et al. Islet autotransplantation after left pancreatectomy for nonenucleable insulinoma. Am J Transplant 2003;3(10):1302–7.

[92] Forster S, Liu X, Adam U, et al. Islet autotransplantation combined with pancreatectomy for treatment of pancreatic adenocarcinoma: a case report. Transplant Proc 2004;36(4): 1125–6.

[93] Leone JP, Kendall DM, Reinsmoen N, et al. Immediate insulin-independence after retransplantation of islets prepared from an allograft pancreatectomy in a type 1 diabetic patient. Transplant Proc 1998;30(2):319.

[94] Wahoff DC, Paplois BE, Najarian JS, et al. Islet autotransplantation after total pancreatectomy in a child. J Pediatr Surg 1996;31(1):132–5 [discussion: 135–6].

[95] Bellin M, Carlson AM, Kobayashi T, et al. Outcome after pancreatectomy and islet autotransplantation in a pediatric population. J Pediatr Gastroenterol Nutr, in press.

[96] Wahoff DC, Leone JP, Farney AC, et al. Pregnancy after total pancreatectomy and autologous islet transplantation. Surgery 1995;117(3):353–4.

[97] Paty BW, Senior PA, Lakey JR, et al. Assessment of glycemic control after islet transplantation using the continuous glucose monitor in insulin-independent versus insulin-requiring type 1 diabetes subjects. Diabetes Technol Ther 2006;8(2):165–73.

[98] Ryan EA, Paty BW, Senior PA, et al. Five-year follow-up after clinical islet transplantation. Diabetes 2005;54(7):2060–9.

[99] Ryan EA, Lakey JR, Paty BW, et al. Successful islet transplantation: continued insulin reserve provides long-term glycemic control. Diabetes 2002;51(7):2148–57.

[100] Johansson BL, Borg K, Fernqvist-Forbes E, et al. Beneficial effects of C peptide on incipient nephropathy and neuropathy in patients with type 1 diabetes mellitus. Diabet Med 2000;17(3):181–9.

[101] Kamiya H, Zhang W, Sima AA. C-peptide prevents nociceptive sensory neuropathy in type 1 diabetes. Ann Neurol 2004;56(6):827–35.

[102] Ekberg K, Brismar T, Johansson BL, et al. Amelioration of sensory nerve dysfunction by C-peptide in patients with type 1 diabetes. Diabetes 2003;52(2):536–41.

[103] Sutherland DE, Gruessner RW, Dunn DL, et al. Lessons learned from more than 1000 pancreas transplants at a single institution. Ann Surg 2001;233:463–501.

[104] Kendall DM, Teuscher AU, Robertson RP. Defective glucagon secretion during sustained hypoglycemia following successful islet allo- and autotransplantation in humans. Diabetes 1997;46:23–7.

[105] Pyzdrowski KL, Kendall DM, Halter JB, et al. Preserved insulin secretion and insulin independence in recipients of islet autografts. N Engl J Med 1992;327(4):220–6.

[106] Berney T, Rudisuhli T, Oberholzer J, et al. Long-term metabolic results after pancreatic resection for severe chronic pancreatitis. Arch Surg 2000;135(9):1106–11.

[107] Carlson AM, Blondet JJ, Gruessner A, et al. Pancreatectomy and autologous islet transplantation: a study of long-term outcomes [abstract]. Pancreas Club Annual Meeting Program Book 2007:21.

[108] Behrman SW, Mulloy M. Total pancreatectomy for the treatment of chronic pancreatitis: indications, outcomes, and recommendations. Am Surg 2006;72(4):297–302.

[109] Angst MS, Clark JD. Opioid-induced hyperalgesia: a qualitative systematic review. Anesthesiology 2006;104(3):570–87.

[110] Chu LF, Clark DJ, Angst MS. Opioid tolerance and hyperalgesia in chronic pain patients after one month of oral morphine therapy: a preliminary prospective study. J Pain 2006; 7(1):43–8.

[111] Gardell LR, King T, Ossipov MH, et al. Opioid receptor-mediated hyperalgesia and antinociceptive tolerance induced by sustained opiate delivery. Neurosci Lett 2006;396(1):44–9.

[112] Liang DY, Liao G, Wang J, et al. A genetic analysis of opioid-induced hyperalgesia in mice. Anesthesiology 2006;104(5):1054–62.

[113] Dogrul A, Bilsky EJ, Ossipov MH, et al. Spinal L-type calcium channel blockade abolishes opioid-induced sensory hypersensitivity and antinociceptive tolerance. Anesth Analg 2005; 101(6):1730–5.

[114] Mercadante S, Arcuri E. Hyperalgesia and opioid switching. Am J Hosp Palliat Care 2005; 22(4):291–4.

[115] Whitcomb DC, Pogue-Geile K. Pancreatitis as a risk for pancreatic cancer. Gastroenterol Clin North Am 2002;31:663–78.

[116] Whitcomb DC. Inflammation and Cancer. V. Chronic pancreatitis and pancreatic cancer. Am J Physiol Gastrointest Liver Physiol 2004;287:G315–9.

[117] Farrow B, Evers BM. Inflammation and the development of pancreatic cancer. Surg Oncol 2002;10:153–69.

[118] Lowenfels AB, Maisonneuve P, Cavallini G, et al. Pancreatitis and the risk of pancreatic cancer. N Engl J Med 1993;328:1433–7.

[119] Langer RM, Mathe Z, Doros A, et al. Successful islet after kidney transplantations in a distance over 1000 kilometers: preliminary results of the Budapest-Geneva collaboration. Transplant Proc 2004;36(10):3113–5.

[120] Rabkin JM, Olyaei AJ, Orloff SL, et al. Distant processing of pancreas islets for autotransplantation following total pancreatectomy. Am J Surg 1999;177(5):423–7.

[121] Rabkin JM, Leone JP, Sutherland DE, et al. Transcontinental shipping of pancreatic islets for autotransplantation after total pancreatectomy. Pancreas 1997;15(4):416–9.

[122] Matsuda T, Suzuki Y, Tanioka Y, et al. Pancreas preservation by the 2-layer cold storage method before islet isolation protects isolated islets against apoptosis through the mitochondrial pathway. Surgery 2003;134(3):437–45.

[123] Fujino Y, Kuroda Y, Suzuki Y, et al. Preservation of canine pancreas for 96 hours by a modified two-layer (UW solution/perfluorochemical) cold storage method. Transplantation 1991;51(5):1133–5.

[124] Fraker CA, Alejandro R, Ricordi C. Use of oxygenated perfluorocarbon toward making every pancreas count. Transplantation 2002;74(12):1811–2.

[125] Tsujimura T, Kuroda Y, Avila JG, et al. Influence of pancreas preservation on human islet isolation outcomes: impact of the two-layer method. Transplantation 2004;78(1):96–100.

[126] Tsujimura T, Kuroda Y, Churchill TA, et al. Short-term storage of the ischemically damaged human pancreas by the two-layer method prior to islet isolation. Cell Transplant 2004; 13(1):67–73.

[127] Contreras JL, Eckstein C, Smyth CA, et al. Brain death significantly reduces isolated pancreatic islet yields and functionality in vitro and in vivo after transplantation in rats. Diabetes 2003;52(12):2935–42.

[128] Hering BJ, Kandaswamy R, Ansite JD, et al. Single-donor, marginal-dose islet transplantation in patients with type 1 diabetes. JAMA 2005;293(7):830–5.

[129] Sutherland DE, Gruessner A, Hering BJ. Beta cell replacement therapy (pancreas and islet transplantation) for treatment of diabetes mellitus: an integrated approach. Endocrinol Metab Clin North Am 2004;33(1):135–48.

[130] Sutherland DER, Goetz FC, Najarian JS. Living-related donor segmental pancreatectomy for transplantation. Transplant Proc 1980;12(Suppl 2):19–25.

[131] Matsumoto S, Okitsu T, Iwanaga Y, et al. Insulin independence of unstable diabetic patient after single living donor islet transplantation. Transplant Proc 2005;37(8):3427–9.

[132] Sutherland DER. Beta cell replacement by transplantation in diabetes mellitus: which patients at what risk, which way (when pancreas, when islets), and how to allocate deceased donor pancreases. Current Opinion in Organ Transplantation 2005;10:147–9.

SURGICAL
CLINICS OF
NORTH AMERICA

ELSEVIER
SAUNDERS

Surg Clin N Am 87 (2007) 1503–1513

Management of Internal and External Pancreatic Fistulas

Katherine A. Morgan, MD, David B. Adams, MD*

*Section of Gastrointestinal and Laparoscopic Surgery,
Medical University of South Carolina, 96 Jonathon Lucas Street,
CSB 211, Charleston, SC 29425, USA*

Modern management of a pancreatic fistula, a well-recognized complication of pancreatic inflammatory disease, requires thoughtful surgical management with a combination of operative and nonoperative strategies. An internal pancreatic fistula may present as pancreatic ascites or as a pancreatic pleural effusion. External pancreatic fistulas generally result after iatrogenic manipulation, most commonly attributable to percutaneous or operative drainage of a pseudocyst or peripancreatic fluid collection. Despite their disparate presentations, internal and external pancreatic fistulas share a common underlying pathophysiology, pancreatic duct disruption. Both require a similar set of priorities for successful management.

A pancreatic fistula is an uncommon disorder. Although the pancreatic duct disruption that underlies a pancreatic fistula can result from any of the multiple causes of pancreatitis, the pattern of duct disruption often correlates with the cause. Gallstone pancreatitis frequently involves pancreatic duct disruption in the neck of the pancreas at the genu ("knee") of the pancreatic duct, where it angles sharply from an anteriorly ascending to a posteriorly transverse course. Alcoholic pancreatitis is less predictable and can involve any part of the duct. Operative trauma generally involves injury to the duct in the tail of the gland, often during splenectomy. Alternatively, a postoperative pancreatic fistula may occur from a leak at the site of pancreatic resection or anastomosis.

Regardless of cause or presentation, a pancreatic fistula is best managed with adherence to several basic tenets. First, stabilization and medical optimization are paramount. This step involves fistula control and nutritional optimization. Second, identification of the anatomy of the pancreatic ductal

---

* Corresponding author.
E-mail address: adamsdav@musc.edu (D.B. Adams).

disruption is essential to decision making. Finally, definitive management of the fistula, nonoperative or operative, is in order.

Stabilization and medical optimization

The initial step in management of the patient with a pancreatic fistula is to ensure control of the pancreatic exocrine secretions. Although pancreatic fluid collections can often be tolerated well for a limited period, the enzymatic secretions can be harmful if activated. Early containment of the potentially dangerous pancreatic secretions can help to avoid erosion and damage to surrounding tissues. Moreover, effective drainage can facilitate possible spontaneous duct closure in many cases. In other cases, it can assist later definitive management.

Nonoperative external drainage of internal pancreatic fistulas should be attempted. Tube thoracostomy is effective in pancreatic pleural fistulas. In most other presentations of pancreatic fistulas, radiographically guided catheters best achieve drainage. When present, peripancreatic fluid collections or pseudocysts may mark the site of pancreatic duct disruption, targeting a site for percutaneous drainage. The skin surrounding the site of an external fistula should be closely protected as well, because pancreatic exocrine fluid, once activated, is erosive.

Patients with a pancreatic fistula are at risk for electrolyte disturbances, particularly related to loss of sodium and bicarbonate in pancreatic exocrine secretions. Patients with a pancreatic fistula may also have considerable risk for profound nutritional deficiency. Patients who have chronic pancreatitis often have attendant chronic malnutrition. With the development of a pancreatic fistula, these patients may develop nausea, anorexia, and poor tolerance of diet. In addition, they have poor absorption of nutrients, particularly of fat and protein, secondary to pancreatic exocrine insufficiency. In patients with a pancreatic fistula, there are severe protein losses from the protein-rich pancreatic secretions. All these obstacles to nutrition occur in the setting of a higher metabolic requirement to heal the fistula site. Thus, total parenteral nutrition (TPN) can be essential to ameliorate catabolism, especially in the initial management of these patients. The goal is to restore protein losses without stimulating further loss of pancreatic exocrine secretions through fistula output. Long-term TPN, however, breeds complication. Patients may incur line sepsis or cholestatic injury to the liver. Therefore, once initially stabilized, patients should be fed with enteral nutrition when possible. Feeding by way of the enteral route maintains enteral mucosal integrity, preventing bacterial translocation, and stimulates the gut-associated lymphoid tissue, allowing for immune protection. Ideally, postpyloric feeds have a theoretic benefit by minimizing pancreatic stimulation and fistula output, although, clinically, gastric feedings may be as effective in the patient whose gut is suitable for enteral alimentation.

Infectious complications need to be addressed early in patient management. Patients with a pancreatic fistula are susceptible to infectious complications because they are often violated with invasive lines and drains and are frequently immunocompromised secondary to protein losses. Evidence of invasive infection should be sought and differentiated from colonization of drains. To prevent serious infection, early and aggressive treatment of positive cultures should be practiced.

Identification of duct anatomy

Once the patient's medical condition has been stabilized, delineation of the anatomy of the ductal disruption is the next priority. Duct size and the location of the duct injury dictate the nonoperative and potential operative decision making. Several radiographic modalities are important in the management of pancreatic fistula. A CT scan is essential in identifying peripancreatic or distant fluid collections and may be used as a guide for nonoperative drainage. The location of fluid collections can be suggestive of the site of duct disruption. A CT scan can help to differentiate small duct chronic pancreatitis from large duct disease (7-mm main pancreatic duct), and therefore define appropriate operative intervention. Magnetic resonance cholangiopancreatography (MRCP) can more precisely image the pancreatic duct. The addition of secretin stimulation increases pancreatic exocrine secretion, and therefore enhances duct imaging by this modality. Often, the duct injury is identified with MRCP. The remainder of the duct can be evaluated for associated strictures or stones, which may guide definitive management. Endoscopic retrograde pancreatography (ERP) is the most sensitive and specific modality to identify pancreatic duct anatomy and the site of disruption. It also offers the opportunity for definitive therapy with endoscopic stenting, sphincterotomy, or nasobiliary drainage. A final imaging modality is a direct fistulogram, often through a percutaneous catheter. A fistulogram is a useful and often overlooked means to evaluate the relation of a fistula site to the main pancreatic duct.

Definitive management of the pancreatic fistula

Once the anatomy of the pancreatic duct and its associated pathologic findings have been identified, definitive management of the fistula is required. Approximately 70% to 82% of fistulas close with nonoperative therapy [1,2]. Initially, the patient is allowed nothing by mouth, with parenteral nutrition only to minimize pancreatic exocrine secretion. In many patients, this simple approach allows closure adequately. In others, adjunctive measures are useful.

Octreotide

Octreotide, a synthetic long-acting somatostatin analogue, inhibits pancreatic stimulation and exocrine secretion. It can be useful in the management of internal and external fistulas. Although octreotide does not cause a fistula to close that would not have otherwise, it may expedite closure and at least limits protein and electrolyte losses during fistula management. Octreotide does not seem to prevent postoperative pancreatic fistula formation after pancreaticoduodenectomy (PD) when given prophylactically at the time of surgery [3,4]. It may, however, be effective in reducing this complication when used after distal pancreatectomy (DP) [5].

Fibrin glue

Fibrin glue has been used to attempt closure of pancreatic fistulas by obliteration of the fistulous track. Although it does not seem to be effective as a sole modality, there are reports of its successful use in conjunction with endoscopic stenting [2]. Fibrin glue does not seem to prevent postoperative pancreatic fistula formation after PD when placed during surgery to seal the pancreatic anastomosis [6]. It may be effective in reducing the fistula rate after DP [7].

Endoscopic therapy

If a pancreatic fistula persists despite proper drainage, nutritional optimization, pancreatic rest, and octreotide use, the next step undertaken is endoscopic therapy. Papillary decompression through sphincterotomy or transampullary stenting allows for preferential flow of pancreatic juice into the duodenum. By decreasing the pressure differential, closure of the ductal defect is facilitated. In the modern era of therapeutic ERP, high rates of nonoperative pancreatic fistula closure are achieved [1].

Operative management

Although conservative therapies are successful in the management of most cases of pancreatic fistula, in those patients with unfavorable characteristics, such as the inability to be cannulated by ERP, a ductal stricture or large defect not amenable to endoscopic therapy, or a disconnected pancreatic duct, surgery is required. Surgical therapy of a pancreatic fistula is dictated by ductal anatomy. The goal of surgery is not only to drain the fistula but to correct the underlying pancreatic duct disorder when possible.

Patients who have large duct disease (pancreatic duct diameter of 7 mm or greater) are successfully managed with lateral pancreaticojejunostomy (LPJ), the classic ductal drainage procedure. The area of ductal disruption should be included in the anastomosis. Often, the duct injury results in a mature pseudocyst that can be incorporated into the LPJ, although correction of the underlying duct disorder with LPJ alone results in cyst eradication [8]. LPJ has low morbidity and mortality rates and is the mainstay in the treatment of dilated duct chronic pancreatitis.

In patients who have nondilated duct chronic pancreatitis, the location of the fistula within the gland becomes important. Those patients with duct injury limited to the pancreatic tail, as seen after splenectomy or nephrectomy, can undergo caudal pancreatectomy. Patients who have disruptions in the pancreatic body do well with DP with or without splenectomy. Often, the inflammation and fibrosis associated with pancreatitis can complicate splenic preservation, resulting in increased operative blood loss that may not be warranted, given the low rate of postsplenectomy sepsis in the adult population. DP can be approached from a medial or lateral approach. A medial approach entails division of the gland over the superior mesenteric vein, which may be treacherous in the setting of acute inflammation. The lateral approach involves mobilization of the pancreas from the retroperitoneum laterally to medially to beyond the area of duct involvement. The pancreatic tissue often can be divided with a stapler, with consideration for stapler reinforcement with biologic tissue support devices. If the pancreas is too thick for stapled apposition because of chronic inflammation, it can be divided and oversewn, with direct ligation of the pancreatic duct if identified. Use of pledgeted monofilament sutures offers a theoretic advantage in closure of the divided pancreatic duct. Closed suction drainage of the divided pancreatic edge is used after the procedure to control postoperative leak. In patients with a disconnected pancreatic duct, which is often seen after acute pancreatic necrosis secondary to gallstone pancreatitis, the neck of the pancreas has undergone autolysis in the region of the genu. In these cases, there is no pancreatic tissue to divide and no duct to ligate after removal of the separated body and tail of the gland, which are the source of the duct leak (Fig. 1).

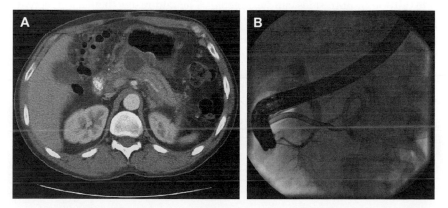

Fig. 1. (A) CT scan of a patient 6 months after a bout of acute pancreatic necrosis secondary to gallstones. Clearly demonstrated is a fluid collection in the neck of the pancreas, where the parenchyma has undergone autolysis. The pseudocyst connects with the main pancreatic duct in the body of the pancreas. (B) ERP of the same patient demonstrates a cutoff at the genu, corresponding to the site of the duct blow-out with autolysis and fibrosis. This patient was managed successfully with DP.

Patients with duct disruptions in the head of the gland can safely avoid a high-risk head resection and undergo a fistula-enterostomy to a Roux-en-y jejunal limb. Although fistula recurrence is possible after this procedure, re-operation at a later date may be safer. Pancreatic fistula-gastrostomy was described by Corachan as early as 1928 [9]. In the modern technique, a per-cutaneous or surgical drain is positioned close to the area of duct disruption to allow a fibrous fistula track to form. At surgery, an anastomosis is then created between the mature fistula track and a Roux-en-y jejunal limb. This technique precludes more extensive dissection required for pancreatic head resection, which can be hazardous in the inflammatory state. Fistula-enter-ostomy has been reported to be successful in 77% to 100% of patients in small series [9,10]. The likely reason for long-term failure in this technique is obliteration of the fistula track with time (Fig. 2).

Internal pancreatic fistula

An internal pancreatic fistula is an uncommon clinical entity occurring in patients who have pancreatitis. Internal pancreatic fistulas occur in patients who have pancreatitis and develop a ductal disruption with leakage of pan-creatic fluid that is not contained by the inflammatory response of the sur-rounding tissues in the retroperitoneum and lesser sac. The exocrine secretions thus track into the free peritoneal or pleural cavities. If the ductal disruption occurs anteriorly, the pancreatic exocrine secretions leak into the free peritoneal cavity and pancreatic ascites occurs (Fig. 3). Alternatively, if the ductal disruption occurs posteriorly, the pancreatic fluid may track through the retroperitoneum into the pleural space, typically on the left side, although both sides can be affected. The end result then is a pancreatic pleural effusion (Fig. 4) [11].

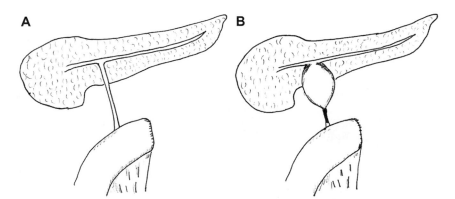

Fig. 2. Mechanism of failure of fistula-enterostomy. The fibrous fistula track obliterates with time.

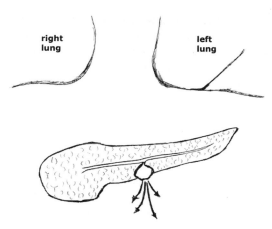

Fig. 3. An anterior pancreatic ductal disruption that is not contained and communicates freely with the peritoneal cavity results in pancreatic ascites.

Pancreatic ascites

Patients who have pancreatic ascites often present with painless abdominal swelling of gradual onset. They may not have a known prior history of pancreatitis. A history of alcohol use is common in this population of patients, and the development of ascites is often presumed to be cirrhotic in origin. Thus, a high index of suspicion is important for appropriate and prompt recognition of the diagnosis. The serum amylase may be mildly elevated, likely secondary to peritoneal absorption. Analysis of the ascitic fluid is diagnostic, with a markedly elevated amylase (greater than 1000 U/dL) and albumin (greater than 3 g/dL unless the serum albumin is extremely low). A CT scan can be useful to identify a calcified pancreas

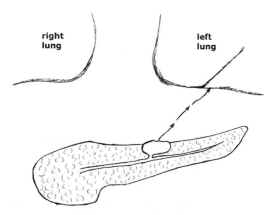

Fig. 4. A posterior pancreatic ductal disruption tracks through the retroperitoneum into the mediastinum or pleural space to result in a pancreatic pleural effusion.

and, in many cases, a pseudocyst, which can then be a target for percutaneous drainage and possible control of the pancreatic duct leak. Pancreatic rest, withholding oral intake, parental nutrition, and octreotide are used. Early endoscopic evaluation of the duct injury and possible therapeutic intervention with sphincterotomy or stenting are warranted. If nonoperative therapy fails, elective surgical intervention should be pursued.

Pancreatic pleural effusion

Patients with pancreatic pleural effusions often present with shortness of breath. Similar to pancreatic ascites, these patients frequently lack a preceding bout of acute pancreatitis to which the duct disruption can be attributed. Often, they have undergone multiple pleural taps with recurrence of the effusion before the diagnosis is considered. Patients may have normal or slightly elevated serum amylase, probably from pleural absorption. Thoracentesis reveals fluid with clearly elevated amylase (greater than 1000 U/dL) and albumin (greater than 3 g/dL). Treatment is drainage with a thoracostomy tube and pancreatic rest with nothing by mouth, parenteral nutrition, and octreotide. Early endoscopic diagnosis and therapy are important. As in pancreatic ascites, if nonoperative therapy fails, surgery is warranted. Surgery addresses the pancreatic duct pathologic findings and does not involve thoracotomy.

External pancreatic fistula

External pancreatic or pancreatocutaneous fistulas usually result after percutaneous drainage of a pancreatic pseudocyst, after operative debridement and drainage of acute pancreatic necrosis, after an operative pancreatic injury, or after a pancreatic resection.

Pancreatic fistula associated with a pseudocyst

An external pancreatic fistula after radiographically guided percutaneous catheter drainage of pancreatic pseudocysts occurs in 15% of cases. Usually, the persistent fistula is secondary to an underlying disorder of the main pancreatic duct (ie, stricture, obstruction) that is in connection with the pseudocyst. The mean length of catheter drainage in patients who develop external pancreatic fistulas by this mechanism is 6 weeks. Early ERP with sphincterotomy or stenting is prudent and can facilitate fistula closure. Most of these fistulas heal without operative intervention; thus, an adequate time period, at least 6 weeks, should be given to allow the fistula to heal before proceeding with surgery. In patients with a dilated main pancreatic duct, however, the fistula is unlikely to close and surgery should be pursued once the patient is optimized from nutritional and infectious standpoints [12].

Pancreatic fistula after debridement of pancreatic necrosis

Severe acute pancreatitis with pancreatic necrosis involves pancreatic duct disruption. The goal of initial operative management is debridement of necrotic tissue and wide drainage. After surgery, most duct disruptions heal with time and adequate drainage. Patients may develop a persistent duct defect, and thus a persistent pancreatic fistula, through one of their surgical drains, however. This fistula is best managed conservatively, because most heal with time. If at 4 weeks, however, high amylase fluid persists, ERP is reasonable for definition of the duct defect and for therapeutic intervention for duct decompression. If the fistula still does not heal despite these measures, operative intervention is warranted.

Pancreatic fistula after operative trauma

The tail of the pancreas can be injured during splenectomy, resulting in a pancreatic fistula. More recently, this injury pattern has been seen with laparoscopic nephrectomy (Fig. 5).

With conservative management, this injury usually heals unless there is underlying duct pathologic change. If surgery is required, caudal pancreatectomy is adequate.

Postoperative pancreatic fistula after pancreatic resection

A postoperative pancreatic fistula after pancreas resection occurs after failure of a pancreatic anastomosis or leak from the divided edge of the pancreas. A pancreatic fistula occurs in 9% to 18% of patients after PD [13] and

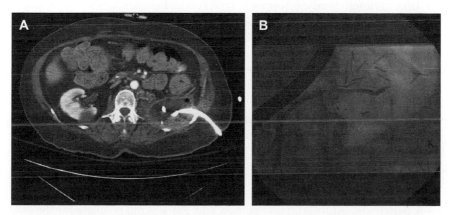

Fig. 5. (*A*) CT scan of a patient who incurred an injury to the tail of the pancreas during a laparoscopic nephrectomy. This fluid collection was percutaneously drained under radiographic guidance. (*B*) ERP of the same patient shows a normal pancreatic duct; thus, this patient was successfully managed with nonoperative therapy (ie, octreotide, endoscopic, stenting, drainage).

Table 1
Postoperative pancreatic fistula

Grade	A	B	C
Clinical conditions	Well	Often well	Ill-appearing/bad
Specific treatment[a]	No	Yes/no	Yes
US/CT (if obtained)	Negative	Negative/positive	Positive
Persistent drainage (after 3 weeks)[b]	No	Usually yes	Yes
Reoperation	No	No	Yes
Death related to POPF	No	No	Possibly yes
Signs of infections	No	Yes	Yes
Sepsis	No	No	Yes
Readmission	No	Yes/no	Yes/no

Drain output of any measurable volume of fluid on or after postoperative day 3 with an amylase content greater than three times the serum amylase activity.

Abbreviations: POPF, postoperative pancreatic fistula; US, ultrasonography.

[a] Partial (peripheral) or total parenteral nutrition, antibiotics, enteral nutrition, somatostatin analogue or minimal invasive drainage.

[b] With or without a drain in situ.

From Bassi C, Dervenis C, Butturini G, et al. Postoperative pancreatic fistula: an international study group (ISGPF) definition. Surgery 2005;138:8–13; with permission.

in 10% to 20% of patients after DP [14]. Risk factors for a fistula include a soft pancreas [13] and a stapled parenchymal closure, prolonged operative time, and multivisceral resection [14]. The postoperative pancreatic fistula rate after PD is not improved by the use of prophylactic octreotide or fibrin glue [3,4,6], but the fistula rate after DP may be improved by these perioperative measures [5,7].

In an effort to allow comparison of surgical experience between centers, an International Study Group on Pancreatic Fistulas (ISGPF) proposed a uniform definition of postoperative pancreatic fistulas and further categorized fistulas according to clinical severity (Table 1) [15]. Postresection fistulas represent a spectrum of disease, with the most being grade A or B, allowing conservative management. Grade C fistulas, however, require more aggressive intervention. In these more severe fistulas, radiographically guided drainage or biliary diversion can often prevent sepsis, but operative intervention with anastomotic revision and wide drainage may be required. In these patients, a damage control approach should be considered.

Summary

A pancreatic fistula is an uncommon and challenging problem for the general surgeon. Protean in presentation, the underlying pathophysiology of a pancreatic duct disruption is consistent. Several basic principles, when followed, simplify management. These tenets include medical stabilization and nutritional optimization, definition of the underlying duct disorder, and, finally, definitive management with or without surgery. With appropriate prompt care, patients can achieve good outcomes.

References

[1] Halttunen J, Weckman L, Kemppainen E, et al. The endoscopic management of pancreatic fistulas. Surg Endosc 2005;19:559–62.

[2] Fischer A, Benz S, Baier P, et al. Endoscopic management of pancreatic fistulas secondary to intraabdominal operation. Surg Endosc 2004;18:706–8.

[3] Yeo C, Cameron JL, Lillemoe KD, et al. Does prophylactic octreotide decrease the rates of pancreatic fistula and other complications after pancreaticoduodenectomy? Results of a prospective randomized placebo-controlled trial. Ann Surg 2000;232:419–29.

[4] Lowy A, Lee JE, Pisters PW, et al. Prospective randomized trial of octreotide to prevent pancreatic fistula after pancreaticoduodenectomy for malignant disease. Ann Surg 1997;226: 632 41.

[5] Montorsi M, Zago M, Mosca F, et al. Efficacy of octreotide in the prevention of pancreatic fistula after elective pancreatic resections: a prospective, controlled, randomized clinical trial. Surgery 1995;117:26–31.

[6] Lillemoe K, Cameron JL, Kim MP, et al. Does fibrin glue sealant decrease the rate of pancreatic fistula after pancreaticoduodenectomy? Results of a prospective randomized trial. J Gastrointest Surg 2004;8:766 74.

[7] Suzuki Y, Kuroda Y, Morita A, et al. Fibrin glue sealing for the prevention of pancreatic fistulas following distal pancreatectomy. Arch Surg 1995;130:952–5.

[8] Nealon W, Walser E. Duct drainage alone is sufficient in the operative management of pancreatic pseudocysts in patients with chronic pancreatitis. Ann Surg 2003;237:614–22.

[9] Voss M, Ali A, Eubanks WS, et al. Surgical management of pancreaticocutaneous fistula. J Gastrointest Surg 2003;7:542–6.

[10] Bassi C, Falconi M, Pederzoli P, et al. Management of pancreatic fistulas. In: Beger HG, Warshaw AL, Buchler MW, et al, editors. The pancreas. 1st edition. Oxford (UK): Blackwell Scientific; 1998. p. 632–49.

[11] Cameron J, Kieffer RS, Anderson WJ, et al. Internal pancreatic fistulas: pancreatic ascites and pleural effusions. Ann Surg 1976;184:587–93.

[12] Adams D, Srinivasan A. Failure of percutaneous catheter drainage of pancreatic pseudocysts. Am Surg 2000;66:256–61.

[13] Lin J, Cameron JL, Yeo CJ, et al. Risk factors and outcomes in postpancreaticoduodenectomy pancreaticocutaneous fistula. J Gastrointest Surg 2004;8:951–9.

[14] Kleeff J, Diener MK, Z'graggen K, et al. Distal pancreatectomy: risk factors for surgical failure in 302 consecutive cases. Ann Surg 2007;245:573–82.

[15] Bassi C, Dervenis C, Butturini G, et al. Postoperative pancreatic fistula: an international study group (ISGPF) definition. Surgery 2005;138:8–13.

ELSEVIER
SAUNDERS

SURGICAL
CLINICS OF
NORTH AMERICA

Surg Clin N Am 87 (2007) 1515–1532

The Management of Pancreatic Trauma in the Modern Era

Anuradha Subramanian, MD[a],*,
Christopher J. Dente, MD, FACS[b],
David V. Feliciano, MD, FACS[b]

[a]Department of Surgery, Michael E. DeBakey Veterans Affairs Medical Center,
Baylor College of Medicine, 2002 Holcombe Boulevard, Houston, TX 77030, USA
[b]Department of Surgery, Grady Memorial Hospital,
Emory University School of Medicine, Atlanta, GA 30303, USA

Pancreatic trauma, while uncommon, presents challenging diagnostic and therapeutic dilemmas to trauma surgeons. Indeed, injuries to the pancreas have been associated with reported morbidity rates approaching 45%. If treatment is delayed, these rates may increase to 60% [1–3]. The integrity of the main pancreatic duct is the most important determinant of outcome after injury to the pancreas [1]. Undiagnosed ductal disruptions produce secondary infections, fistulas, fluid collections, and prolonged stays in the intensive care unit and hospital [1,4]. This article analyzes the epidemiology, diagnostic approaches, options for nonoperative and operative management, and outcome after blunt and penetrating pancreatic trauma.

Epidemiology

Injuries to the pancreas occur in approximately 5% of patients with blunt abdominal trauma [1–4], 6% of patients with gunshot wounds to the abdomen [5], and 2% of patients with stab wounds to the abdomen [6]. Because of the proximity of the pancreas to multiple important structures, isolated pancreatic injuries are rare. Most patients with pancreatic injuries sustain multiple other significant injuries, which compounds an already high mortality rate [6–10]. After blunt abdominal trauma, injuries to the pancreas are most commonly associated with trauma to the duodenum, liver, and spleen.

---

* Corresponding author.
E-mail address: anu.mouse@gmail.com (A. Subramanian).

0039-6109/07/$ - see front matter © 2007 Elsevier Inc. All rights reserved.
doi:10.1016/j.suc.2007.08.007
surgical.theclinics.com

Conversely, victims of penetrating trauma most frequently have concomitant injuries to the stomach, major vascular structures, liver, colon, spleen, kidney, and duodenum [11]. Ilahi and colleagues [12] reported on 40 patients with blunt pancreatic injuries, and this group had a mean Injury Severity Score (ISS) of 29 ± 13. Similarly, Vasquez and colleagues [6] described 62 patients with penetrating pancreatic trauma with a mean ISS of 28 ± 17. Additionally, Asensio and colleagues [10] reported on 18 patients who underwent pancreatoduodenectomy for combined pancreatoduodenal injuries with a mean ISS of 27 ± 8. In this series, there was an average of 2.7 associated nonvascular injuries and 0.89 associated vascular injuries per patient.

Diagnosis

Grading system

To standardize the diagnosis and treatment of pancreatic injuries, the American Association for the Surgery of Trauma (AAST) published a pancreas Organ Injury Scale (OIS) in 1990 (Table 1). This scale involves five grades, which are determined by the presence or absence of ductal disruption and by the anatomic location of injury. In general, grade I or II injuries are treated with relatively straightforward management techniques, whereas grade III or higher injuries often require resection.

Serum amylase levels

Isolated pancreatic injury may present with few abnormal physical findings; therefore, early diagnosis may be difficult [8]. Unfortunately, initial serum levels of amylase are neither sensitive nor specific for predicting an injury to the pancreas. Jones [13] reported that up to 35% of patients with complete transection of the main pancreatic duct may have normal serum amylase levels. If the amylase level is abnormal, however, further investigation with a contrast-enhanced abdominal CT scan or endoscopic

Table 1
Pancreas Organ Injury Scale of the American Association for the Surgery of Trauma

Grade	Injury	Description
I	Hematoma	Minor contusion without duct injury
	Laceration	Superficial laceration without duct injury
II	Hematoma	Major contusion without duct injury or tissue loss
	Laceration	Major laceration without duct injury or tissue loss
III	Laceration	Distal transection or parenchymal injury with duct injury
IV	Laceration	Proximal transection or parenchymal injury involving ampulla
V	Laceration	Massive disruption of pancreatic head

Data from Moore EE, Cogbill TH, Malangoni MA, et al. Organ injury scaling II: pancreas duodenum, small bowel, colon, and rectum. J Trauma 1990;30:1427–9.

retrograde cholangiopancreatography (ERCP) is warranted. Although the usefulness of an isolated amylase value is suspect, reports in literature have suggested a role for serial or delayed measurement of amylase levels. Indeed, Takishima and colleagues [14] reported that all their 73 patients with blunt injuries to the pancreas had elevated serum amylase levels when drawn at least 3 hours after the initial trauma.

CT

Most patients with penetrating abdominal trauma associated with hypotension, peritonitis, or evisceration proceed to the operating room without much diagnostic workup. In the hemodynamically stable patient with blunt trauma in whom there is a suspicion of pancreatic trauma, additional diagnostic studies are warranted. A contrast-enhanced CT scan is the initial imaging study of choice, realizing that the overall accuracy of CT for diagnosis of pancreatic injuries is only fair [15]. Ilahi and colleagues [12] demonstrated an overall sensitivity of only 68% with a correct injury grade in less than 50% of the 40 patients in their series. Newer generation multi-slice scanners may have better accuracy, although few data exist. Indeed, an AAST-sponsored multicenter review of the accuracy of grading pancreatic injuries with new-generation CT scanners is currently underway. Findings suspicious for an injury to the pancreas include the following: a hematoma surrounding the pancreas, fluid in the lesser sac, or thickening of the left anterior Gerota's fascia. CT scans can also demonstrate parenchymal lacerations or transections of the main pancreatic duct and can be used to follow the course of posttraumatic pancreatitis or a phlegmon [11,16].

Endoscopic retrograde cholangiopancreatography

If a CT scan is equivocal or a small parenchymal laceration is present, ERCP is the most reliable method to use in defining continuity of the main pancreatic duct accurately [1,2,8,16,17]. ERCP can precisely localize the site of a ductal injury by demonstrating extravasation or a cutoff, especially in patients with delayed presentations [8]. A group from Japan documented a classification of pancreatic injuries according to findings on ERCP (Table 2) [18]. An advantage of this modality is that in addition to being diagnostic, ERCP-placed stents may be useful as an adjunct to nonoperative management of proximal pancreatic duct injuries in the appropriate setting [16]. Disadvantages of ERCP include the risks of endoscopy, exacerbating a smoldering pancreatitis, and sepsis from overfilling of a disrupted duct [19,20]. In addition, ERCP can be used as a complement to surgical treatment of proximal pancreatic injuries, as is discussed elsewhere in this article. Unfortunately, in some centers, this imaging and treatment modality is not readily available in emergent and even urgent situations [1].

Table 2
Classification of pancreatic injuries by endoscopic retrograde cholangiopancreatography

Grade	Description
I	Normal main pancreatic duct on ERCP
IIa	Injury to branches of main pancreatic duct on ERCP with contrast extravasation inside the parenchyma
IIb	Injury to branches of main pancreatic duct on ERCP with contrast extravasation into the retroperitoneal space
IIIa	Injury to the main pancreatic duct on ERCP at the body or tail of the pancreas
IIIb	Injury to the main pancreatic duct on ERCP at the head the pancreas

Data from Takishima T, Hirat M, Kataoka Y, et al. Pancreatographic classification of pancreatic ductal injuries caused by blunt injury to the pancreas. J Trauma 2000;48:745–52.

Dynamic secretin-stimulated magnetic resonance cholangiopancreatography

Dynamic secretin-stimulated (DSS) magnetic resonance cholangiopancreatography (MRCP) is a variation on standard MRCP and may rival ERCP in diagnostic accuracy. Like ERCP, DSS MRCP provides dynamic information as to whether there is continuing leakage from an injured main pancreatic duct. Gillams and colleagues [20] illustrated the technique, which includes standard MRCP, followed by an imaging sequence immediately after administration of secretin (0.1 mL/kg) intravenously over 20 seconds. The sequence is then repeated at 2-minute intervals for 7 minutes after secretin administration. They also reported on eight patients with traumatic pancreatic injuries who were all successfully treated with management decisions based on results of the DSS MRCP. Unlike ERCP, this imaging modality is noninvasive; however, it can illustrate the entire pancreatic parenchymal and ductal anatomy as well as pathologic fluid collections and ductal disruptions [20]. MRCP may be an appropriate substitute to ERCP in certain cases, but its disadvantages include the time needed for a study to be completed and the inability to perform therapeutic maneuvers. Because of the length of the procedure, it is not considered suitable for multiply injured patients. Also, although MRCP may miss an injury to a nondilated acutely injured main pancreatic duct, it may be more useful in a chronic or delayed setting, because a previous injury often appears as a stricture with distal ductal dilatation [2].

Exploratory laparotomy

In those patients who are taken emergently to the operating room for abdominal trauma, pancreatic injuries are diagnosed at exploration. When evaluating an injury to the pancreas, it is important to establish the continuity of the main pancreatic duct. Injury to this structure may be obvious, such as in the patient with a complete transection of the head, neck, or body or an extensive laceration in the area of the duct. Injury can be more subtle, however, occasionally requiring a dose of secretin (1 unit/kg administered intravenously) to demonstrate leakage of clear pancreatic fluid. Any of these findings predicts the existence of an injury to the main pancreatic duct with a high degree of accuracy [7,10]. In the authors' experience, simple examination of the area of injury for several minutes with loupe magnification reveals clear pancreatic fluid leaking in most injuries that involve the pancreatic duct. Also, intraoperative ultrasound (IOUS) can be used to help diagnose a parenchymal or ductal laceration [21]. Finally, intraoperative pancreatography, which is discussed in the section on ductal transection, may also be used to detect an injury to the main pancreatic duct [11].

Nonoperative management

There are occasional patients who present with blunt abdominal trauma, hyperamylasemia, and a small peripancreatic hematoma or evidence of posttraumatic pancreatitis on a subsequent CT scan. If there is no evidence of a ductal injury on fine-cut CT, nonoperative management is acceptable, although it may be wise to perform ERCP to establish normal ductal anatomy definitively. As with nonoperative management of blunt injuries to the liver or spleen, serial physical and laboratory examinations (ie, hemoglobin, amylase, lipase) are required. A continued increase in serum amylase levels or change on physical examination mandates an abdominal operation or repeat imaging with CT or ERCP [8,14].

Endoscopically placed stents

Endoscopically placed stents have been used occasionally as definitive management of isolated injuries to the proximal pancreatic duct in hemodynamically stable patients or in those with associated severe injuries to the brain or severe intracranial hypertension. If the stent is placed immediately at the time of initial ERCP, the chance of successful nonoperative treatment with this modality is the greatest [16]. In some centers, however, the lack of immediate availability renders this management modality not an option [2]. Finally, because of the small size of the pancreatic duct distal to the ampulla, stenting would ordinarily not be used in this location [22].

Operative treatment

Indications

The indications for operative management in patients with blunt or penetrating abdominal trauma with high suspicion of injury to the pancreas include the following: peritonitis on physical examination, hypotension and a positive (anechoic fluid present in the abdomen) focused surgeon-performed ultrasound examination of the abdomen, and evidence of disruption of the pancreatic duct on fine-cut CT or on ERCP [2,8].

Isolated injuries to the pancreas without ductal involvement

General principles and exposure

As previously described, most patients with pancreatic trauma have associated injuries to other organs or vascular structures, and injury to those nearby structures should raise suspicion of an injury to the pancreas [6,8–11]. During laparotomy for blunt or penetrating trauma, the initial priorities are control of active hemorrhage and control of gross gastrointestinal contamination. These maneuvers are generally undertaken before evaluation of the pancreas. Once a pancreatic injury is identified, however, the principles for management are well established and include hemostasis, debridement of dead tissue with anatomic resection as appropriate, and wide drainage [7]. After exposure, the choice of management technique depends on the following: the presence or absence of injury to the main pancreatic duct; the location of the ductal injury, if present, and the presence or absence of a concomitant duodenal injury; and, finally, the patient's hemodynamic status. Treatment options, resectional and nonresectional, are described here and are also summarized in Table 3 [11].

Complete exposure of the pancreas necessitates opening of the lesser sac with cephalad retraction of the posterior wall of the stomach and caudad retraction of the transverse mesocolon. In patients with penetrating trauma,

Table 3
Treatment options for isolated pancreatic injuries based on the American Association for the Surgery of Trauma pancreas Organ Injury Scale

AAST grade	Treatment options
I	Observation
	Omental pancreatorrhaphy with simple external drainage
II	Simple external drainage
	Omental pancreatorrhaphy and drainage
III	Distal pancreatectomy ± splenectomy
	Roux-en-Y distal pancreatojejunostomy
IV	Pancreatoduodenectomy
	Roux-en-Y distal pancreatojejunostomy
	Anterior Roux-en-Y pancreatojejunostomy
	Endoscopically placed stent
	Simple drainage in damage control situations
V	Pancreatoduodenectomy

exposure of the region of the pancreas in the track of the missile or knife generally suffices. Conversely, in patients with blunt injury to the upper abdomen, the entire pancreas must be exposed for proper evaluation. The head, body, and tail of the pancreas each must be systematically and meticulously inspected by sight and by palpation [11]. In penetrating and blunt abdominal trauma, all peripancreatic hematomas or areas of bile staining should be explored [1,6,10]. An extended Kocher maneuver is used to expose the anterior and posterior aspects of the head and neck of the pancreas. For examination of the anterior body and tail, entrance into the lesser sac by means of division of the gastrocolic ligament is performed as described previously. After dividing the retroperitoneum inferior to the pancreas and then by lifting of its lower edge, the posterior aspect of the body can also be visualized. For total exposure of the posterior tail of the pancreas, the spleen must be mobilized and the tail should be dissected out of the retroperitoneum using blunt and sharp dissection [11].

Simple external drainage

In the hemodynamically stable patient, pancreatic contusions (AAST grade I), minor capsular injuries, and traumatic pancreatitis can be treated without drainage [7,11]. Most other injuries require drainage of some sort. Furthermore, in damage control situations, to avoid lengthy complex procedures, there has been a renewed interest in simple drainage of more complex injuries [6]. Indeed, the potential complication of a controlled pancreatic fistula is acceptable and may be associated with less morbidity and mortality than a complex reconstruction in a coagulopathic patient [1,4,9]. Because of the risk for pancreas-related septic complications associated with open or sump drainage, closed suction drainage is preferred. Drains should be left in place until output is minimal while the patient is tolerating enteral nutrition [6].

Pancreatorrhaphy and drainage

Pancreatic lacerations not involving the duct (AAST grade I and grade II) are often associated with parenchymal bleeding. In cases in which the edges of the lacerations have been oversewn, however, repeat laparotomy generally reveals necrosis of these suture lines. This necrosis can lead to late complications, such as fistulas or pseudocysts. An alternative, and possibly a better option, after confirming that there is no injury to the main pancreatic duct is to sew a piece of viable omentum directly into the laceration. The omental plug is able to absorb small amounts of pancreatic fluid and avoids the problem of local pancreatic necrosis caused by sutures. Wide drainage should be performed because of the obvious risk for a fistula from a minor pancreatic duct [11].

Isolated pancreatic injuries with ductal involvement

General principles

All hematomas overlying the pancreas should be explored because they may obscure a transection of the main pancreatic duct (Fig. 1) [11]. In rare cases, if a ductal injury is unable to be confirmed by local examination as described previously, some centers recommend intraoperative ERCP or some form of surgeon-performed pancreatogram. Because of associated technical limitations, however, these methods should be reserved for patients in whom the extent of resection is to be directed by the findings [1]. Operative techniques to perform a pancreatogram if endoscopy is not available include surgical duodenotomy with cannulation of the ampulla of Vater and a retrograde pancreatogram after distal pancreatectomy. The major drawback of the former is the need for formal biliary sphincteroplasty for cannulation of the duct. This can be a lengthy and challenging endeavor and, fortunately, is rarely indicated. Conversely, the main disadvantage of the latter technique is that the duct at this level is usually small and challenging to visualize and cannulate in the young patient with trauma. If cannulation is successful, however, pancreatography is quite accurate in demonstrating the location and complexity of injury to the proximal pancreatic duct [11]. The authors have little enthusiasm for this overaggressive diagnostic approach, especially if it would require sacrifice of a normal spleen.

Ductal transection in the neck, body, or tail of the pancreas

Distal pancreatectomy

In a case of transection of the pancreas to the left of the mesenteric vessels (AAST grade III), a distal pancreatectomy should be performed [1,4,8,11].

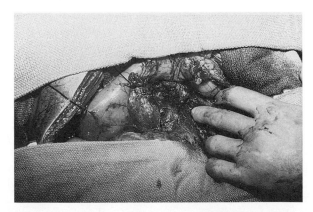

Fig. 1. Transection of the neck of the pancreas secondary to blunt trauma. (*From* Feliciano DV. Abdominal trauma. In: Schwartz SI, Ellis H, editors. Maingot's abdominal operations. 9th edition. East Norwalk (CT): Appleton & Lange; 1989. p. 497; with permission.)

Ideally, an attempt at splenic salvage should be considered, but this is not often feasible in multiply injured patients. If resection is delayed, as in a damage control situation, or is performed in the presence of posttraumatic pancreatitis, fibrosis and inflammation make resection a difficult undertaking [1,8,11].

In the hemodynamically stable patient with an isolated pancreatic injury, especially a child 10 years of age or younger, splenic salvage should be considered. First, the splenic artery and vein should be exposed and isolated with vessels loops or umbilical tapes. This allows for expeditious vascular control if either vessel is injured during the mobilization of the pancreas. The transection of the pancreas can then be completed, if necessary, with division of the remaining parenchyma. Next, with cephalad retraction of the splenic vessels and caudal retraction of the pancreatic specimen, multiple small branches between these structures are exposed. After ligation with sutures or metal clips and division of all the branches, the body and tail of the pancreas can be removed with salvage of the spleen (Fig. 2) [11].

If the patient is hemodynamically unstable, an expeditious distal pancreatectomy with splenectomy should be performed. In this case, the splenic branch vessels should be isolated, ligated, and divided starting approximately 1 to 2 cm proximal or distal to the area of ductal disruption (Fig. 3). This method minimizes splenic bleeding during mobilization and places the ligated ends of the splenic vessels away from a potential postoperative pancreatic fistula from the stump of the pancreas. Splenic mobilization should then be accomplished by dividing the splenorenal and splenophrenic ligaments. A combination of blunt and sharp dissection should be used toward the midline of the body. The spleen and tail of the pancreas can then be mobilized medially as a unit. Next, the short gastric

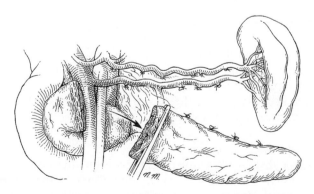

Fig. 2. Distal pancreatectomy with splenic salvage should be considered in the hemodynamically stable patient with an isolated pancreatic injury. The arrow illustrates the detachment of distal pancreas.

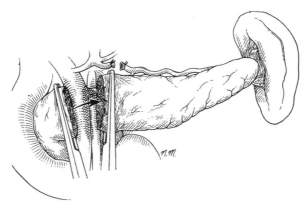

Fig. 3. Distal pancreatectomy is most commonly performed after ductal transection in the neck of the pancreas or to the left of the mesenteric vessels. The arrow illustrates the detachment of distal pancreas. (*From* Cushman JG, Feliciano DV. Contemporary management of pancreatic trauma. In: Maull KI, Cleveland HC, Feliciano DV, et al, editors. Advances in trauma and critical care. St. Louis (MO): Mosby; 1995. p. 323; with permission.)

vessels are isolated, ligated, and divided starting from the proximal greater curvature of the stomach. Finally, the division of the splenocolic ligament completes the mobilization of the spleen, and the splenectomy can then be performed with the distal pancreatectomy as described previously [23].

Although the management of the pancreatic stump is controversial, the authors recommend that, if possible, the end of the stump be tailored with anterior and posterior oblique planes of transection, creating a "fish-mouth" appearance. These two surfaces can then be opposed with continuous or interrupted horizontal mattress sutures. As mentioned previously, overly tight suturing of the edges can cause early necrosis and late complications of a fistula or pseudocyst. Alternatively, closure of the stump with 4.8-mm staples is used more commonly because it is a simple reliable technique that may avoid necrosis of the parenchyma under sutures. A segment of the gastrocolic omentum can also be mobilized and sewn to the pancreatic stump, potentially to seal small ductal branches not controlled by the staples [11]. Despite various descriptions in literature, no method of closure of the main pancreatic duct at the stump has been shown to influence the incidence of postoperative fistulas [6,9].

Roux-en-Y distal pancreatojejunostomy

A Roux-en-Y distal pancreatojejunostomy is an alternative to distal pancreatectomy, but it is rarely performed (five times in the senior author's 29-year experience). The most appropriate indication is in the hemodynamically stable patient who has a transection of the pancreas at the neck or just to the right of the mesenteric vessels and few associated injuries. A distal pancreatectomy is less appealing in this situation, because it requires 75% to 80% of the pancreas to be resected, which results in an abnormal glucose tolerance test result or frank hyperglycemia in at least 50% of patients on long-term follow-up [11,13].

If this unusual procedure is to be performed, the first step is completion of the pancreatic transection by ligation and division of remaining pancreatic attachments. Next, if it is visible, the proximal main pancreatic duct is isolated and ligated with permanent suture. A short segment of the distal end is then mobilized off the superior mesenteric vessels and portal vein by ligating and dividing small posterior pancreatic branches. This should be performed to the extent that elevation of the distal end by approximately 2.5 to 3 cm can be accomplished. Next, a Roux segment of jejunum, 40 to 45 cm distal to the ligament of Treitz, is created and mobilized through the transverse mesocolon to the right of the middle colic vessels. An end-to-end Roux-en-Y distal pancreatojejunostomy can now be completed in two layers with at least a 2-cm circumferential serosal cuff around the end of the pancreas. Finally, drains are left to control potential leakage from the proximal stump and distal pancreatojejunostomy [11].

Anterior Roux-en-Y pancreatojejunostomy

In the rare patient, a penetrating wound through the pancreatic duct at the head of the pancreas preserves the parenchyma posterior to the transected duct. In these cases, several investigators have recommended performance of an anterior Roux-en-Y pancreatojejunostomy. A Roux limb is mobilized in the fashion described previously and anastomosed in an end-to-side fashion over the site of injury. Unfortunately, sutures have a tendency to pull through the normal soft pancreatic parenchyma that is present in most young healthy patients with trauma. An inner continuous row of absorbable suture is placed from the edge of the injured parenchyma through the full-thickness wall of an enterotomy made at the end of the Roux limb. A second layer of interrupted silk sutures is placed between the capsule of the pancreas and the seromuscular layer of the jejunal limb. Leaks are common after this procedure; thus, extensive drainage is recommended [11]. The authors do not perform this procedure.

Ductal transection of the head of the pancreas

Resection

Extensive trauma to the head of the pancreas usually creates combined pancreatoduodenal injuries and is discussed here.

Endoscopically placed stents

As mentioned previously, endoscopically placed stents have been inserted in hemodynamically stable patients with isolated proximal ductal injuries

[16,22]. As noted previously, these are most commonly used when the patient has a significant traumatic injury to the brain or other severe injures precluding complex operative repair. The authors have no experience with this technique in the absence of surgical exploration, and it should be used with caution.

Combined pancreatoduodenal injuries

General principles and exposure

Combined pancreatoduodenal injuries often require complex management and have a significant risk for morbidity and mortality that may be related to associated injuries. Postoperative fistulas, abscesses, and hemorrhage occur commonly after this injury complex [10,11]. As with the management of isolated pancreatic injuries, control of hemorrhage and gastrointestinal contamination must occur first. Then, after adequate exposure and identification of the injuries, a decision must be made on the choice of procedure based on the extent of the pancreatic and duodenal injuries, the hemodynamic status of the patient, and the expertise of the surgeon [11].

The entire pancreas and duodenum must be thoroughly and methodically examined. As mentioned previously, all areas of bile staining and peripancreatic or periduodenal hematomas should be explored [1,6,10]. An extended Kocher maneuver, entrance into the lesser sac, division of the retroperitoneum inferior to the pancreas, and mobilization the spleen are needed to expose the entire pancreas and the first, second, and third portions of the duodenum [11].

Simple primary repair and drainage

In approximately 25% of the patients with combined pancreatoduodenal injuries, small duodenal injuries can be repaired primarily and moderate injuries to the pancreas can be widely drained [11]. Drainage of the primarily repaired duodenal injury is not recommended.

Complex repair

In some patients with some combined pancreatoduodenal injuries, each organ can be treated separately, and if this is the case, multiple options exist for each repair. The pancreatic injury can be treated with the aforementioned omental pancreatorrhaphy, distal pancreatectomy, or a Roux-en-Y distal pancreatojejunostomy. A duodenal injury may require a transverse duodenorrhaphy, resection with end-to-end anastomosis, or Roux-en-Y jejunal limb to repair (mucosa-to-mucosa) a large defect in the wall of the duodenum [11]. Jejunal "patch" procedures using serosa-to-mucosal opposition should not be employed.

Diversion procedures

In many patients, however, injuries to the pancreas and duodenum are extensive and require combined management. Indeed, when there is significant concern about the possibility of a postoperative fistula from the injured pancreas or duodenum, a diversion procedure is probably wise. Three such procedures have been described in the past 95 years

Duodenal diverticulization

Duodenal diverticulization was first described in 1968 by Berne and colleagues [24,25] from Los Angeles County Hospital/University of Southern California. This six-part procedure includes the following: (1) truncal vagotomy, (2) antrectomy with gastrojejunostomy, (3) duodenal closure, (4) tube duodenostomy, (5) drainage of the common bile duct, and (6) external drainage. The rationale for this procedure was the known decrease in morbidity and mortality when fistulas occurred from the end of the isolated duodenal stump as compared with a lateral fistula from a duodenum still in continuity with the stomach. Unfortunately, the disadvantages of this approach, as it was classically described, are many and include sacrifice of the normal distal stomach and pylorus, postvagotomy sequelae, manipulation of a normal-sized common bile duct, and the time required to complete the procedure. Approximately 20 years after duodenal diverticulization was first described, Kline and colleagues [26] suggested that drainage of the common bile duct and vagotomy could be safely omitted and thought that this was attributable to the common availability of histamine-2 (H2) receptor antagonists. Although this avoids potential long-term biliary complications, this extensive procedure is still rarely performed by the authors.

"Triple-tube" approach

Stone and Fabian from Grady Memorial Hospital/Emory University first described the "triple-tube" approach in 1979. Primarily indicated for duodenal drainage in a combined pancreatoduodenal injury, it involves the placement of a gastrostomy tube for proximal decompression, a retrograde duodenostomy tube inserted by way of the jejunum for decompression of the repaired duodenum, and an antegrade jejunostomy tube for enteral feeding [27]. The disadvantages of this approach are obvious and include the time required to complete the procedure and the potential for postoperative leaks from three fresh ostomies. Furthermore, in the damage control situation, the presence of multiple tubes complicates the management of the open abdomen and, in the authors' experience, the tubes have a tendency to pull away from the abdominal wall as bowel edema resolves, leading to fistulas and leaks.

Pyloric exclusion with gastrojejunostomy

The technique was first described by Berg [28] in 1909 and revivified by Vaughan and colleagues [29] in 1977. In this technique described by Martin and colleagues [30] in 1983, the pyloric muscle ring is closed with a number 1 polypropylene suture through a dependent gastrotomy. An antecolic gastrojejunostomy is then performed using this gastrotomy. This should allow for temporary diversion while the duodenal and pancreatic injuries heal. Fortunately, in 95% of cases, the exclusion reopens in 2 to 3 weeks. Although this technique is somewhat more time-consuming than the triple-tube technique, the authors prefer this method for severe combined injuries not requiring a Whipple procedure.

Resection

As mentioned previously, pancreatoduodenectomy is indicated when there is extensive trauma to the head of the pancreas, a severe combined pancreatoduodenal injury, or destruction of the ampulla of Vater (Fig. 4) [10]. In the hemodynamically stable patient, this procedure can be performed at the time of the original trauma laparotomy. In most of the patients who are hypothermic, acidotic, or coagulopathic, a damage control procedure is indicated. In this instance, the pancreatoduodenectomy or the reconstruction after a prior pancreatoduodenectomy should be performed at the reoperation. This operation has been used in approximately 10% to 11% of combined pancreatoduodenal injuries in the past and has a mortality rate of 30% to 40% [6,10]. In a recent article, Asensio and colleagues [10] reported on 18 patients who underwent a standard pancreatoduodenectomy after upper abdominal trauma. All 18 patients had an unreconstructable injury or

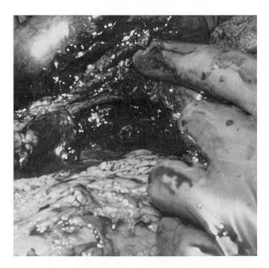

Fig. 4. Devascularization of the duodenal C-loop and maceration of the head of the pancreas mandated pancreatoduodenectomy in this victim of a motor vehicle crash. (*From* Feliciano DV. Abdominal trauma. In: Schwartz SI, Ellis H, editors. Maingot's abdominal operations. 9th edition. East Norwalk (CT): Appleton & Lange; 1989. p. 498; with permission.)

devitalization of the head of the pancreas, including the main pancreatic duct, duodenum, intrapancreatic common bile duct, and ampulla of Vater. Five patients (28%) were treated with staged reconstructive procedures. Similar to previous reports, 12 patients (67%) survived.

Complications and outcome

Complication rates after operative treatment of pancreatic injuries range from 26% to 86% [1,3,6,9,16,31]. Interestingly, higher AAST OIS scores have not translated into higher overall risks for complications [9]. Recently, Tyburski and colleagues [4] from Detroit Receiving Hospital assessed the risk factors for infectious complications after pancreatic trauma. They grouped complications into general nosocomial and trauma-related infections, and the latter included wound infections, truncal cellulitis, abdominal abscesses, fasciitis, and fistulas. They noted an almost threefold increase in the incidence of infection in the patients with pancreatic injury as compared with those without. They also stated that regardless of the type of pancreatic repair, drainage procedure, or resection performed, no difference in the rate of infectious complications was noted.

In many series, the most common postoperative infectious complication and the leading cause of morbidity in patients with injuries to the pancreas is an intra-abdominal abscess [2–4,6,9]. With this particular complication, a higher grade of pancreatic injury and the presence of an associated injury to the colon increase the incidence [4,6,9]. These abscesses, which most commonly occur in the left upper quadrant or left subphrenic space, can generally be treated with CT-guided drainage or a rare reoperation [2,11].

A pancreatic fistula is the most common "pancreatic" complication after operative repair of a major injury [1,6]. The literature reports an incidence of pancreatic fistulas after trauma ranging from 5% to 37% [1,4,6,8,16,31]. As stated previously, the method of ligation of the main pancreatic duct after a distal pancreatectomy does not influence the rate of formation of a postoperative fistula [6]. Most series report spontaneous closure within 4 months in 50% to 100% of patients. Occasionally, a patient requires a delayed distal pancreatectomy (none in senior author's series) [1,6,8]. Also, an anterior Roux-en-Y pancreatojejunostomy has occasionally been used to treat a persistent fistula from the main pancreatic duct in the head or the neck of the pancreas [11]. Conservative management of pancreatic fistulas includes initial bowel rest and total parenteral nutrition (TPN). Enteral nutrition may be initiated in patients with low-output fistulas as long as the fistula output does not substantially increase. Somatostatin analogue administered subcutaneously has not been proved to shorten the healing time of a postoperative fistula, although it may decrease the daily output [6].

A postoperative fistula may also lead to a pseudocyst. In addition, pseudocysts can form as a late complication of a missed injury to the pancreatic duct, often after blunt abdominal trauma [6]. Indeed, the incidence of postresection fluid collections in the left upper quadrant or pancreatic pseudocysts after trauma has been as high as 30% in some series [22]. Although some fluid collections may resolve spontaneously, persistent pseudocysts should be treated to prevent hemorrhage, perforation, infection, or obstruction of the bowel or bile duct [6,22]. Percutaneous drainage is safe, effective, and an acceptable option for initial management of fluid collections or traumatic pseudocysts. If a fluid collection or a suspected pseudocyst persists after percutaneous drainage, timely investigation by means of ERCP to rule out injury to the main pancreatic duct is recommended. A persistent pseudocyst with a distal ductal injury warrants a distal pancreatectomy or internal drainage if the cyst wall is mature. If the proximal duct is injured, Lin and colleagues [22] describe the following three options in a published protocol: placement of a stent by means of ERCP, internal drainage, and resection. The main principle of the stent is to restore continuity of the main pancreatic duct, and therefore allow the pseudocyst to drain into the newly repaired duct. If ERCP reveals a ductal obstruction and a stent is unable to be passed, surgery is required [3]. Internal drainage by means of a cystogastrostomy or cystoenterostomy can be performed if the wall of the pseudocyst is mature. If the wall is not mature, open external drainage or resection is necessary [11,22].

Occasionally, patients may present with late posttraumatic pancreatitis, which is caused by obstructive pancreatic fibrosis or a stricture in the duct. This disease process is confirmed by histologic features consistent with chronic pancreatitis and fibrosis after delayed resection of an injured pancreas [1]. Treatment, like any other form of pancreatitis, includes proximal bowel rest and TPN or jejunal feeds [6]. The use of stents in the management of posttraumatic pancreatitis is rare and is generally unnecessary unless the main pancreatic duct is disrupted or strictured [22].

A known complication of stents placed in the main pancreatic duct is stricture, which may occur because of inflammation from the stent itself, occlusion of the stent, or occlusion of ductal side branches. Situations that increase the likelihood of a stricture include the use of longer stents and prolonged or repeated stenting. Lin and colleagues [2] recommend using Teflon stents, which have multiple lateral holes for drainage of side branches and exchanging them every 3 weeks.

Summary

Even in the modern trauma center, pancreatic trauma remains a source of significant morbidity and mortality. Fortunately, it remains relatively uncommon. When pancreatic trauma does occur, however, it is rarely isolated, and it is the associated injuries that are directly responsible for much of the morbidity. ERCP has been used more frequently to assist in diagnosis and, on occasion, for definitive management of ductal discontinuity in patients with contraindications to laparotomy. To render this treatment modality successful with a reduced incidence of strictures, shorter stents and frequent exchanges are recommended. Early operative intervention is warranted in most patients with confirmed or suspected ductal injury, because undiagnosed ductal disruptions carry considerable morbidity. Indeed, the integrity of the main pancreatic duct is key in the management and outcome of patients with pancreatic trauma. Simple external drainage and distal pancreatectomy are commonly performed operative procedures and have a favorable outcome most of the time. Pancreatoduodenectomy is indicated in those select patients with extensive combined pancreatoduodenal injuries who are hemodynamically stable with few associated injuries. Postoperative complications after repair of major pancreatic injuries include intra-abdominal abscesses, postoperative fistulas, and an occasional pancreatic pseudocyst. Many of these complications may be treated successfully without reoperation.

References

[1] Wind P, Tiret E, Cunningham C, et al. Contribution of endoscopic retrograde pancreatography in management of complications following distal pancreatic trauma. Am Surg 1999; 65(8):777–83.

[2] Lin BC, Chen RJ, Fang JF, et al. Management of blunt major pancreatic injury. J Trauma 2004;56(4):774–8.

[3] Wolf A, Bernhardt J, Patrzyk M, et al. The value of endoscopic diagnosis and the treatment of pancreas injuries following blunt abdominal trauma. Surg Endosc 2005;19:665–9.

[4] Tyburski JG, Dente CJ, Wilson RF, et al. Infectious complications following duodenal and/ or pancreatic trauma. Am Surg 2001;67(3):227–31.

[5] Feliciano DV, Burch JM, Sput-Patrinely V, et al. Abdominal gunshot wounds. An urban trauma center's experience with 300 consecutive patients. Ann Surg 1988;208(3):362–70.

[6] Vasquez JC, Coimbra R, Hoyt DB, et al. Management of penetrating pancreatic trauma. An 11-year experience of a level-1 trauma center. Injury 2001;32:753–9.

[7] Cushman JG, Feliciano DV, et al. Contemporary management of pancreatic trauma. In: Maull KI, Cleveland HC, Feliciano DV, et al, editors. Advances in trauma and critical care, vol. 10. St. Louis (MO): Mosby; 1995. p. 309–36.

[8] Buccimazza I, Thomason SR, Anderson F, et al. Isolated main pancreatic duct injuries spectrum and management. Am J Surg 2006;191:448–52.

[9] Rickard MJFX, Brohi K, Bautz PC. Pancreatic and duodenal injuries. Keep it simple. ANZ J Surg 2005;75:581–6.

[10] Asensio JA, Petrone P, Roldan G, et al. Pancreaticoduodenectomy. A rare procedure for the management of complex pancreaticoduodenal injuries. J Am Coll Surg 2003;197(6): 937–42.

[11] Feliciano DV. Abdominal trauma. In: Schwartz SI, Ellis H, editors. Maingot's abdominal operations. 9th edition. East Norwalk: Appleton & Lange; 1989. p. 457–512.

[12] Ilahi O, Bochicchio GV, Scalea TM. Efficacy of computed tomography in the diagnosis of pancreatic injury in adult blunt trauma patients. A single-institutional study. Am Surg 2002;68(8):704–8.

[13] Jones RC. Management of pancreatic trauma. Am J Surg 1985;150:698–704.

[14] Takishima T, Sugimoto F, Hirata M, et al. Serum amylase level on admission. Ann Surg 1997;226:70–6.

[15] Udekwu PO, Gurkin B, Oller DW. The use of computed tomography in blunt abdominal injuries. Am Surg 1996;62(1):56–9.

[16] Lin BC, Liu NJ, Fang JF, et al. Long-term results of endoscopic stent in the management of blunt major pancreatic duct injury. Surg Endosc 2006;20:1551–5.

[17] Gupta A, Stuhlfaut JW, Fleming KW, et al. Blunt trauma of the pancreas and biliary tract. A multimodality imaging approach to diagnosis. Radiographics 2004;24(5):1381–95.

[18] Takishima T, Hirat M, Kataoka Y, et al. Pancreatographic classification of pancreatic ductal injuries caused by blunt injury to the pancreas. J Trauma 2000;48:745–52.

[19] Ragozzino A, Manfredi R, Scaglione M, et al. The use of MRCP in the detection of pancreatic injuries after blunt trauma. Emerg Radiol 2003;10:14–8.

[20] Gillams AR, Kurzawinski T, Lees WR. Diagnosis of duct disruption and assessment of pancreatic leak with dynamic secretin-stimulated MR cholangiopancreatography. AJR Am J Roentgenol 2006;186:499–504.

[21] Hikida S, Sakamoto T, Higaki K, et al. Intraoperative ultrasonography is useful for diagnosing pancreatic duct injury and adjacent tissue damage in a patient with penetrating pancreas trauma. J Hepatobiliary Pancreat Surg 2004;11:272–5.

[22] Lin BC, Fang JF, Wong YC, et al. Blunt pancreatic trauma and pseudocyst: management of major pancreatic duct injury. Injury 2007;38(5):588–93.

[23] Wisner DH. Injury to the spleen. In: Moore EE, Feliciano DV, Mattox KL, editors. Trauma. 5th edition. New York: McGraw-Hill; 2004. p. 663–86.

[24] Berne CJ, Donovan AJ, Hagen WE. Combined duodenal pancreatic trauma. Arch Surg 1968;96:712–22.

[25] Berne CJ, Donovan AJ, White EJ, et al. Duodenal 'diverticulization' for duodenal and pancreatic injury. Am J Surg 1974;127:503–7.

[26] Kline G, Lucas CE, Ledgerwood AM, et al. Duodenal organ injury severity (OIS) and outcome. Am Surg 1994;60(7):500–4.

[27] Stone HH, Fabian TC. Management of duodenal wounds. J Trauma 1979;19:334–9.

[28] Berg AA. Duodenal fistula. Its treatment by gastrojejunostomy and pyloric occlusion. Ann Surg 1907;45:721–9.

[29] Vaughan GD III, Frazier OH, Graham DY, et al. The use of pyloric exclusion in the management of severe duodenal injuries. Am J Surg 1977;134:785–90.

[30] Martin TD, Feliciano DV, Mattox KL, et al. Severe duodenal injuries. Treatment with pyloric exclusion and gastrojejunostomy. Arch Surg 1983;118:631–5.

[31] Lopez PP, Benjamin R, Cockburn M, et al. Recent trends in the management of combined pancreatoduodenal injuries. Am Surg 2005;71(10):847–52.

ELSEVIER
SAUNDERS

SURGICAL
CLINICS OF
NORTH AMERICA

Surg Clin N Am 87 (2007) 1533–1541

Index

Note: Page numbers of article titles are in **boldface** type.

Moving?

Make sure your subscription moves with you!

To notify us of your new address, find your **Clinics Account Number** (located on your mailing label above your name), and contact customer service at:

E-mail: elspcs@elsevier.com

800-654-2452 (subscribers in the U.S. & Canada)
407-345-4000 (subscribers outside of the U.S. & Canada)

Fax number: 407-363-9661

Elsevier Periodicals Customer Service
6277 Sea Harbor Drive
Orlando, FL 32887-4800

*To ensure uninterrupted delivery of your subscription, please notify us at least 4 weeks in advance of move.

ELSEVIER